Sick jokes

Manchester University Press

SOCIAL HISTORIES OF MEDICINE

Social Histories of Medicine is concerned with all aspects of health, illness and medicine, from prehistory to the present, in every part of the world. The series covers the circumstances that promote health or illness, the ways in which people experience and explain such conditions, and what, practically, they do about them. Practitioners of all approaches to health and healing come within its scope, as do their ideas, beliefs and practices, and the social, economic and cultural contexts in which they operate. Methodologically, the series welcomes relevant studies in social, economic, cultural and intellectual history, as well as approaches derived from other disciplines in the arts, sciences, social sciences and humanities. The series is a collaboration between Manchester University Press and the Society for the Social History of Medicine.

To buy or to find out more about the books currently available in this series, please go to: https://manchesteruniversitypress.co.uk/series/social-histories-of-medicine/

Sick jokes

Visual histories of humour, health and the body

Edited by

Christine Slobogin,
Katie Snow and Laura Cowley

Manchester University Press

Published by Manchester University Press
Oxford Road, Manchester, M13 9PL

www.manchesteruniversitypress.co.uk

British Library Cataloguing-in-Publication Data
A catalogue record for this book is available from the British Library

ISBN 978 1 5261 8797 0 hardback

First published 2026

EU authorised representative for GPSR:
Easy Access System Europe, Mustamäe tee 50, 10621 Tallinn, Estonia
gpsr.requests@easproject.com

Typeset
by Cheshire Typesetting Ltd, Cuddington, Cheshire

Dedications

For Cindy Slobogin, who taught me to love art – Christine Slobogin

For Rory Ivor Snow, who can find the funny in anything – Katie Snow

For Sue Cowley, who was a good patient but a far better teacher – Laura Cowley

A note on the cover image

When deciding which image from this volume to put on the cover, we knew that we wanted something that captured one of the book's central themes: the use of humour as a means of reclaiming power from the medical systems or diagnoses that so often leave us feeling powerless. Marc Geller's photograph of Tom Shearer does exactly that, with Tom's personality – embodied in his smiley face tattoo and steady gaze – posing a pointed challenge to medical and cultural assumptions about what it means to be, or to joke about being, 'sick'. The context in which this portrait (one of many, discussed in Jo Michael Rezes's Chapter 6, in this volume) was taken also suggests the importance of laughing in the faces of death and danger, of creating community and of sharing experience – other prominent themes throughout *Sick Jokes*.

We are very aware of the ethical quandaries of sharing patient photographs, especially on a book cover, publicly viewable on shelves and on screens. While we cannot get consent from Shearer for this specific use of his photograph, we have received permission from Geller. The portrait was taken by Geller on assignment for the American LGBT magazine *The Advocate* in 1991, to accompany an interview about Shearer and Beowulf Thorne's radically funny zine *Diseased Pariah News*. Geller stated in an email to us that he felt 'Tom's bravery in creating such a zine comes through in the way he faced the camera'. While we cannot know how Shearer or Thorne imagined these portraits might circulate after their deaths, the photographs belong to a project and artistic friendship that was itself public-facing. Geller's photographs were made for a story about two editors whose zine invited, and often unsettled, wide publics to laugh in the face of darkness, and Geller has affirmed his support for this new use of the image.

With this photograph on the cover, a person picking up this book or browsing for it online has to make eye contact with Tom. As Rezes writes about this photograph in their chapter,

> Power resides in Shearer's direct, unwavering gaze into the camera. He does not look away, not into a middle-distance of metaphysical abstraction, but at us, the viewers. This is not a look of resignation; it is knowing charged with irony. Shearer's eyes, framed by both a smiley-face tattoo and Kaposi's lesions, challenge the genre of AIDS deathbed photography by refusing to take up its usual emotional cues ... Shearer insists we laugh and grieve with his image on different terms. This is an image for those who can read the joke and feel the intimacy in it. Shearer is both performer and patient, camp icon and dying friend, holding eye contact with a public that too often looked away or looked only to feel righteous sadness ... His look is the punchline, an invitation into a world of queer resistance and humour aesthetic that *Diseased Pariah News* built. Even at death's door, his body speaks back – eyes daring you to make him the 'butt' of any joke.

We hope that this photograph draws people into this volume while also showing Shearer as he wanted to be perceived. We hope that we have done him – and other patients, artists and jokers – justice.

Christine Slobogin, Katie Snow and Laura Cowley

Contents

Figures

Contributors

Soha Bayoumi is a political theorist and historian whose work examines the intersection of health and social justice and the medicine–politics nexus, with a regional focus on the Middle East and a particular interest in postcolonial and gender studies. Her research and teaching focus on medicine and authoritarianism; gendered aspects of healthcare; and the visual cultures of medicine, science and technology (including, among other things, cinema and comics). She is a teaching professor in the Medicine, Science and the Humanities programme at the Johns Hopkins University's Krieger School of Arts and Sciences and an affiliate faculty member of the Department of the History of Medicine at the Johns Hopkins School of Medicine. She is the editor-in-chief of the *Journal of Middle East Women's Studies* (*JMEWS*) and associate editor of the *Journal of Islamic and Muslim Studies* (*JIMS*).

Peder Clark is a cultural and social historian of drugs and health in modern Britain. His research on ecstasy (MDMA) and the drug's risks and pleasures in late twentieth-century Britain has been supported by a Wellcome Trust Fellowship. More broadly, he is interested in visual culture, class, gender and everyday life. He received his PhD from the London School of Hygiene and Tropical Medicine in 2019, and is the co-author of *Placing the Public in Public Health in Post-War Britain, 1948–2012* (Palgrave Macmillan).

Laura Cowley is an artist-researcher and PhD student at Birkbeck, University of London, where her Wellcome Trust funded project explores the use of visual humour in the work of disabled artists.

She was previously a Leverhulme Trust painting scholar at the Royal College of Art.

Georgia Haire is a historian of health and medicine. Her research focuses on gendered experiences of health, sexual and pelvic pain, self-help and everyday healthcare. Currently, she is working as a postdoctoral research fellow on Pelvic Health and Public Health in Twentieth Century Canada, a Canadian Institutes of Health Research (CIHR) funded project based at Vancouver Island University, which explores how pelvic health issues became matters of growing public health concern. Her research strand examines experiences of vaginismus in Canada, from the 1960s to the 2000s.

Allison Morehead is Professor of Art History and in the Graduate Program in Cultural Studies at Queen's University, Canada. Morehead is the author of *Nature's Experiments and the Search for Symbolist Form* (The Pennsylvania State University Press, 2017), the curator and editor of *Lifeblood – Edvard Munch* (MUNCH, 2025) and the co-editor (with Fiona Johnstone and Imogen Wiltshire) of *Art and the Critical Medical Humanities* [Series: Critical Interventions in the Medical and Health Humanities] (Bloomsbury, 2026).

Jo Michael Rezes is a theatremaker and educator in the Greater Boston Area. Their dissertation 'Tastes Like AIDS: Sweet Aesthetics, Bitter Humor and Viral Performances of HIV/AIDS' centres flavour in the study of HIV/AIDS media. They have published work in Polari Press, *Refinery29*, and *Texas Theatre Journal* with chapters in *Milestones in Queer US Theatre* (Routledge), *Queers at the Table* (Arsenal Pulp Press) and *The Methuen Drama Book of Trans Plays* (vol. 3). Online, Jo is a TED official speaker and runs an online cooking show (Jiffy Mae's Sick Kitchen) with a cookbook in development featuring recipes found in queer, chronically ill (and online) food cultures. Having held teaching appointments at Boston College, Emerson College and Harvard University, Rezes currently serves as the Associate Director of Education at The Theater Offensive – leading their nationally recognised True Colors programmes for LGBTQIA+ youth. They are a proud Vassar College alum and hold a PhD in Theatre & Performance from Tufts University. Learn more: JMRezes.com

Jeffrey S. Reznick is Senior Historian at the National Library of Medicine, National Institutes of Health. He is author or editor of several books, including *Through High Windows* (Universitas Press, 2025), *Circulating Now, Full Circle: From the Historical Collections of the National Library of Medicine* (with Elizabeth A. Mullen; Virginia Tech Publishing, 2024), and *War and Peace in the Worlds of Rudolf H. Sauter: A Cultural History of a Creative Life* (Anthem Press, 2022).

Christine Slobogin is an art historian of medicine and Assistant Professor of Health Humanities and Bioethics at the University of Rochester, where she teaches medical and master's students. Her first book, titled *Putting Plastic Surgery on Paper: How Art and Archives Defined Second World War Reconstructive Surgery in Britain*, was published in June 2025.

Callum D. Smith is an interdisciplinary historian of British politics and society post-1780, with a particular interest in visual culture, drinking studies, sociability and radicalism. He is currently Head of Online Learning at Aberystwyth University, and an Honorary Research Fellow in the department of History at the University of Bristol. Callum has previously held a lectureship in Modern History at the University of Bristol, and teaching and research positions at the universities of Bath and Aberystwyth. His monograph entitled *The Foxite Whigs and Visual Culture, 1780–1810: Radical Sociability* was published in 2025.

Katie Snow is a medical historian with wide research interests in the history of the body and visual culture. She has taught across History, English and Medicine, including in an anatomy school. Katie is currently a Research Fellow on the Wellcome-Trust funded project 'Drinking Culture: The Cultural Reception of Developments Related to Alcohol in Ireland, 1700–1900' at University College Dublin. Her first monograph, on representations of breasts in caricature, is due to be published by Rutgers University Press.

Rebecca Whiteley is a British Academy Postdoctoral Fellow in the Department of History at the University of Birmingham. Her research resides in the intersections of visual and material cultures, and medical and social history. She is particularly interested in printed images, books and medical models. Her first book, *Birth Figures*, examines the many lives of early modern midwifery illustrations. She is currently working on a history of the print cultures of sex and medicine in mid-nineteenth-century Britain, from medical illustrations to satirical prints to pornography.

Acknowledgments

We would like to express our sincere gratitude to our contributors for their generous scholarship and collegial spirit throughout the process of putting together this edited volume. The chapters collected here were borne of a shared passion for art, humour and medicine, and we are certain that the imaginative material that they bring to light will inspire future research in the visual medical humanities.

This work has been enriched by the award of a Book Development Prize from The Society for the Social History of Medicine, which supported our authors in overcoming the financial barriers increasingly associated with the fair publication of images within scholarly research. We are grateful for the expert guidance of the editorial and production team at Manchester University Press, and for the support provided by Meredith Carroll, David Cantor, Humairaa Dudhwala and Annabel Holland in particular.

We are deeply thankful to the *Confabulations: Art Practice, Art History, Critical Medical Humanities* collective for their early enthusiasm and feedback on the project, to Johns Hopkins University's Center for Medical Humanities & Social Medicine for hosting our first symposium with our authors, to Keren Hammerschlag for her thoughtful reading of our introduction and proposal, to our anonymous peer reviewers and to David Cantor. Each of these people and groups offered careful and constructive insights that undoubtedly improved the manuscript.

Finally, we are indebted to the artists whose work inspired this scholarship. Thank you.

Introduction

Christine Slobogin, Katie Snow and Laura Cowley

From medieval marginalia to modern cartoons, videos and performances, humorous visual art depicting medicine and the body has prompted us to suspend – or perhaps, more productively, lean into – our discomfort around that which is typically deemed unfunny or inappropriate.[1] These representations have laid bare the stark realities of death, disability, sickness, injury, medical mistreatment and institutional injustice. Instances of medical humour can trigger a complex array of embodied and emotional responses: surprise, relief, recognition, anger, hurt, shame, despair, cynicism – each of which finds routine and potentially problematic expression in laughter. But where does the power reside in visual jokes, how is that power determined and who defines it? What insights and functions can visual humour offer the medical realm that spoken or written forms cannot? And, perhaps most importantly: what practical, political and psychological purposes do these visual jokes serve, both within and beyond the medical world?

By working at the intersection of humour studies, medical history and the history of art and visual culture, this volume begins to unravel these knotty questions and, in doing so, reconciles scholarship in these three fields.[2] This book reveals visual humour as a deeply human response to life's uncertainties, the body's complexities and medicine's limitations. In what follows, we see how humorous or satirical visual culture can make bodily or medical experiences more understandable, while also opening space for critical reflection, emotional response and moments of levity. We also see from the material analysed in this volume how visual culture complicates histories of health and medicine, asking questions that are potentially uncomfortable and unresolvable, challenging or messy. In this way, *Sick Jokes* is attentive to what William Viney, Felicity Callard and Angela Woods frame as the 'capabilities and responsibilities' of the critical medical humanities as it works to entangle itself with, rather than serve, solve or antagonise, clinical and biomedical culture.[3]

The chapters in this volume engage with philosophies of humour; histories of medicine, disease, emotion and the body; gender, class, disability and race; and histories of art and visual culture. Turning to humour to think through the emotional excesses generated when art and medicine collide, the authors in this volume show how visual culture has offered a particularly embodied – and yet oftentimes comfortably removed – perspective on both everyday and exceptional experiences of health and the body. With traits like text-image coupling, physical exaggeration and intertextual allusion, the visual humour explored in these chapters provides unique and entertaining insights into the experiences of illness and health, medical treatments and tools, public health communications, injury, addiction, disfigurement, disability and death.

Attentive to questions of power and positionality, this volume sheds light on the complex subjectivity of visual humour. Many of the images discussed will not be funny – initially or ever – to readers. On the other hand, some of this material has made us editors laugh out loud in the archive or while reading these chapters. The context in which the joke is constructed and told – by whom and at the expense of whom – is a vital consideration. Almost every joke, whether spoken, written or visual, establishes an in-group and an out-group. As editors and academics analysing jokes, we acknowledge our position as members of the out-group, a position that demands critical awareness and sensitivity, but which also affords critical distance. We do not intend to mock or deride the bodies, behaviours, communities or healthcare providers featured as subjects of humour in this volume; rather, we interrogate the social contexts that set them up as the butts of jokes. This approach allows for deep understanding of the diverse uses and abuses of comedy as it interacts with visual depictions of the body, medicine and difference, both today and in the past.

The recent surge of interest in the visual cultures of medicine – with enthusiasm for research with visual culture at the centre, rather than as supplementary to traditional medical history – has demonstrated that situating images and other visual media in their cultural and historical contexts enriches our understanding of the porous relationship between the body and society.[4] Visual representations can affirm our understanding of place, people and period, but they can also contradict such knowledge, inviting us to rethink accepted social, cultural, political and medical notions. The inherently subjective nature of both humour and art breeds intellectual challenges as well as opportunities. Unavoidable interpretative differences in humour and art suggest that these images resist fixed meaning, but it is precisely within this ambiguity that original thought thrives. The meaning in humour also shifts greatly depending on the media through which it is transmitted: this collection features visuals from comic strips, live performance, photographs, postcards, zines, videos and drawings. Different types of humour are more readily associated with each of these mediums, and what is funny in one may not be in another. As chapters such as Laura Cowley's (Chapter 7) show, many nuances of humour are lost or obscured as they are translated into different mediums (e.g. live performance to video documentation), with the intention and feeling behind 'jokes' particularly at risk. Despite drawing together diverse methods and disciplines, and highly subjective source material, this volume produces a cohesive narrative: visual humour pictures, critiques and reimagines the powers, risks, joys and absurdities of medicine and the body.

The visual material covered in this volume is necessarily limited in scope, with focus falling predominantly on Western prints, drawings, photographs, zines, performance art and cartoons. These sources skew towards the visual culture of Britain, particularly England, with the context of English language texts and captions – inextricable from the delivery of many of the visual jokes examined here – tying the chapters together. Although this geographic leaning narrows the diversity of material in this volume, it also offers a valuable critical opportunity to explore a distinct perspective: the very particular brand of both British visual culture and British humour as they combine and relate to the body and to medicine.[5] The witty, dry and often dark countenance of British jokes finds fertile ground in bodily, grotesque metaphors and in medical encounters. As the following chapters show, even within this particular brand of British and, more widely, Western humour, there is great diversity in its visualisations and perspectives. While the chapter submissions that we received largely shaped these limits, these geographical and material parameters also lend this volume a clearer intervention in the field of the critical medical humanities.

The temporal scope of *Sick Jokes* is also delimited, focusing on the modern period from the early nineteenth century to the present day. Humour theorist John Morreall suggested that the meaning of 'humour' today emerged alongside medical research advances in the eighteenth century, as we came to redefine the nervous system as electrochemical and not made up of transmitted fluids.[6] Focusing on this modern period, the chapters in this volume therefore obliquely suggest that the emergence and popularity of visual medical humour also parallels this modernisation and the professionalisation of the field of medicine, as a period when medical humour became more visible.[7]

The material discussed here covers many fields and concerns within health and medicine: alcoholism and drug use; obstetrics; dentistry; death; surgery; infectious diseases and pandemics; disability; and medical communications. This volume not only triangulates the three fields of medical history, art history and humour which, until now, have not been examined together in such breadth and depth, but it is also considers how humour can be handled and mishandled in the varied fields included here in order to both illuminate and obscure perceptions, understandings and experiences of health, ill health and medical systems.

Art and humour

Humour, art historian Wendy Wick Reaves reflected, is a 'slippery subject ... elemental, universal, and yet extraordinarily difficult to define'.[8] This ambiguity, coupled with hierarchical qualms about modes like graphic satire's perceived 'lowness' as an artistic form, has previously deterred art historians from treating visual humour as a serious object of study. 'The arbiters of the fine art world,' Wick Reaves continued, 'dealers, critics, and art historians – seldom want to grapple with humour. Comic or satirical art is ignored, and the humorous elements of fine art are deftly sidestepped.'[9] Humour, however, serves as a powerful historiographical lens for understanding how people in different cultures and societies perceive and engage with the world around them. It functions both as a mirror to reflect social behaviour, and as a tool for critique and affirmation. Since Wick Reaves's comments, scholars have worked to dispel the myth of visual humour as, in Jennifer A. Greenhill's words, an extraneous 'amusement' or foil to 'more pressing' artistic mediums and matters. The artistic impulse 'to strike the funny bone' or play 'the entertainer' can be, Greenhill argues, a reaction to modern demands for levity amidst widespread unease: a case of 'cracking jokes to make the medicine of "culture" go down more easily'.[10]

Yet humour strategies such as caricature and irreverence are nothing new – in parodic images of satyrs on ancient Greek vases to twenty-first-century satirical sketches on TikTok, we can see artists turn to comedy to register, remark on and remake the human experience.[11] To recover the meanings in visual humour is to recover political, cultural and also bodily contexts, to monitor the changing afflictions, preoccupations, joys and truths that colour the world in which we live (and laugh). Overlooking or looking down on visual humour risks stymying understanding of the cultural agency of art as it both takes and changes the temperature of the debates, moods and tastes that engender its creation. The artistic aspiration to humour is, to borrow again from Greenhill, as 'high-stakes' an endeavour as Romantic portraiture or documentary photography; moving audiences to laughter, relief or wry recognition requires exhaustive cultural knowledge, sharp wit and an instinctive sense of what is appropriate (even in its very inappropriateness).[12]

While, as Wick Reaves noted, 'researching the art in humor and the humor in art' presents methodological challenges – particularly around interpretation – it can help us to think otherwise about cultures and environments of health.[13] In places, the work in this volume is torn between appreciation or contempt on the one hand,

and critical analysis on the other. Encounters with art and humour are deeply personal and political, and this complexity only intensifies when applied to bodily or medical contexts. The intimate nature of visual jokes prompts us to examine our own individual senses of humour, values and worldviews, but also to consider ourselves in relation to others. The images within this volume might prompt questions like: Is this actually funny or amusing? What is the joke, and is it clever? Would I 'get' it without guidance? Who thinks this is funny, and do I want to be more or less like them? What does my reaction to this image say about me? Having read the analysis that accompanies the images, you may feel moved to a different perspective, closer to or more distant from the joker, artwork and joke itself. Some of the visuals in this volume are not fun or funny, or at least not straightforwardly so. Some set out to provoke, relishing in the unexpected and the absurd. Others lay out their visual gags like an instruction manual, holding the viewer's hand and encouraging them to find humour in everyday and exceptional experiences of health and medicine.

The futility of explaining a joke is not lost on art historians, who have recognised that deciphering visual humour can dilute its impact and obscure its implications. 'Nothing ruins a good joke like an explanation of why it is funny,' Temi Odumosu warned in her study of Black bodies in caricature, 'and even more so when the artfulness of its construction is picked to shards.'[14] 'When the emotion of humour is taken seriously', Wick Reaves similarly mourned, 'the fun can quickly evaporate.'[15] Of course, as Odumosu's work shows, this work is vital for jokes that exploit, bully and deride. Unpicking visual jokes can expose hate but also, as this volume shows, can destabilise it. The subversive power of art and humour is visible in the chapters that relate how marginalised groups have been supported by visual jokes as they platform different perspectives, affirm dignity and bolster belonging. Indeed, the enduring popularity of visual humour can be partly attributed to its capacity to bring people together. From the eighteenth-century 'golden age' of graphic satire where people would gather to view prints pasted in shop windows to more recent practices of 'social' consumption like sharing memes online, visual media has long helped to form group identities.[16] Satire in particular fosters feelings of inclusion and exclusion, in the process providing sharp insights into collective thought, ideological values and social power structures. It is perhaps for this reason that so much research in what is now referred to as the visual medical humanities settled its gaze early on satirical print culture, finding plain crossover between art and medicine in graphic representations of bodily difference, clinical spaces and places, medical (un)professionals, disease and death.[17] Since then, the field has become capacious, with studies spanning a diverse spectrum of visual, material and curatorial sources and methods and taking into account a wealth of different perspectives on the role of the medical humanities across art, history and medical contexts.[18] Following Fiona Johnstone's 'Manifesto for a Visual Medical Humanities' (2018) and Johnstone and Suzannah Biernoff's 'What Can Art History Offer the Medical Humanities?' (2024) and amidst concurrent calls to reverse and entangle the conceptual frameworks that underpin the critical medical humanities, further scrutiny has fallen on how art and medicine might come together to produce new cultural knowledge, rather than aiming for evidential analysis.[19]

In this vein, the chapters in this volume do not venture to intervene in, or resolve, the often problematic visual cultures that they survey, but rather to ask questions about their impulses and aims. Accuracy in representation or interpretation is not the goal when it comes to art analysis – to search for clear answers, Mark Philp warns, is 'arguably to misread the nature' of humorous visual mediums like satire.[20] While Fiona Haslam has argued that visual humour had to be 'based on the truth if its message were to be understood and passed on effectively', the most productive work lies in noticing how artists twist or depart from the 'truth' as it plays out in other medical media including contemporary medical testimonies, treatises and imaging.[21] If early thinking around humour and art struggled to reconcile its levity or acerbity with its seriousness as a cultural artefact, then the chapters in this volume position it as a unique point from which to ask weighty questions about – but also laugh in the face of – addiction, death, sex, medical impropriety, disability, disease and contagion. If, as Alun Withey argued, histories of medicine get 'straight to the heart of [a] culture and the beliefs of its people', then histories of humour and art are comparably insightful.[22] Whether articulating anxieties, relieving tensions, highlighting injustices, condemning bodily compulsions, mocking health movements or calling for accountability, visual humour engages with the complexities of health and medicine in a distinctly social fashion. Sitting at the nexus of art, humour and medicine, the sources in this volume hold a – not always faithful, and rarely flattering – mirror up to self and society, and dare us to rethink our place within it.

Medicine's approach to humour

The often retold, combined and liquid etymological histories of humour and the medicalised body emerge from the Hippocratic Corpus, where man's nature was expressed as consisting of 'humours', or bodily fluids. A healthy person was a person without extremes, consisting of balanced liquid content. Imbalance and separation of the humours could lead to a sick complexion that was choleric, melancholic, sanguine or phlegmatic in excess. These states were not inevitable but could be controlled through intervention and careful management, for example, by changing your habits with the seasons or with age.[23] These humoral states were physical, but also came to describe mental states and personality types, enjoying remarkable persistence in the expression of temperament as described by Galen, second-century physician to Marcus Aurelius. By the sixteenth century, humour came to mean whim, eccentricity and mood, and became thereafter tied to an idea of the comic. Humour as used in modern parlance is slippery in its definition – as seen in our discussion of theories of humour in the next section of this introduction – but can be broadly expressed as all things amusing, witty or comical. For this volume, where humour meets the medical, this humour is not only examined as discourse, around power, agency and identity, but also as an expression of the excesses and inevitabilities of the body, producing a medical humour that is often scatological and macabre.

Humour has been examined as corporeal by sociologists and psychologists adjacent to medical research, who approach the study of humour through the biological motivations of laughter and play.[24] Sociologist Cate Watson joked that if evolutionary psychologists theorise that laughter preceded speech, then perhaps slapstick – itself a visual and embodied type of humour – is the earliest source of laughter, and that she must therefore be allowed to theorise that we came down from the trees laughing at someone who had first fallen, perhaps injuring themselves.[25] These evolutionary psychology theories embroil us again in the changing definition of 'humour' and its relationship with the almost violent physicality of laughter, where laughter is both prosocial behaviour and abject humiliation.

Theories on the biological and social functions of laughter align themselves naturally with claims that humour and laughter are linked to good health. This is most clearly parsed in Part II of this volume, in which those experiencing or ruminating on death, disfigurement, disease and disability use humour in a palliative manner, or to subvert the expected reactions to their bodily situations. Immanuel Kant found medicinal use for laughter, writing that it 'comes out of a feeling of health, it furthers the business of living … and thus shows that the soul can become a physician for the body'.[26] This theory has had significant staying power; one can quote either *Proverbs* 17:22's claim that merriment is as good as medicine or William McDougall's *A New Theory of Laughter* (1903), which asserts that laughter maintains psychological health.[27] The increased professionalisation and institutionalisation of medicine has afforded researchers opportunity to test these theories, sometimes showing that humour has measurable but limited benefits in small sample groups.[28] Despite the difficulty of measuring the healing power of the comic, there seems to be a vested interest in the medical value of a good sense of humour, perhaps because it offers us control of our own health outcomes through pleasure.

Claims that laughter is itself medicine are given more weight in patient anecdotes. Morreall has noted that the popularity of the humour and health movement is in part attributed to journalist and researcher Norman Cousins's *Anatomy of an Illness as Perceived by the Patient: Reflections on Healing and Regeneration* (1979), where Cousins described his self-administered laughing cure, which led to a miraculous improvement of his life-threatening disease.[29] There are also plentiful examples of patients exploring heightened medical experiences by producing visual comedy, for example Miriam Engelberg's darkly observed *Cancer Made Me a Shallower Person: A Memoir in Comics* (2006), and Marisa Acocella Marchetto's graphic novel *Cancer Vixen* (2006).[30] What these patient-led uses of humour have in common is their re-situation and re-evaluation of a patient experience beyond the clinic, resisting the medicalisation of their sick or disabled bodies. This patient-led humour appears to upend the prototypical power relationship between medical patient and practitioner – but more can be found on *who* gets the chance to make these jokes in Soha Bayoumi's Chapter 10 at the end of this volume.

Medical humour is, of course, not solely the purview of the patient. Morreall noted the circulation of jokes by nurses in the late Doug Fletcher's *Journal of Nursing Jocularity*, a quarterly publication serving over 30,000 nurses with the opportunity to share humorous stories alongside nursing insights.[31] Scholars have variously approached humour used by health professionals, usually limited to doctors and nurses, framing their insider joking strategies as gallows humour that allows them to express their anxieties and anger and cope with their highly stressful jobs.[32] Humour has been approached as a risky but worthwhile and positive communicative bridge between professionals and patients, bringing clarity and promoting empathy. In psychotherapy, humour can produce trust, providing a moment of empathy in the shared experience of a joke, creating a comfortable space for working through difficult and painful experiences. Moving again beyond viewing humour as a coping mechanism, doctors, nurses and other healthcare professionals can deploy humour as a disruptive tool in medical environments.[33]

If this humour has power, it follows that its use may also be fraught. Medical professionals often occupy positions of both superiority and ambivalence, and their humour can therefore cause great hurt and harm – as shown in one instance by Jenna Healey's investigation of famed physician William Osler's racist and sexist joking hoaxes.[34] The authors in this volume pay particular attention to this often exploited power dynamic. In Part I, for example, Rebecca Whiteley's chapter explores Victorian anxieties about medical impropriety as depicted in mid-nineteenth-century prints, with humour emerging as a means to identify and process the enduring and unsettling power of the (male) physician. In Part II, Christine Slobogin's chapter examines the power dynamics and ethics of visual humour used by medical professionals and by patients in surgical spaces, attending to the role that positionality played in such expressions. Laura Cowley's chapter ventures far beyond the clinical encounter, tracing how twenty-first-century disabled artists have used satirical performances to critique and confront fears about medical professionals colluding with eugenicist policy. The inclusion of disability – a concept that disability scholars have resisted describing as either visual or medical – in a collection about visual humour and health makes an argument for the importance of shared research between health and medical humanities and disability studies.[35]

The power and the positionality of the medical joke is inherently inflected by the joke-teller's lived experience – as shown by many of the chapters in this volume. This work closely builds on scholarship from disability studies, where for example, John Callahan, an American cartoonist, is theorised as being able to produce biting comedy about stereotypes around disability because he was himself quadriplegic.[36] This is despite his work regularly being met with accusations of insensitivity. Research has also confirmed that the families of disabled people, while finding social benefits from humour, were more reluctant to joke about disabilities beyond their experience, reflecting their uncertain status as both insiders and outsiders, with and without permission to engage in humour.[37] This again suggests the importance of the humorist's positionality to successful humorous communications. The question of permission and authority is necessarily re-framed when it comes to laughing about death. No one, after all, can truly joke about being dead from the perspective of lived experience; yet as several chapters in *Sick Jokes* demonstrate, attempts can still be made. Despite protestations that the encounter with the medical, and particularly with debility and dying, is universal, the social acceptability of joking and laughter in these spaces is constantly contested and in flux. By juxtaposing diverse perspectives on medical care, addiction, death, disfigurement, disease and disability, this volume investigates who can and who does make medical jokes.

Theories of humour

In order to understand what novel theories of humour might be suggested by the chapters of this book, one must first understand the three established theories within humour studies. Within the worlds of art and of medicine, as well as at their intersection, the three primary ways of categorising and thinking about humour – the relief theory, the incongruity theory and the superiority theory – can be useful lenses through which to analyse both 'high' and 'low' pieces of visual culture. Some authors in this volume will contextualise their material with one or more of these theories, whereas others will use broader cultural frameworks beyond the philosophy of humour.

None of these theories work as a catch-all for the breadth and variety of styles and purposes of humour, jokes and cartoons; rather these accepted theories offer ways of organising and categorising instances of humour in a porous and moveable manner.[38] Theories of humour are helpful in some respects, but in others, trying to pigeonhole a joke into the relief, incongruity or superiority model of humour takes away some of the cultural amorphousness that these gags exemplify and on which they rely.[39] While the established theories of humour are helpful for a basic understanding of the primary ways in which humour operates, oftentimes they do little to elucidate the nuances that exist when humour hinges upon the historical vulnerabilities of the body or power dynamics of medical care. They also risk spoiling the joke by over-explaining it (a tendency of academics and scholarly writers, in any context). And yet, figuring out which theory of humour applies can be a useful exercise when parsing out the functions of a joke in the wider society or medical culture within which it exists or existed.

When telling jokes in situations of addiction, illness, injury, death or disability, it is the 'relief' or 'release' theory that first seems to be most pertinent, as it explains jokes that are said or drawn in order to release nervous energy or to diffuse tension. Relief humour can be useful in situations from the most banal – such as an awkward interaction with a colleague – to the most traumatic – such as a terminal diagnosis. Jokes that fall into this theory of humour can also be referred to as 'gallows humour', 'morbid humour' or 'black comedy'. The articulation of this theory can be traced to the early eighteenth century in Lord Shaftesbury's essay 'Sensus Communis: The Freedom of Wit and Humour' (1709), but it is more obvious in the work of Herbert Spencer and later Sigmund Freud.[40] Freud's approach to this theory of humour, as may be expected, related to the sublimation of socially improper impulses of violent or sexual natures through the accepted vehicle of the joke.[41] Jokes or cartoons that conform to the relief theory of humour are methods of dealing with difficult thoughts or situations, which can and often do arise from malfunctions of the body or of the medical care system – as shown by several of the case studies written about by the authors in this volume, particularly in Part II, 'Dying laughing'.

There already exists scholarship on the historical applications of the relief theory of humour, particularly in relation to violent episodes in history, such as the Holocaust and 9/11.[42] Traumatic events such as these feed into and/or parallel physical and medical traumas and anxieties; therefore many of the takeaways of the scholars writing on these topics can be applied to this volume's area of interest.[43] Both the violent and the medical are tense situations that require release, in which the balance of propriety is exceedingly precarious. While in some situations the humour can be inopportune or even offensive, in other cases the humour can be a relief, making the literal or metaphorical pill easier to swallow.

The incongruity theory may provide a similar release, but the construction of the joke differs. Cartoons or jokes that utilise the incongruity theory play on the absurdity of two or more things placed together that do not seem to belong, perhaps like medical care and humour in the first place. Think: a monkey dressed as a nurse, a mime at a funeral or cooked spaghetti in lieu of surgical tools in the operating theatre. This theory of humour arose in Immanuel Kant's *Critique of Judgment* (1790) and was picked up by Arthur Schopenhauer and William Hazlitt.[44] This surreal formulation of humour also brings us back to black comedy and the relief theory, as Surrealist extraordinaire André Breton is the one who coined the term 'l'humour noir'.[45] Jokes that make use of the incongruous can perhaps tell us the most about the social context in which they were created: with these types of jokes, there must be a shared understanding of what is *usual* in order for there to be a shared understanding of what is *un*usual and why that is funny.[46] As is the case with many of the visual jokes in this volume, reverse engineering can be performed on an incongruous joke in order to glean what was classified as the norm in a medical setting or group. Additionally, there are many processes, practices or protocols within medical systems in many countries (particularly in the United States) that are incongruous in themselves and that therefore provide excellent fodder for these types of jokes.[47]

The oldest theory of humour, yet the one least applicable – perhaps surprisingly – to the topics and themes of this volume, is the superiority theory, most famously articulated by Thomas Hobbes in the seventeenth century.[48] In this formulation, humour functions to assert supremacy over the butt of the joke. While as an overarching theory of humour it has largely fallen out of favour, the idea of laughing *at* someone is still an important one to acknowledge and explore, especially when the politics of the body and health are at stake.[49] We can see this theory in action most clearly in this volume in its political usage: when looking at satirical print representations of the failing, alcoholic body of Richard Brinsley Sheridan (the subject of Callum Smith's chapter), viewers feel themselves superior to the pickled, wasted and ineffectual body and political power of this ailing man.

These three theories of humour – based in Western philosophy and regrettably excluding approaches to humour from other cultures – may prove useful, but there are potential other 'theories' of humour that one can see emerging through the chapters of this book. In addition to potential for relief, incongruity or superiority, this volume also puts forward two major themes or possibilities within medically inflected humour: that of community building and of communicating information.[50] Community building is apparent in Christine Slobogin, Jo Michael Rezes, Laura Cowley and Peder Clark's chapters, with many disparate groups taking solace and making social connections through humorous visualisations of the body's vulnerabilities. The latter additional theory of humour is evident in Part III of this volume: 'Comical health communications'. All three of the authors in this final section – Jeffrey Reznick, Peder Clark and Soha Bayoumi – show that humour is vital in communicating health information. In fact, in the cases discussed by these authors, humour is more effective in getting medical information across than 'straight' public health materials. These additional theories on the emotional and practical uses of humour do not replace the theoretical frameworks of humour developed by philosophers in the last several centuries; rather they complement them, working in conjunction or alongside the needs for relief, incongruity or superiority.

Reading *Sick Jokes*

In three parts, this book explores vital aspects of the humorous visual culture of medicine: its materiality and widespread audience in print form, its flippancy in the face of bodily or medical challenges and its role in communicating health information. These chapters also largely show that these types of jokes are more commonly found in ephemera such as prints, drawings and performance pieces rather than in more canonical artistic mediums like painting or sculpture. Taken together, these chapters encourage the reader to see and interrogate the humorous in the body and in medicine, asking *why* the pathologised body or the medical encounter is funny, who that visual joke benefits or harms and what social role this material culture serves. As seen in particular with the final chapter, these questions, and these forms of humour, are still present and relevant today.

The chapters in Part I explore how British print media pathologised and politicised transgression from the early nineteenth century through to the mid-twentieth century. Tracing representations of addiction, professional impropriety and prosthetic intervention, they show how art, medicine and humour came together to tell stories of – and intervene in – debates about excess, whether that be related to overconsumption, sexual misconduct or physical matter out of place.

Callum D. Smith opens Part I ('Pathologies and power in print') with a case study on Richard Brinsley Sheridan (1751–1816), a Whig politician and infamous drunkard who was pilloried across graphic satire. Drawing connections between medical and political power, Smith shows how the perceived alcoholic excesses of Sheridan's body were translated into widespread visual metaphors that warned viewers of the grotesque constitutional, as well as personal, consequences of overindulgence. Turning to satires by James Gillray and George Cruikshank as well as lesser discussed caricaturists such as William O'Keefe, Smith showcases how artists engaged with medical observations on the consequences of habitual intoxication, working conditions like rhinophyma, bloating, palsy and vomiting into their tragicomic representations of the drunkard in decline. Drawing on Julia Skelly's theoretical concept of the 'Grim Chuckle', Smith frames this dark, embodied form of humour as a mechanism for release – offering catharsis both for those who saw themselves reflected in Sheridan, and for those relieved to be nothing like him.[51] Peppering his analysis with humorous anecdotes on Sheridan's intemperance from the parliamentary men who worked – and drank – alongside him, Smith places satirical visual culture at the centre of pathological and political reckonings on the dangers of excess.

Chapter 2 takes us into the Victorian period, with Rebecca Whiteley focusing on comical, satirical and pornographic portrayals of the doctor as a sexual actor. With print media serving to critique medical power as well as to diffuse its threat, Whiteley considers how contemporary discourses around the professionalisation of medicine collided with well-founded anxieties about (male) medical impropriety, intervention and intimacy. Whiteley's analysis sets the stage for a theme that appears several times throughout this volume: the sexual undertones (or overtones) of medical humour (see also chapters by Georgia Haire, Allison Morehead, Christine Slobogin and Jo Michael Rezes). Exploring how the Victorian popular imagination grappled with its conflicted perception of the doctor as an authoritative professional figure on the one hand and as an invasive, potentially predatory character on the other, Whiteley shows how print media intensified cultural scrutiny of both physicians and the medical encounter. Amid the mid-century boom in printed visual culture, a proliferation of pornographic flap prints, advertisements, periodical illustrations and even paintings turned their gaze toward the figure of the doctor. His 'medico-sexual' power, Whiteley argues, was a source of both fascination and fear, with the motif of medical impropriety likely provoking a nervous laugh – nervous not due to the incongruity of sexual seduction or assault in a medical encounter, but because such scenarios were all too imaginable, perhaps even expected.

The lewd and the comic are visited again in Chapter 3, as Georgia Haire examines depictions of dentures and dentistry in British seaside postcards from the mid- to late-twentieth century. Considering these cheap, ephemeral and widespread print media in their social, economic and cultural contexts, Haire demonstrates how visual jokes about dental prostheses and their users were shaped by, and helped reinforce, prejudiced attitudes related to class, gender and sex. Making visible a site often excluded from medical histories of the body, Haire's theorising on the place of the mouth in humorous visual culture situates its analysis within developments in dental treatment in the National Health Service across the twentieth century. By looking at these visual jokes about the body and its medico-dental needs and prostheses, Haire's chapter brings the history that Smith and Whiteley told of the visual jokes of power and pathology in prints of the nineteenth century into the twentieth. Theorising teeth and the mouth brings a vital perspective to thinking about humour and the body, as dentists and dental care are often excluded from medical histories and medical cultural analysis, even though oral health is often a marker or a harbinger of overall health.

Pathological politicians, lecherous doctors and false teeth are perhaps unsurprising as targets for visual jokes. In Part II, the similarly familiar but fraught subjects of death, disfigurement, disease and disability come under comic treatment, with dark humour variously surfacing as a coping mechanism, as a provocation or as a tool to build community feeling, support and understanding. Chapters 4–7 examine how artists, physicians, patients and performers have used medical humour to represent these conditions, often countering the emotions of anger, hopelessness or sadness that are socially and culturally presumed as 'natural' responses. With grotesque and carnivalesque depictions at the forefront, these chapters on 'Dying laughing' present four distinct approaches to understanding the significance of visual humour in giving representation to embodied experiences that are often left unpictured.

Many prominent artists have ruminated on the death and ageing of both their own bodies and those of others. In Chapter 4, Allison Morehead takes Edvard Munch (1863–1944) – specifically his 1915 lithograph *Dance of Death*, in which the artist portrays himself cuddling up to a skeleton – as a way to understand iconographies of death as they relate to humour, gender and power. Theories of the grotesque (particularly that of Charles Baudelaire, whose poems Munch illustrated) serve as a potent way to understand a type of visual humour that commonly deals with the body. Munch was an artist entrenched in the world of medicine, and viewing his work with a pathologised grotesque mode in mind helps us to see a critical medical humour within his *oeuvre*. Morehead's sustained exploration of this method of humour, originating from one lithograph, explodes out the medicalised cultural meanings of three artistic iconographies: the dance of death, death and the maiden and the self-portrait with death.

The grotesque mode of making the body humorous also appears in Christine Slobogin's discussion of the tube pedicle procedure in mid-century plastic surgery wards. The tube pedicle is a plastic surgery technique, popular in the twentieth century, in which a rolled piece of flesh from the patient's own body is used to reconstruct body parts (particularly noses, chins and ears). The tube pedicle, which is both part of the patient's body and separate from it, can be seen as a grotesque – and perhaps phallic and sexually suggestive – protuberance or as an enlarged body part, much like that which commonly appeared in caricatures and satirical prints of the eighteenth and nineteenth centuries. Slobogin shows that understanding the positionality of the joke teller is especially important when the tube pedicle is the vehicle of the humour. The relative power or lack thereof of plastic surgeons, medical artists and the patients themselves is teased out through the ways in which the tube pedicle is or is not visualised in a humorous way by these groups. Slobogin shows that the surgeons tended to be the most irreverent with jokes about this fleshy apparatus, medical artists tended to depersonalise it and patients tended to make it invisible.

Moving from disfigurement to disease, in Chapter 6 we see how people with HIV/AIDS used visual jokes to negotiate the social stigma of visible symptoms. Jo Michael Rezes analyses the ironically titled zine *Diseased Pariah News* (1990–99), published in California, whose editors, illustrators and contributors produced darkly humorous features about food, sex and survival. Their niche brand of dark comedy, which did not shy away from bodily functions and malfunctions, reveals a community that shared health tips and meal recipes – for example an illustrated feature titled 'GET FAT, don't die!'. Through this humour they challenged emerging conventions for visual representations of people with AIDS. Rezes examines historical contexts and makes comparative analyses with other visual constructions of HIV/AIDS as a racialised and sexualised 'wasting disease', using illustrations from *Diseased Pariah News*, Therese Frare's famous photograph of David Kirby, images of 'othered' African bodies from Ugandan public health campaigns and journalistic photography from the Biafran War. From this analysis, humour emerges as a way for people with AIDS to powerfully deconstruct the ways in which their lives and deaths had been made visible elsewhere.

Chapter 7 also looks at dark humour about medicine and death from a politically engaged community, turning to an ironic performance by Katherine Araniello (1965–2019) and Aaron Williamson (b. 1960), a duo of disabled artists from the UK who performed as the Disabled Avant-Garde. Laura Cowley analyses video documentation of their performance *Assisted Passage* (2007), a pretend, satirical protest. In this piece, Araniello starred as a 'medical model cripple', ostensibly raising support for her own medically assisted suicide. The audience of this performance did not discern the insincerity of the Disabled Avant-Garde, despite the artists' heightened performances and use of carefully ridiculous posters. Araniello and Williamson documented this failure, showing that their audience was unable to countenance their humour and ill-equipped to engage with disability arts critically. Sustained irony was leveraged by these artists to resist medicalisation, expose the ubiquity of socially constructed expectations of disability and make these ideas newly absurd.

Part III, 'Comical health communications', examines a more instrumental use of visual jokes. Humour can be a useful tool in the field of public health, to be applied by institutional bodies, health activists and individuals in affected communities to communicate health information to their audiences.[52] In these contexts, humour can be the spoonful of sugar that helps the medicine go down, to borrow from Mary Poppins. Drawn jokes and humorous delivery can bring audiences of doctors or potential healthcare recipients in, facilitating a transfer of information that might improve their practice or save their lives. Visuals help to ease the transmission of these often difficult communications, as humour does. As in Part II, analysis of humour still reveals power relations and offers opportunities to examine the ties that bind communities. In this final section, authors address humour dynamics as influenced by gender, class, regional identities and race, exploring why joking might sometimes be the key to successful communication, and why this tool is not available to all people equally.

In Chapter 8, Jeffrey Reznick analyses the sarcastic, witty humour used by medical communication experts Lois and Selma DeBakey. The sisters commissioned cartoons and produced educational films, encouraging American doctors and other health professionals to be clearer in their language. Their humour aimed to demonstrate why medical jargon (what they termed 'Medicant') and metaphorical language were ineffective. The cartoons they commissioned comically illustrate how easily thoughtless language could be misinterpreted by patients – for example, think of all of the potential meanings of 'the patient has lost a kidney'. Reznick's analysis situates the DeBakeys' professional lives and humour in the context of their medically famous family – they were the surgeon Michael DeBakey's sisters. Reznick explores the sisters' pedagogical use of dry humorous imagery, pointing out the multilayered, gendered complexity of lecturing to well-educated and often haughty clinicians. Humour helped to reach this hard-to-reach audience.

Cartoons also prove effective in the health communication campaigns of activist and charity groups. Peder Clark brings us to Manchester, England, to look at the illustrated characters of Peanut Pete and Tough Shit Thomas, among others: an unlikely ensemble of public health advocates created by Lifeline, a harm reduction charity. Rather than using the visual scare tactics more common in the 1990s era of the war on drugs, these cartoon characters took bawdy British humour – in a lineage with the seaside postcards from Haire's chapter – into nightclubs and onto the streets of northern

England to address ways to stay safe while partying and while using or addicted to drugs. Working with archival material as well as oral history interviews with former Lifeline staffers, Clark shows that humour functioned well in this context of health communication because it took into account the class, regional identity, gender identities and day-to-day experiences of the targeted audience.

This volume ends with a rumination on a topic that any reader of this book (at least in the first few years of its existence) will have experienced: the use of humour in the visual communication of the realities and best practices in the time of COVID-19. As Soha Bayoumi shows, these 'pandemic funnies' were found in news outlets, webcomics and comic books, made by both professional and amateur artists and designers. Executing a functional analysis of the vast corpus of COVID-19 comics produced in the early days of 2020 and 2021, Bayoumi argues that humour played several key roles in visual communications around the pandemic: it was didactic, it was cathartic and it was critical, with a significant overlap of these functions in some comics. All three forms of humour are displayed in the visuals analysed throughout the chapters of this volume, and this final entry shows how all of these functions of humour appeared in the visuals of COVID-19. In this chapter, Bayoumi also coins the term 'cosy comics' to define the particular subset of COVID-19 comics that were domestically focused and leaned heavily on the 'cute' factor for their humour. Bayoumi argues that, ironically, the deathly serious context of the COVID pandemic reinvigorated the use of humour in the field of graphic medicine, but with a caveat. Bayoumi shows that some people – those with relative privilege – were better able to use humour in their COVID comics; for others, particularly frontline workers and artists of colour, humour was less available to them in their depictions of the twin pandemic of COVID-19 and racial injustice.

These insights from Bayoumi end our volume on a particularly salient note, throwing into sharp focus the Western- and white-centric sources of *Sick Jokes*. This again prompts questions about positionality, inviting us to consider how some of the visual jokes featured here found form and resonance precisely because their creators and audiences occupied positions secure enough to make and appreciate them. Much more work is needed at this intersection, but we hope that *Sick Jokes* inspires more global scholarship on the role of visual humour within the critical medical humanities. The demographic dynamics of joking relating to race, gender and class – and their junctions – remain underexplored.

These chapters do not purport to construct any sort of 'complete' visual history of humour and health, nor any unequivocal theory of humour (for example, there could be another entire volume with a more 'medical history from below' perspective that looks at how patients themselves have used visual humour). Yet these chapters provide diverse examples of the key roles that visual humour plays in medical or medicalised contexts. There are continuing comic threads among all of these pieces: the infelicities of the body and medical treatments lending themselves to a grotesque humour that turns the unsettling or the 'ugly' on its head; the sexual nature of many medical jokes; humour as a way for physicians and patients alike to wrest power in medical settings and wider society; and many more. Throughout the volume, laughter and the visual joke emerge also as tools for community building and communication, used across medicalised spaces or mediums to improve information transmission and to ease or even heighten discomfort.

Taken together, the chapters that follow showcase the role of visual culture as it works with and against contemporary notions of humour, offering embodied and emotional visions of the body, (ill) health and medicine. From the dark humour that typically resides in depictions of sickness, death and disability, to the tongue-in-cheek jokes that help ease medical communication, visual histories of humour and health not only shed light on how we care for each other, but also propose humour itself as a radical method of care. The work in this volume underscores the activist potential of humorous art, showing how its deployment in medicalised contexts takes on layered political significances – both holding up a mirror to society and seeking to remake it. Ultimately, this volume weaves together art and visual culture, humour studies and the history of medicine in order to reveal the multivalent and multilayered purposes of visual humour in medical and medicalised contexts.

Notes

1 This work was supported by the Wellcome Trust [223350/Z/21/Z].
2 Previous works that have studied this intersection have largely been compilations of cartoons with minimal captions or historical/archival work added. For example, see Georges C. Benjamin, Theodore M. Brown, Susan Ladwig and Elyse Berkman (eds), *The Quest for Health Reform: A Satirical History* (American Public Health Association Press, 2013); Gideon Bosker (ed.), *Medicine is the Best Laughter* (Mosby, 1995). A recent, more in-depth, piece at this intersection: Chuan Hao (Alex) Chen, 'Narrating Humor and Persuasion in Biological Safety Cartoons', in E. Thomas Ewing and Priyanka Ganguly (eds), *Challenging Stories: Exploring the Intersections Between Health and the Humanities* (Virginia Tech Publishing, 2024), pp. 86–125.
3 William Viney, Felicity Callard and Angela Woods, 'Critical medical humanities: Embracing entanglement, taking risks', *Medical Humanities* 41:1 (2015), 7.
4 Marsha Morton and Ann-Marie Akehurst (eds), *Visual Culture and Pandemic Disease Since 1750: Capturing Contagion* (Routledge, 2023); Axel Fliethmann and Christiane Weller (eds), *Anatomy of the Medical Image: Knowledge Production and Transfiguration from the Renaissance to Today* (Brill, 2021); Fiona Johnstone, Allison Morehead and Imogen Wiltshire (eds), *Art and the Critical Medical Humanities* (Bloomsbury, 2026).
5 For studies on the particularities of English/British humour: J.B. Priestley, *English Humour* (William Heinemann, 1976). Eric G. Linfield and Egon Larsen (eds), *Laughter in a Damp Climate: An Anthology of British Humour* (Herbert Jenkins, 1963); Juliette Pattinson and Linsey Robb (eds), *British Humour and the Second World War: 'Keep Smiling Through'* (Bloomsbury, 2023).
6 John Morreall, *Comic Relief: A Comprehensive Philosophy of Humour* (John Wiley & Sons, 2009), p. 73.
7 For early modern humour histories: Joy Wiltenburg, *Laughing Histories: From the Renaissance Man to the Women of Wit* (Routledge, 2022).
8 Wendy Wick Reaves, 'The Art in Humor, the Humor in Art', *American Art* 15:2 (2001), 1, 4.
9 Wick Reaves, 'The Art in Humor', 4.
10 Jennifer A. Greenhill, *Playing It Straight: Art and Humor in the Gilded Age* (University of California Press, 2012), p. 2.

11 For more on the comedy of ancient Greek ceramics, see Alexandre G. Mitchell, *Greek Vase-Painting and the Origins of Visual Humour* (Cambridge University Press, 2009).
12 Greenhill, *Playing It Straight*, p. 5.
13 Wick Reaves, 'The Art in Humor', 1.
14 Temi Odumosu, *Africans in English Caricature: Black Jokes, White Caricature 1769–1819* (Harvey Miller Publishers, 2017), p. 41.
15 Wick Reaves, 'The Art in Humor', 5.
16 For more on the production and consumption of graphic satire in the eighteenth century, see for example James Baker, *The Business of Satirical Prints in Late-Georgian England* (Palgrave Macmillan, 2017), pp. 59–78.
17 See Sander L. Gilman, *Health and Illness: Images of Difference* (Reaktion Books, 1995); Fiona Haslam, *From Hogarth to Rowlandson: Medicine in Art in Eighteenth-century Britain* (Liverpool University Press, 1996); Roy Porter, *Bodies Politic: Disease, Death and Doctors in Britain,1650–1900* (Reaktion Books, 2001); Cindy McCreery, *The Satirical Gaze: Prints of Women in Late Eighteenth-Century England* (Clarendon Press, 2004); Corinna Wagner, *Pathological Bodies: Medicine and Political Culture* (University of California Press, 2013); Angela Rosenthal, David Bindman and Adrian W.B. Randolph (eds), *No Laughing Matter: Visual Humours in Ideas of Race, Nationality and Ethnicity* (Dartmouth College Press, 2016); Noelle Gallagher, *Itch, Clap, Pox: Venereal Disease in the Eighteenth-Century Imagination* (Yale University Press, 2018).
18 See for example the chapters in Victoria Bates, Alan Bleakley and Sam Goodman (eds), *Medicine, Health and the Arts: Approaches to the Medical Humanities* (Routledge, 2014).
19 Fiona Johnstone, 'Manifesto for a Visual Medical Humanities', *BMJ Medical Humanities Blog*, 31 July 2018, https://blogs.bmj.com/medical-humanities/2018/07/31/manifesto-for-a-visual-medical-humanities/; Fiona Johnstone and Suzannah Biernoff, 'What can art history offer the medical humanities?', *Medical Humanities* 50 (2024), 529–38; Helen Scott-Fordsmand, 'Reversing the medical humanities', *Medical Humanities* 49 (2023), 347–60; Viney, Callard and Woods, 'Critical Medical Humanities: Embracing Entanglement, Taking Risks'; Des Fitzgerald and Felicity Callard, 'Entangling the Medical Humanities', in Angela Woods and Anne Whitehead (eds), *The Edinburgh Companion to the Critical Medical Humanities* (Edinburgh University Press, 2016), pp. 35–49.
20 Mark Philp, 'Nervous Laughter and the Invasion of Britain 1797–1805', in Mark Knights and Adam Morton (eds), *The Power of Laughter*

and Satire in Early Modern Britain: Political and Religious Culture, 1500–1820 (Boydell & Brewer, 2017), p. 189.

21 Haslam, *From Hogarth to Rowlandson*, p. xv.

22 Alun Withey, *Physick and the Family: Health, Medicine and Care in Wales 1600–1750* (Manchester University Press, 2011), p. 1.

23 Jouanna Jacques, 'The Legacy of the Hippocratic Treatise *The Nature of Man:* the Theory of the Four Humours', trans. Neil Allies, in Philip van der Eijk (ed.), *Greek Medicine from Hippocrates to Galen: Selected Papers* (Brill, 2012), p. 335.

24 Matthew Gervais and David Sloan Wilson, 'The evolution and functions of laughter and humor: A synthetic approach', *The Quarterly Review of Biology* 80:4 (2005), 395–430.

25 Cate Watson, *Comedy and Social Science: Towards a Methodology of Funny* (Routledge, 2015), p. 21.

26 Peter L. Berger, *Redeeming Laughter: The Comic Dimension of Human Experience* (Walter de Gruyter, 1997), p. 23.

27 John Morreall, 'Applications of Humor: Health, the Workplace, and Education', in Victor Raskin (ed.), *The Primer of Humor Research* (Mouton de Gruyter, 2008), p. 452.

28 Rod A. Martin, 'Humor and Health', in Victor Raskin (ed.), *The Primer of Humor Research* (Mouton de Gruyter, 2008), p. 501; Kei Hayashi et al., 'Laughter is the Best Medicine? A Cross-Sectional Study of Cardiovascular Disease Among Older Japanese Adults', *Journal of Epidemiology and Community Health* 26:10 (2016), 546–52; Luís Carlos Lopes-Júnior et al., 'Effectiveness of hospital clowns for symptom management in paediatrics: systematic review of randomised and non-randomised controlled trials', *British Medical Journal* 371 (2020), https://doi.org/10.1136/bmj.m4290.

29 Norman Cousins, *Anatomy of an Illness as Perceived by the Patient: Reflections on Healing and Regeneration* (Norton, 1979); Morreall, 'Applications of Humor: Health, the Workplace, and Education', p. 452.

30 Miriam Engelberg, *Cancer Made Me a Shallower Person: A Memoir in Comics* (Harper Collins, 2006); Marisa Acocella Marchetto, *Cancer Vixen: A True Story* (Knopf, 2014).

31 Morreall, 'Applications of Humor: Health, the Workplace, and Education', p. 453.

32 Vera Robinson, *Humor and the Health Professions: The Therapeutic Use of Humor in Health Care*, 2nd edition (Slack Books, 1991), quoted in Victor Raskin, *The Primer of Humor Research* (Mouton de Gruyter,

2008), p. 453; Katie Watson, 'Gallows Humor in Medicine', *Hastings Center Report* 41:5 (2012), 37–45.

33 Slobogin has previously suggested that in the tightly hierarchical context of the twentieth-century surgical ward, jokes, and particularly visual humour, can disrupt gender and class roles associated with the status of healthcare workers and their patients, including not just doctors and nurses, but also hospital orderlies. Christine Slobogin, *Putting Plastic Surgery on Paper: How Art and Archives Defined Second World War Reconstructive Surgery in Britain* (University of Rochester Press and Boydell & Brewer, 2025), pp. 151–86.

34 Jenna Healey, '"A Vile Custom": The Strange Career of William Osler's "Professional Notes"', *Journal of the History of Medicine and Allied Sciences* 80:2 (2025), 105–25.

35 Rosemarie Garland-Thomson, *Extraordinary Bodies: Figuring Physical Disability in American Culture and Literature* (Columbia University Press, 2017), p. 6.

36 Beth Haller and Sue Ralph, 'John Callahan's Pelswick cartoon and a new phase of disability humor', *Disability Studies Quarterly* 23:3/4 (Summer/Fall 2003), 4–16.

37 Alicja Rieger, 'Humor and other types of fun: Explorations of the functions of humor among families of children with disabilities', *Research and Practice for Persons with Severe Disabilities* 29:3 (2005), 194–209.

38 In his introduction, Morreall traces how these theories have come in and out of fashion for humour theorists. This book looks at all three of these theories equally while understanding that their borders are permeable, their uses are many and their necessity is not absolute. John Morreall, 'Introduction', in *The Philosophy of Laughter and Humor* (State University of New York Press, 1987), pp. 3–6.

39 A succinct and clear summary of these three theories and their histories appears in John Morreall's chapter in *The Primer of Humor Research*, although a reader should beware that he cites his own previous work rather than providing helpful footnotes to the writers and theorists about whom he speaks. John Morreall, 'Philosophy and Religion', in Victor Raskin (ed.), *The Primer of Humor Research* (Mouton de Gruyter, 2008), pp. 211–29. See also: John Morreall (ed.), *The Philosophy of Laughter and Humour* (State University of New York Press, 1987).

40 Anthony Ashley Cooper, Earl of Shaftesbury, *Sensus Communis: An Essay on the Freedom of Wit and Humour. In a Letter to a Friend* (Egbert Sanger, 1709); Herbert Spencer, 'The Physiology of Laughter',

in *Illustrations of Universal Progress: A Series of Discussions* (D. Appleton & Company, 1875), pp. 194–209.

41 Sigmund Freud, *Jokes and Their Relation to the Unconscious*, trans. Joyce Crick (Penguin Random House, 2003 [1905]).

42 Steve Lipman, *Laughter in Hell: The Use of Humor During the Holocaust* (Jason Aronson, 1991); Paul Lewis, *Cracking Up: American Humor in a Time of Conflict* (The University of Chicago Press, 2006).

43 In fact, on the first page of *Cracking Up: American Humor in a Time of Conflict* (2006), Paul Lewis compares an improv troupe doing an skit on the theme of 'terrorists' to a clown appearing in a hospital room to 'cheer up' a post-operative teenaged girl. Lewis, *Cracking Up*, pp. 1–2.

44 Some humour scholars trace this theory back even further to Francis Hutcheson's 1750 *Reflections on Laughter*, which was initially a critique of Hobbes's superiority theory of humour. Francis Hutcheson, *Reflections upon Laughter and Remarks Upon The Fable of the Bees* (R. Urie, 1750); Simon Critchley, *On Humour* (Routledge, 2002), p. 3; Hutcheson also appears in Morreall's edited volume *The Philosophy of Laughter and Humor*, where Hutcheson is described as having 'at least the beginnings of an Incongruity Theory of humour'. John Morreall, 'Francis Hutcheson (1694–1746)', in *The Philosophy of Laughter and Humor* (State University of New York Press, 1987), p. 26; Immanuel Kant, *Kant's Critique of Judgement*, 2nd edition, ed. J.H. Bernard (Macmillan, 1974 [1790]); Arthur Schopenhauer, *The World as Will and Idea*, trans. R.B. Haldane and J. Kemp, vol. 1, 3rd edition (Kegan Paul, Trench, Trübner & Co, 1891 [1818/1819]), pp. 76–80; William Hazlitt, 'On Wit and Humour', in *Lectures on the English Comic Writers*, 3rd edition (John Templeman, 1819), pp. 1–55.

45 André Breton, *Anthology of Black Humor*, trans. Mark Polizzotti (City Lights Books, 1997 [1940]).

46 Critchley, *On Humour*, p. 4.

47 See: Benjamin, Brown, Ladwig and Berkman, *The Quest for Health Reform*.

48 Thomas Hobbes, *Leviathan, or The Matter, Forme, & Power of a Common-Wealth Ecclesiasticall and Civill* (Andrew Crooke, 1651), p. 40; Thomas Hobbes, 'Human Nature: Or the Fundamental Elements of Policy', in *The English Works of Thomas Hobbes of Malmesbury*, ed. William Molesworth, vol. 4 (John Bohn, 1840 [1684]), pp. 45–7.

49 In his 1987 edited volume, humour philosopher John Morreall noted that the theorising behind the superiority theory is overall sloppy and that it held too much of a hold on humour studies for centuries

(it was the only developed theory of humour until the mid-eighteenth century). Morreall, *The Philosophy of Laughter and Humor*, pp. 3–4; Morreall, 'Philosophy and Religion', p. 211.

50 Humour is a marker of belonging and not belonging for social groups, and is inflected by national and racial identity. Sander Gilman has discussed how racialised, religious diaspora groups, and particularly Jewish men in the West, have met demands to affirm their civic status through humour since the eighteenth century. Sander Gilman, '"Jewish Humour" and the terms by which Jews and Muslims join Western civilization', *Year Book – Leo Baeck Institute* 57:1 (2012), 53–65.

51 Julia Skelly, 'The politics of drunkenness: John Henry Walker, John A. Macdonald, and graphic satire', *Canadian Art Review* 40:1 (2015), 71–84.

52 Amy Clare Schumacher, 'Humor in Public Health Messaging: Past, Present, Future' (PhD thesis, University of Iowa, 2017); Lars Cernerud and Henny Olsson, 'Humour seen from a public health perspective', *Scandinavian Journal of Public Health* 35:3 (2004), 396–8.

References

Acocella Marchetto, Marisa. *Cancer Vixen: A True Story*. Knopf, 2014.

Baker, James. *The Business of Satirical Prints in Late-Georgian England*. Palgrave Macmillan, 2017.

Bates, Victoria, Alan Bleakley and Sam Goodman (eds). *Medicine, Health and the Arts: Approaches to the Medical Humanities*. Routledge, 2014.

Benjamin, Georges C., Theodore M. Brown, Susan Ladwig and Elyse Berkman (eds). *The Quest for Health Reform: A Satirical History*. American Public Health Association Press, 2013.

Berger, Peter L. *Redeeming Laughter: The Comic Dimension of Human Experience*. Walter de Gruyter, 1997.

Bosker, Gideon (ed.). *Medicine is the Best Laughter*. Mosby, 1995.

Breton, André. *Anthology of Black Humor*. Translated by Mark Polizzotti. City Light Books, 1997 [1940].

Cernerud, Lars, and Henny Olsson. 'Humour seen from a public health perspective'. *Scandinavian Journal of Public Health* 32:5 (2004), 396–8.

Chen, Chuan Hao (Alex). 'Narrating Humor and Persuasion in Biological Safety Cartoons'. In Thomas Ewing and Priyanka Ganguly (eds),

Challenging Stories: Exploring the Intersections between Health and the Humanities. Virginia Tech Publishing, 2024.

Cooper, Anthony Ashley, Earl of Shaftesbury. *Sensus Communis: An Essay on the Freedom of Wit and Humour. In a Letter to a Friend*. Egbert Sanger, 1709.

Cousins, Norman. *Anatomy of an Illness as Perceived by the Patient: Reflections on Healing and Regeneration*. Norton, 1979.

Critchley, Simon. *On Humour*. Routledge, 2002.

Engelberg, Miriam. *Cancer Made Me a Shallower Person: A Memoir in Comics*. Harper Collins, 2006.

Fitzgerald, Des, and Felicity Callard. 'Entangling the Medical Humanities'. In Angela Woods and Anne Whitehead (eds), *The Edinburgh Companion to the Critical Medical Humanities*. Edinburgh University Press, 2016.

Fliethmann, Axel, and Christiane Weller (eds). *Anatomy of the Medical Image: Knowledge Production and Transfiguration from the Renaissance to Today*. Brill, 2021.

Freud, Sigmund. *Jokes and Their Relation to the Unconscious*. Translated by Joyce Crick. Penguin Random House, 2003 [1905].

Gallagher, Noelle. *Itch, Clap, Pox: Venereal Disease in the Eighteenth-Century Imagination*. Yale University Press, 2018.

Garland-Thomson, Rosemarie. *Extraordinary Bodies: Figuring Physical Disability in American Culture and Literature*. Columbia University Press, 2017.

Gervais, Matthew, and David Sloan Wilson. 'The evolution and functions of laughter and humor: a synthetic approach'. *The Quarterly Review of Biology* 80:4 (2005), 395–430.

Gilman, Sander L. *Health and Illness: Images of Difference*. Reaktion Books, 1995.

Gilman, Sander L. '"Jewish Humour" and the terms by which Jews and Muslims join Western civilization'. *Year Book – Leo Baeck Institute* 57:1 (2012), 53–65.

Greenhill, Jennifer A. *Playing It Straight: Art and Humor in the Gilded Age*. University of California Press, 2012.

Haller, Beth, and Sue Ralph. 'John Callahan's Pelswick cartoon and a new phase of disability humor'. *Disability Studies Quarterly* 23:3/4 (2003), 4–16.

Haslam, Fiona. *From Hogarth to Rowlandson: Medicine in Art in Eighteenth-century Britain*. Liverpool University Press, 1996.

Hayashi, Kei, Ichiro Kawachi, Tetsuya Ohira, Katsunori Kondo, Kokoro Shirai and Naoki Kondo. 'Laughter is the best medicine? A cross-sectional study of cardiovascular disease among older Japanese adults'. *Journal of Epidemiology and Community Health* 26:10 (2016), 546–52.

Hazlitt, William. *Lectures on the English Comic Writers*. 3rd edition. John Templeman, 1819.
Healey, Jenna. '"A Vile Custom": The Strange Career of William Osler's "Professional Notes"'. *Journal of the History of Medicine and Allied Sciences* 80:2 (2025), 105–25.
Hobbes, Thomas. 'Human Nature: Or the Fundamental Elements of Policy'. In William Molesworth (ed.), *The English Works of Thomas Hobbes of Malmesbury*. Volume 4. John Bohn, 1840 [1684].
Hobbes, Thomas. *Leviathan, or The Matter, Forme, & Power of a Common-Wealth Ecclesiasticall and Civill*. Andrew Crooke, 1651.
Hutcheson, Francis. *Reflections upon Laughter and Remarks Upon the Fable of the Bees*. R. Urie, 1750.
Johnstone, Fiona. 'Manifesto for a Visual Medical Humanities'. *BMJ Medical Humanities Blog* 31 July 2018, https://blogs.bmj.com/medical-humanities/2018/07/31/manifesto-for-a-visual-medical-humanities/.
Johnstone, Fiona, and Suzannah Biernoff. 'What can art history offer the medical humanities?' *Medical Humanities* 50 (2024), 529–38.
Johnstone, Fiona, Allison Morehead and Imogen Wiltshire (eds). *Art and the Critical Medical Humanities*. Bloomsbury, 2026.
Jouanna, Jacques. 'The Legacy of the Hippocratic Treatise *The Nature of Man*: The Theory of the Four Humours'. In Philip van der Eijk (ed.), *Greek Medicine from Hippocrates to Galen: Selected Papers*. Translated by Niel Allies. Brill, 2012.
Kant, Immanuel. *Kant's Critique of Judgment*. Second edition. Edited by J.H. Bernard. Macmillan, 1974 [1790].
Lewis, Paul. *Cracking Up: American Humor in a Time of Conflict*. The University of Chicago Press, 2006.
Linfield, Eric G., and Egon Larsen (eds). *Laughter in a Damp Climate: An Anthology of British Humour*. Herbert Jenkins, 1963.
Lipman, Steve. *Laughter in Hell: The Use of Humor During the Holocaust*. Jason Aronson, 1991.
Lopes-Júnior, Luís Carlos, Emma Bomfim and Karin Olson, et al. 'Effectiveness of hospital clowns for symptom management in paediatrics: systematic review of randomised and non-randomised controlled trials'. *British Medical Journal* 371 (2020). doi: 0.1136/bmj.m4290.
Martin, Rod A. 'Humor and Health'. In Victor Raskin (ed.), *The Primer of Humor Research*. Mouton de Gruyter, 2008.
McCreery, Cindy. *The Satirical Gaze: Prints of Women in Late Eighteenth-Century England*. Clarendon Press, 2004.
Mitchell, Alexandre G. *Greek Vase-Painting and the Origins of Visual Humour*. Cambridge University Press, 2009.
Morreall, John (ed.). *The Philosophy of Laughter and Humor*. State University of New York Press, 1987.

Morreall, John. 'Applications of Humor: Health, the Workplace, and Education'. In Victor Raskin (ed.), *The Primer of Humor Research*. Mouton de Gruyter, 2008.

Morreall, John. 'Philosophy and Religion'. In Victor Ruskin (ed.), *The Primer of Humor Research*. Mouton de Gruyter, 2008.

Morreall, John. *Comic Relief: A Comprehensive Philosophy of Humour*. John Wiley & Sons, 2009.

Morton, Marsha and Ann-Marie Akehurst (eds). *Visual Culture and Pandemic Disease Since 1750: Capturing Contagion*. Routledge, 2023.

Odumosu, Temi. *Africans in English Caricature: Black Jokes, White Caricature 1769–1819*. Harvey Miller Publishers, 2017.

Pattinson, Juliette, and Linsey Robb (eds). *British Humour and the Second World War: 'Keep Smiling Through'*. Bloomsbury, 2023.

Philp, Mark. 'Nervous Laughter and the Invasion of Britain 1797–1805'. In Mark Knights and Adam Morton (eds), *The Power of Laughter and Satire in Early Modern Britain: Political and Religious Culture, 1500–1820*. Boydell & Brewer, 2017.

Porter, Roy. *Bodies Politic: Disease, Death and Doctors in Britain, 1650–1900*. Reaktion Books, 2001.

Priestley, J.B. *English Humour*. William Heinemann, 1976.

Raskin, Victor. *The Primer of Humor Research*. Mouton de Gruyter, 2008.

Rieger, Alicja. 'Humor and other types of fun: Explorations of the functions of humor among families of children with disabilities'. *Research and Practice for Persons with Severe Disabilities* 29:3 (2005), 194–209.

Robinson, Vera. *Humor and the Health Professions: The Therapeutic Use of Humor in Health Care*. Second edition. Slack Books, 1991.

Rosenthal, Angela, David Bindman and Adrian W.B. Randolph (eds), *No Laughing Matter: Visual Humours in Ideas of Race, Nationality and Ethnicity*. Dartmouth College Press, 2016.

Schopenhauer, Arthur. *The World as Will and Idea*. Third edition, volume 1. Translated by R.B. Haldane and J. Kemp. Kegan Paul, Trench, Trübner & Co, 1891 [1818/19].

Schumacher, Amy Clare. 'Humor in Public Health Messaging: Past, Present, Future'. Unpublished doctoral thesis, University of Iowa, 2017.

Scott-Fordsmand, Helen. 'Reversing the Medical Humanities'. *Medical Humanities* 49 (2023), 347–60.

Slobogin, Christine. *Putting Plastic Surgery on Paper: How Art and Archives Defined Second World War Reconstructive Surgery in Britain*. University of Rochester Press and Boydell & Brewer, 2025.

Spencer, Herbert. 'The Physiology of Laughter'. In *Illustrations of Universal Progress: A Series of Discussions*. D. Appleton & Company, 1875.

Viney, William, Felicity Callard and Angela Woods. 'Critical medical humanities: Embracing entanglement, taking risks'. *Medical Humanities* 41:1 (2015), 2–7.

Wagner, Corinna. *Pathological Bodies: Medicine and Political Culture*. University of California Press, 2013.

Watson, Cate. *Comedy and Social Science: Towards a Methodology of Funny*. Routledge, 2015.

Watson, Katie. 'Gallows humor in medicine'. *Hastings Center Report* 41:5 (2012), 37–45.

Wick Reaves, Wendy. 'The Art in Humor, the Humor in Art'. *American Art* 15:2 (2001), 2–9.

Wiltenburg, Joy. *Laughing Histories: From the Renaissance Man to the Woman of Wit*. Routledge, 2022.

Part I

Pathologies and power in print

1

'Uncorking' Richard Brinsley Sheridan: Alcohol, the body and political decline in visual culture

Callum D. Smith

'Men of all ages drink abominably', wrote Sir Gilbert Elliot, 'Sheridan excessively'.[1] By the late eighteenth century, alcohol was integral to politics, particularly among the Foxite Whigs, a political faction centred around Charles James Fox, known for their tactical use of insular and porous sociability and for their notoriously excessive drinking.[2] This chapter explores the relationship between alcohol, the body, morality and politics in the late eighteenth and early nineteenth centuries, focusing on the heaviest Foxite imbiber, Richard Brinsley Sheridan (1751–1816), during his political decline.[3] Despite frequent contemporary allusions to Sheridan's 'Six-Bottle Man' status, an in-depth study of alcohol's role on his health, career and character is overdue.[4] Sheridan's relationship with alcohol is best summarised by his own retort: warned that alcohol would destroy the coat of his stomach, he replied, 'well then my stomach might just digest in its waistcoat'.[5] By the end of his career, Sheridan was commonly depicted in visual culture in the midst of vomiting, and this chapter is concerned with how the physical effects of excessive consumption were used to illustrate a subject's decline, illness, corruption and political unsuitability in caricature.[6] Sheridan will serve as a case study to explore the wider significance of how excessive consumption was perceived by his contemporaries and the voting public, how it affected his political career and his health, how it became the subject of satirical culture and how these interrelated.

The focus of this investigation on Sheridan makes it male-centric, with masculine sociability a dominant theme. As others have shown, female sociability was equally nuanced in the period.[7] Cultural perceptions and gender norms were key factors that shaped drinking behaviours, including the public drinking by Sheridan's contemporaries. Venues often dictated types of drinkers; taverns, coffeehouses and social clubs were predominantly, though not exclusively, male spaces.[8] Ian Newman's work introduces the Crown & Anchor tavern as one such Foxite venue for both 'political dining of the masculine associational world' and 'mixed-company forms of gathering' suitable for fashionable female sociability.[9] Within these spaces, drinking rituals like toasting reinforced social bonds, loyalty and mutual respect.[10] Contemporary notions of honour and public persona were closely tied to excessive consumption. Masculinity was often measured by a man's ability to drink heavily without losing composure; these were the revered Six Bottle Men.[11] In contrast, perceived excessive drinking by women such as Georgiana Cavendish, Duchess of Devonshire reflected moral failure and loss of status. During the 1784 General Election, satirical prints attacked her alleged inebriation, inter-class mingling and sexual promiscuity.[12] Engaging in sociable drinking without succumbing to excess maintained honour, a concept Mark Hailwood terms 'good fellowship' in a masculine context. This involved both informal and formal regulations, such as everyone paying their share, and the expectation that, despite heavy drinking, one remained in control of body and mind and kept pace with their peers.[13] The line between 'good fellowship' and excessive drunkenness will be assessed through political caricature, revealing how the medium portrayed excessive alcohol consumption and how this related to the public and political self. Though alcoholism as a term is anachronistic, and was not coined until 1852, it will be used in this chapter to denote the concept of alcohol addiction and uncontrolled excessive consumption.[14]

Two key questions underpin this chapter: what exactly is funny about drunkenness, and how did visual satire package and weaponise alcoholism?[15] Julia Skelly's 'Grim Chuckle' framework, rooted in Sigmund Freud's theory of laughter as tension release, will be used to analyse depictions of Sheridan.[16] A form of dark or gallows humour, the 'Grim Chuckle' is a response to subjects generally considered serious, distressing or taboo – in this case alcoholism. The function of the intended laughter in these satirical prints is to change or influence the viewer's perception of drunkenness and the drinker. Jokes and satire often draw upon taboo subjects or suppressed impulses, confronting these issues in a comical context, allowing repressed feelings to be safely addressed.[17] Audience responses are dual in nature: they may recognise their own experiences with alcohol while rejecting the depicted drinker's actions. Laughter in this context can be both uncomfortable and a form of catharsis.

Audiences might also deplore such alcoholic excess, and in this context Thomas Hobbes's 'superiority theory' is relevant to the satirical depiction of addiction.[18] Laughter, under this model, results from feeling superior – experiencing a 'sudden glory' in relation to someone else's mistakes, flaws or failings; there is an underlying element of competition or conflict.[19] In the context of alcoholism, this might manifest in jokes that highlight the foolishness, lack of control or 'bad fellowship' of the alcoholic, providing a sense of superiority as well as the aforementioned relief for the audience. The notion of superiority is particularly interesting when one considers the audience of caricature, and the status of the medium's depicted subjects in relation to the work of art historian Diana Donald. Donald views caricature as 'the art of the excluded', expressing not 'powerlessness but contempt for the mighty'; indeed, politics was not only seen from below but attacked from below through the medium of caricature.[20] It was, in Vic Gatrell's words, 'people's art', which not only acted as a tool of expression but also encouraged homo-sociability.[21]

Caricature's audience was often depicted as a diverse crowd peering into a print shop window; the most cited example is James Gillray's *Very Slippy Weather* (1808), which portrays such a crowd viewing hanging prints for free through a shop window.[22] Gillray's portrayal holds some truth, as Tamara Hunt shows that between 1770 and 1820, between seventy-five and one hundred 'individuals or firms published prints'.[23] Thus, anyone passing by could view caricatures for free. It is commonly assumed that such a free display and its visual allure was designed specifically for the illiterate lower orders, however this assumption is reductive. As H.T. Dickinson notes, 'these claims are very easily made, but rather difficult to verify'.[24] Roy Porter further cautions that viewing pictures as 'baby-food' for those unable to digest real words misinterprets the role of visual imagery in the emerging commercial culture.[25]

But the relatively high cost of caricatures did restrict their purchasing audience. Robert Hume suggests that between 1688 and 1801, only about 3 per cent of families could afford more than the bare minimum of 'cultural' products such as commercial art.[26] However, this does not mean the remaining 97 per cent had no access to political caricatures. Print 'consumption' took many forms, though most were centred in London. Beyond print shops, pirated and rented volumes also allowed for dissemination among the lower orders.[27] Scholars rely on Donald and Dickinson's estimates of caricature print runs, averaging 500–1,500 copies, though Eirwen Nicholson's study reveals variations, with popular prints reaching as many as 16,000 copies.[28] Costs also varied: Donald's estimate of one shilling for coloured prints and sixpence for uncoloured ones is commonly cited, but Nicholson notes that more sophisticated works by renowned artists fetched higher prices.[29] Caricatures' mission of 'attacking from below' fits Hobbes's 'superiority theory', creating a temporary power reversal between caricature's predominantly lower-middle order audience and its largely aristocratic subjects. Sheridan's privileged social position must therefore be considered in assessing his bodily, political and moral depictions.

Born in Dublin in 1751 into the middle orders, Sheridan pursued a career as a playwright and purchased the Drury Lane Theatre in 1776, before pursuing a political career. His bridging of the theatrical and political realms made him a frequent target for satirists; Marc Baer claims that one in ten Sheridan prints referenced the theatre.[30] Yet, it was Sheridan's role as a purveyor of entertainment to the aristocracy that gained the middle-order Irishman entry into the elite Whig world. The Foxites, largely male aristocrats with a few middle-order men of 'great talents', spent most of their careers opposing the conservative government of William Pitt the Younger.[31] Sheridan's place in their circle was solidified by his appointments to the Literary Club in 1777 and Brooks's in 1778.[32] Given Sheridan's Irish heritage, stereotyping in caricature was relatively common, despite James Kelly's work revealing that the

Irish 'propensity for excessive drinking' had 'little basis in reality'.[33] In visual culture, heavy Irish drinking was often signified by Irish Whiskey punch, and in Sheridan caricatures, its inclusion dragged him into the realms of the middling and lower orders. Symbolically, punch was a communal drink favoured by the 'middling sorts'; its presence in a scene indicated that the guests drank both physically and metaphorically from the same bowl.[34]

Aside from his social connection with the Foxites, Sheridan was politically tied to Fox's faction, being elected to Stafford in 1780 and holding a Treasury post during Fox's brief 1783 coalition with Lord North.[35] In the late 1780s, Sheridan grew more involved with radical movements, through connections with the Society of the Friends of the People and the United Irishmen.[36] After Pitt's death in 1806, Sheridan was made Treasurer of the Navy during the fifteen-month 'Ministry of all the Talents'.[37] However, his political fortunes soon declined. Following Fox's death in September 1806, he was overlooked as Fox's Westminster successor in favour of Lord Percy.[38] Though he eventually secured the Westminster seat, Sheridan's incumbency was short-lived; he lost his seat in the 1807 election to Francis Burdett and Lord Cochrane, leading him to admit to his 'total ruin as a public man'.[39] The extent to which his alcohol consumption, and its reported impact on his health, visualised this 'total ruin' is of particular interest.

Unsurprisingly, and given his surname, the most common caricature reference to Sheridan's alcoholism was the inclusion of 'sherry', be it a bottle of the alcoholic namesake, or used as an epithet. Among the most known pictorial uses of the sherry signifier is Gillray's 1805 *Uncorking Old Sherry* (Figure 1.1) in which an alcohol-pickled head of Sheridan ('sherry') is about to be released by an uncorking Pitt. The 'pickled' nature of the 'old' head is likely a swipe at Sheridan's preserved and stale position in political life. Similarly, the choice of alcohol used to represent the bottled Foxites is deliberate and pointed, while Sheridan is 'sherry'; Erskine is 'Spruce Beer', a drink known for its volatile and frothy nature; while Fox is 'true French wine'. French alcohol, be it wine, port or brandy was consistently used in caricature to emphasise the Foxites' Francophilia.[40]

Gillray's depiction is relatively rare: despite the print's clear links to alcohol, Sheridan, by nature of being trapped within the bottle,

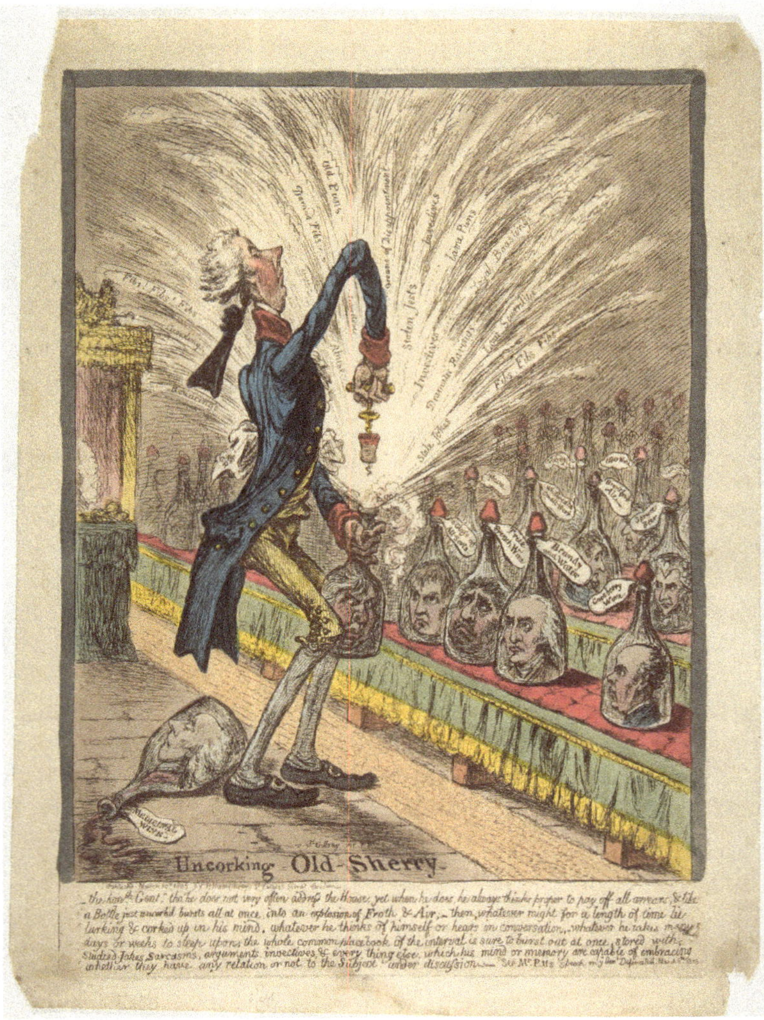

Figure 1.1 James Gillray, *Uncorking Old Sherry*. Published by Hannah Humphrey, 10 March 1805, hand-coloured etching.

is not depicted in a state of excessive consumption or drunkenness. *Uncorking Old Sherry* does situate Sheridan at the front of the Foxite drinking vanguard; however, he is the volatile bottle which Pitt has chosen to uncork. Even as an isolated head, the effects of

Sheridan's drinking are visible from his red, blotchy skin and nose (sometimes referred to as rhinophyma), a characteristic not shared by the majority of the other bottled Foxites. Though the exact cause of this condition is not fully known, colloquial terms for the condition – 'whiskey nose' and 'gin blossom'- reveal the enduring association between the condition and excessive drinking.[41] Beyond the obvious comic function of associating 'Sherry' with alcohol and excess, there were deeper symbolic functions to Sheridan's consistent portrayal as an excessive alcoholic.

'The drinking man's disease': The physical effects of excess

To understand how Sheridan's drinking was caricatured and received by the viewing public, it is necessary to chart the period's understanding of alcohol, addiction and disease. Roy Porter argued that despite the belief that doctors only began viewing habitual drunkenness as a medical issue in the nineteenth century, evidence suggests an awareness of its dangers in the earlier eighteenth century.[42] As Skelly notes, 'even if terms such as "addiction" and "alcoholism" only came into popular use in the late nineteenth and early twentieth centuries', the concept of addiction is not a recent phenomenon. Though anachronistic, these terms have value in contextualising our understanding of eighteenth-century alcohol consumption and reliance.[43] The perils of overindulgence were also understood alongside medical praise for alcohol, which commonly attributed any ill-effects to abuse by individuals rather than moderate consumption. Indeed, in 1773 Dr Peter Shaw praised wine as the 'grand remedy' for ailments like gout, hypochondria and venereal disease, advising patients to 'take a hearty glass and be merry with your friends'.[44] Erasmus Darwin wrote of the physical effects of alcohol on unaccustomed drinkers, suggesting those familiar with heavy drinking were less prone to ill effects: 'mark what happens to a man who drinks a quart of wine or of ale ... He loses the use both of his limbs and of his understanding. He becomes a temporary idiot, and has a temporary stroke of the palsy.'[45] The visual comic potential of such 'temporary idiocy', and indeed loss of manliness or 'Good Fellowship', was not lost on caricaturists. Satirical depictions of excess in 'hard drinkers' like Sheridan drew on symptoms listed by Matthew Baillie and his contemporaries, including flatulence, dyspepsia, dropsy, gout and cirrhosis. Dr Robert Willan categorised these effects into three phases in 1803: beginning with 'stomach discomforts', progressing to 'serious diseases' like convulsions or dropsy and finally leading to 'mental derangement'.[46]

In prints depicting Sheridan's drunkenness one can therefore expect to see such consequences caricatured, and one can presume an awareness among the viewing public of the alcoholic cause of such actions. Indeed, in Gillray's *Uncorking Old Sherry* there are hints at Sheridan's lapses into 'idiocy' or loss of control in the explosion of words frothing from the bottle: 'Bouncings!', 'lame puns', 'egotism'. These contribute to Sheridan's image as an 'uncontrolled' excess-favouring politician. The text below the print further supports this image by commenting on his tendency to take 'days or weeks to sleep upon issues', or to speak in Parliament 'whether [his words] have any relation or not to the subject under discussion'.[47] These are not descriptions of a statesman in full control of his actions, though they are undeniably comical.

Perhaps the most visceral physical manifestation of Sheridan's drinking in caricature, and of excessive consumption more broadly, was projectile vomiting. Unlike more subtle characteristics of over-imbibing, vomiting was a visible symbol of excess, the implication being that the consumer either does not know their limits or has chosen to exceed them. This was certainly the case in W. O'Keeffe's *Frontispiece to The Rising Sun, Vol. III* (Figure 1.2).[48] Published in June 1807 following the collapse of the Ministry of All the Talents, in which Sheridan held the minor role of Treasurer of the Navy, the print centres around an imagined final supper of the ministry. Sheridan had narrowly won the Westminster seat in 1806, though the collapse of the ministry led to another contest in which Sheridan would ultimately lose his short-held seat.[49] Having over-imbibed, Sheridan has fallen from his chair and lies vomiting excessively upon the floor, mirroring the spilling bottle to his left.

The vomit itself is noteworthy; pink in colour, it appears to be red wine or port, and the quantity flowing from Sheridan's body indicates the excess consumed. Willan's phases of degeneration are

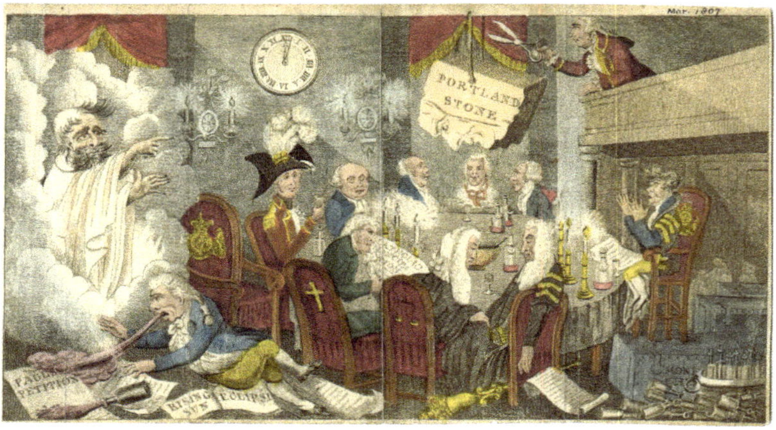

Figure 1.2 W. O'Keeffe, *Frontispiece to The Rising Sun, Vol. III*. Published by Benjamin Appleyard, 1 June 1807, hand-coloured etching.

visualised: his loss of muscle control (palsy), flailing legs (convulsions) and distended stomach (dropsy).[50] The next phase, 'mental derangement', is implied.[51] Sheridan is the most inebriated, but not the only one; glasses are drained, and five decanters are nearly empty. A mountain of empty bottles adds to the scene's debauchery. While Sheridan vomits, Erskine, Ellenborough and Derby are asleep. George III prepares to release the 'Portland Stone', while a ghostly Fox's warning goes unheard.[52] Yet again the Foxites' reputed passion for overindulgence and conviviality is depicted as taking precedence over statesmanship and as having allowed the Talents ministry to fall unnoticed by its own ministers. Incapacitated by alcohol, Sheridan falls to the floor and grasps at Fox's ghostly feet, possibly indicating a desire to join his former mentor in the afterlife.

This fallen-drunk portrayal of Sheridan continued into the early nineteenth century, most notably in Charles Williams's *The Opening of Pandora's Box* (1812). While once more depicted in a fallen state of drunkenness in the mythological scene, Sheridan is not solely responsible for his state in this instance. A nude and drunken Silenus – a companion to the wine god Dionysus in Greek mythology, known for encouraging ecstasy, drunken joy and dancing – drags Sheridan away from his broken decanter.

The value of Williams's caricature lies in its symbolic portrayal of responsibility. Unlike in O'Keeffe's print, Sheridan is not solely responsible for his intoxication, rather he is a victim of greater forces, symbolised in this instance by Silenus, with the demon of addiction fuelling Sheridan's consumption. Although the physical effects of drinking might have been understood, the reasons and motivations behind such drinking – the Silenus – were less clear and depended on a range of factors including social status and gender.[53] To fully understand the psychological and sociological nuances of depictions of Sheridan's drinking, one must first delve deeper into contemporary notions of disease and personal responsibility.

The psychological effects of excess

Though the 'disease' concept of alcoholism had been gaining momentum by the end of the eighteenth century, as Porter identified, it was not until about 1804 that drunkenness became regarded as a disease in Britain.[54] Dr Thomas Trotter's medical thesis of that year stated that the 'habit of drunkenness was a disease', specifically a disease of the mind, not dissimilar to delirium.[55] The 'physiological theory of disease' was still largely endorsed by the eighteenth-century medical community. Disease was therefore viewed as a 'legacy of classical humoralism' and the individual's constitution, and the actions affecting their constitution, deemed responsible for their physical and physiological conditions. In this context, drinking was specifically viewed as an excess associated with 'extremes of the passions'.[56] There was therefore a notion that it was the continued surrender to the vice of alcohol and drunkenness that led to alcohol addiction and reliance. In this model, pioneered by William Buchan in 1776, alcoholism was considered an excess rather than a disease.[57] By the end of the eighteenth century, however, notions of disease had altered, and the 'ontological theory' gained traction. Diseases were increasingly being viewed more as 'real entities' that could be medically classified and understood. This development coincided with the birth of psychiatry and developments in conceptions of 'madness'.[58] As Porter summarised, these advances engendered social and medical perceptions that 'dependence essentially flowed not from a poisoned stomach but from a poisoned consciousness'.[59]

Despite the early nineteenth-century conception of alcoholism, in Sheridan's late eighteenth-century heyday, social class remained a key factor in understanding alcoholism. Elite alcohol dependence was medicalised, while lower-order drinking was seen as the 'vice of the poor'.[60] Dana Rabin argues that a distinction existed between the drunkenness of the wealthy and the plebeian lower orders. Sheridan's intoxication was viewed as a 'private vice', removed from society.[61] The prints assessed thus far all take place in Parliament or the sphere of insular sociability. For the rest of society, as Rabin explores, drunkenness was 'a sin which turns a man wholly to sin', initiating a 'chain of sin' including lost productivity, violence and theft. Plebeian drunkenness was seen as encouraging 'political mischiefs' and societal breakdown.[62] This 'chain of sin' framework can be applied to Sheridan's portrayal in *Frontispiece to The Rising Sun, Vol. III*, where his drinking led to a loss of productivity, bodily function and respectability. Caricaturists mirrored this sequence in their consistent depictions of Sheridan's excess, adding link after link to this visual chain of addiction.

By the 1780s, the once 'hermetically sealed' world of insular Foxite sociability was fracturing.[63] Amelia Rauser's work reveals that politicians' personal lives were increasingly scrutinised, citing the Westminster Election of 1784 as a turning point against the 'libertine profligacy' of privileged politicians, as new political values and public awareness emerged and such behaviour became less tolerated.[64] Depictions of Sheridan's drinking must therefore be viewed in this context. Though hailing from the middle orders, to the average caricature viewer Sheridan was associated with the debauchery of his aristocratic companions.[65] He was often depicted as the heaviest drinker, with the least control over his actions. Fiona Haslam and Corinna Wagner argue that during the period, neglect of health and body maintenance had both private and public consequences and was seen as unstatesmanlike. In visual culture, depictions of disease and illness such as *Frontispiece to The Rising Sun, Vol. III* and *The Opening of Pandora's Box* could be seen as 'just desserts for past sins'.[66] Haslam's work argues that gouty, swollen bodies provided critics and caricaturists 'with innumerable opportunities to deride' subjects for their debauched lives and political incapacity.[67] Such figures were presented as needing political remedies, often suggesting removal from office. Sheridan's vomiting depictions can thus be read as criticism of his libertine profligacy and perhaps an explanation for his political decline. If he was seen as literally too drunk to stand, what hope was there for him to successfully stand in an electoral context?

The moral effects of excess

Beyond publicising the physical effects of Sheridan's addiction, these satirical prints can be read as reflecting wider contemporary views on health, disposition and responsibility. Disease, illness and addiction had a symbolic visual function beyond the comic, portraying personal or professional character defects. Artists used these portrayals to invoke sympathy or distaste, signify health deterioration and represent flaws in decision-making and competency.[68] Physical and developing mental ailments were linked to moral and, in Sheridan's case, political failings. Contemporary thinking, as evidenced in the work of Roy Porter and Noelle Gallagher, highlights that even if predisposed to illness one could follow a 'regimen' to balance tendencies and avoid exacerbating issues with indulgent behaviours.[69] Similarly, Roy and Dorothy Porter argued that the early modern 'holistic' health approach traced ailments to 'personal problems in the character or habits of the individual'.[70] Gallagher claims that literary satire was presented in the early modern period as 'a kind of medicine for the mind or soul', treating moral corruption like 'a course of physic treated bodily illness'.[71]

Satire was certainly used in this context as an intended corrective treatment or, indeed, an attack on Sheridan's moral character. Specifically, Sheridan was often depicted as a corrupting presence as a mentor to the Prince of Wales, portrayed in the *The Royal Sneak* (1813) (Figure 1.3) published by John Johnston, and Charles Williams's *The Modern Calypso* (1812). In the former print, Sheridan follows the Prince in fleeing from a potential encounter with his estranged wife, the Princess of Wales. Within the scene,

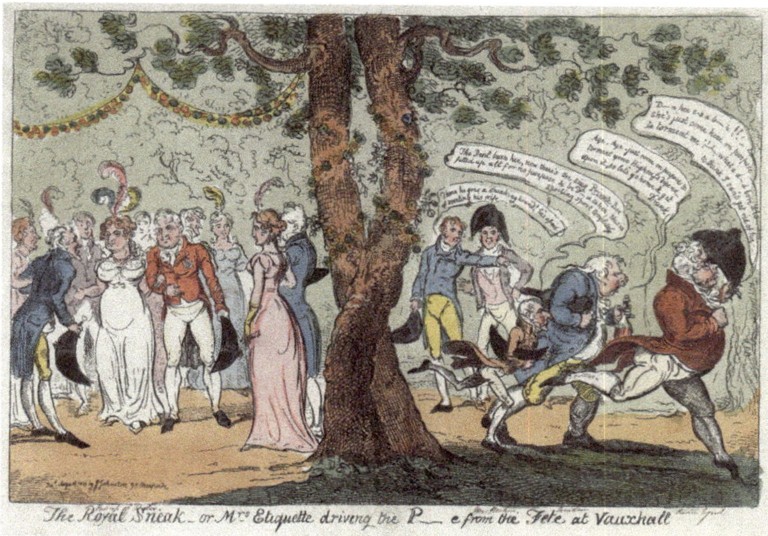

Figure 1.3 G.M. Woodward, *The Royal Sneak – or Mrs Etiquette Driving the P— from the Fête at Vauxhall*. Published by J. Johnston, August 1813, hand-coloured etching.

Sheridan's addiction is once again signified by his red blotchy skin, yet a more obvious symbol of his alcohol reliance is his stealing of both a decanter and a magnum of wine. His intentions are made clear in the final line of his speech: 'so let's go home and get drunk'. Similarly, in the imagined classical scene *The Modern Calypso*, Sheridan advises the Prince, who has taken on the role of Odysseus, to remain on the island of Ogygia under the spell of Calypso. Sheridan's motivation for remaining trapped on the island is again revealed by his dialogue and his uncontrolled hiccupping: 'We had better stay here, hic come let's have some, hic more Nectar ….' Both scenes symbolically portray Sheridan as first and foremost serving his own addiction; in the latter print he is willing to be trapped upon the island for eternity, so long as his supply of wine remains abundant. There is also an underlying assumption that the Prince has become the epitome of excess and debauchery because of Sheridan's mentorship: in *The Modern Calypso* the Prince attests to this and describes Sheridan as 'Mentor, the Guide of my youth …'

Alcohol was also used during the 1810s as a conduit and signifier of Sheridan's financial corruption, debt and mismanagement. Having demolished his Drury Lane Theatre in 1791 to renovate, Sheridan's financial investment was lost because of a fire at the theatre in 1809. To reopen the venue, Sheridan borrowed heavily from fellow Foxite and brewer Samuel Whitbread, who granted the loan on the condition that Sheridan would withdraw from all management of the building. In one resulting caricature, *Management-or-Butts & Hogsheads* (1812), Sheridan is depicted as syphoning off and intercepting his share of the profit from the new theatre from large casks or hogsheads of Whitbread ale. Sheridan's financial corruption is thus intrinsically linked with alcohol; he has accumulated masses of debt and has all but lost his theatre, yet still he tries to profit through stealing ale (a signifier for wealth in the scene) from under Whitbread's nose. The underlying accusation is that Sheridan will likely 'waste' any profits he accrues on his addiction. Even as the fire ravaged Drury Lane in 1809, alcohol remained ever-present. When asked why he drank a glass of wine while watching his investment burn, Sheridan is reported to have said: 'A man may surely be allowed to take a glass of wine by his own fireside.'[72]

Such visual representations of addiction were inherently rooted in medical, moral and political discourses, and caricature by its very nature is reliant on excess or the 'exaggeration of physical traits and behavioural tics'.[73] When reading such visual depictions of excess or addiction one must critically examine the anxieties behind the image, that is, understanding that at the first glance such images 'trigger a set of beliefs and assumptions about addiction that are not questioned'.[74] Skelly's recent work has questioned the 'long-held belief that addiction is legible from the body'. Discussing the case of Oscar Wilde, Skelly's assertion that the blaming of alcohol in textual and visual sources for Wilde's death constructed 'a narrative in which ... excesses killed him, thereby making him responsible for his own death' is directly relevant to Sheridan's portrayal.[75] The caricatures explored here certainly portray a man on the road to alcohol-fuelled self-destruction. Sheridan's death was not directly ascribed to alcoholism; the cause of death was 'disease in the stomach, which from its feeble state rejected nourishment'.[76] Yet modern research highlights the correlation between excessive and habitual alcohol consumption and stomach cancer.[77] Sheridan's final years were marked by alcohol-induced bodily failure, such as reddened skin, bloating and vomiting. Having explored the context of pre-alcoholism and alcoholism, the questions remain about how the contemporary viewing public reacted to or consumed such depictions of excess; as Skelly puts it, 'what exactly is funny about drunkenness?'[78]

Skelly's 'Grim Chuckle' may hold the key to understanding the symbolic portrayal of Sheridan as an excessive alcoholic in political caricature. Despite the creator's intention, Skelly argues that the response of the viewer to a depiction of drunkenness is the 'Grim Chuckle' – a form of laughter rooted in dark humour and the Freudian theory of 'laughter as a release of psychic or emotional tension'.[79] Laughter, in this context, has the potential to alter the way in which the viewer perceives drunkenness and the depicted drinker. The 'Grim Chuckle' is a means of releasing anxiety 'as part of a process of identification or recognition, which may be simultaneously accompanied by a rejection of the drinker'. According to Skelly, through recognising their own experiences with alcohol in the experiences of another, the response is to laugh uncomfortably or to laugh with abandon as a form of catharsis.[80] Skelly's theory is closely linked to the 'Release Theory'.[81] The notion that laughter is not always joyous or optimistic, but a release of something darker and deeper is relevant to the case of Sheridan. The depiction of a public figure engaging in excess to the point of bodily failure is starkly incongruous. According to the incongruity theory of humour, this mismatch between expectations or preconceptions and the disappointing reality causes laughter, even if that reality has adverse effects for the audience. In this instance the supposed seriousness of a statesman and the indignity and debauchery of his behaviour, is not just humorous, but the laughter itself offers a cultural criticism of not only his actions, but those of his political circle.[82]

Building on Mike Goode's work, Skelly focuses on caricature's influence beyond rational persuasion. Goode examines how caricature shaped its own audience, creating an identifiable catalogue of social and political characters akin to a modern-day soap opera. He argues that caricatures trained viewers to consume and discuss prints and to recognise their subjects.[83] Whereas Dickinson argued that caricatures' primary motive was the 'persuasion' of its public, Goode questions the very concept of eighteenth-century 'persuasion'.[84] Though caricature 'undoubtedly' aimed to alter public opinion, it did so through modes that its audience would not necessarily have understood as 'persuasive' – through 'name-calling and distortion'. Viewing caricatures as merely persuading audiences is too simplistic; rather, they shaped public opinion through exaggerated, coarse comic effects intended to appeal to a taste for the absurd and carnivalesque.[85] Goode also suggests that bodily distortion in caricature could have been taken more literally than assumed, supported by the influence of eighteenth-century physiognomy, namely Johann Kaspar Lavater's work.[86] Goode further credits caricature's ability to cause laughter – bodily distortion being key – as its primary mode of altering opinion: 'the medium literally sought to sway public opinion by convulsing people's bodies with laughter'.[87]

The complex case of Sheridan has shown that excessive consumption was used as a symbol of his political incapacity by the early nineteenth century, with his inability to maintain a form of 'good fellowship' emphasised. By the end of his career alcohol had evidently taken precedence over politics and there were clear associations between Sheridan's moral corruption and alcohol. Sheridan's immoral mentorship of the Prince of Wales and the financial mismanagement of his Drury Lane theatre were both depicted as being driven by alcohol addiction. Though caricature also allowed for a softer gaze: in the more symbolic and metaphorical *Frontispiece to The Rising Sun, Vol. III* and *The Opening of Pandora's Box*, he was depicted as not being in control of his alcoholism; rather he was a victim of both the literal and metaphorical Silenus of addiction. Not actively choosing to corrupt his body and career, he was a victim of disease.

The extent to which audiences needed to be persuaded of Sheridan's addiction to alcohol in caricature by the early nineteenth century is interesting. Skelly's notion that graphic satire was able to offer an alternative version to the 'official' image of an individual, which in the political sphere could function as a system of checks and balances, holds water in relation to Sheridan's public image.[88] While Sheridan's 'Six-Bottle Man' status was certainly known among his circles of social and political acquaintance, there were few public allusions in the press to any addiction. Caricature therefore offers a unique lens through which to view Sheridan's political and personal public image and reveals what lay 'well below the surface of what could be publicly admitted'.[89] Of the three recorded instances of Foxite drunkenness in Mabell, Countess of Airlie's memoir, all related solely to Sheridan: 'he thinks Sheridan must have been drunk', 'Sheridan was very drunk', and 'Sheridan rather drunk rolling about in another corner'.[90] Similarly, in another account, Sheridan is recorded as having consumed 'five bottles of port, two of madeira, and one of brandy', the result being that 'he was not able to raise his head from his pillow, nor did he get out of bed until seven o'clock'. That evening, however, he 'again drank very deep'.[91] As Lord Byron once wrote, he had seen Sheridan 'drunk, with all the world; his intoxication was that of Bacchus'.[92]

This chapter has contributed to our understanding of the relationship between alcohol, addiction and the body politics in the period, with the case of Sheridan conveying the symbolic significance of the art of alcoholism. The power of images of disease and alcoholism were clearly understood by caricaturists, and through their art we are left with a portrait of Sheridan as a political, moral and financial failure by the early nineteenth century. As viewers of caricature, we are led to believe that the root cause of all these shortcomings was the ever-present spectre of alcohol. Perhaps what Sheridan's case conveys most is the transformation that took place at the turn of the century, whereby the old guard of libertine profligates gave way to a more professional political order. This was certainly the image put forward by Gillray in his 1809 *Pillars of the Constitution* (Figure 1.4), in which Sheridan and the Duke of Norfolk stumble drunkenly from Brooks's club. More bloated and red-faced than in any previous depiction, Sheridan leads Norfolk, who has stashed a bottle of port for the journey, into a new day at three o'clock in the morning. These, Gillray states, are the 'pillars of the constitution', and one could add, the last vestiges of the six-bottle men. Of the six-bottle men of Sheridan's time, James Parton asked in 1877, 'where are they?' The answer by the mid-nineteenth century was, 'gone, quite gone'.[93]

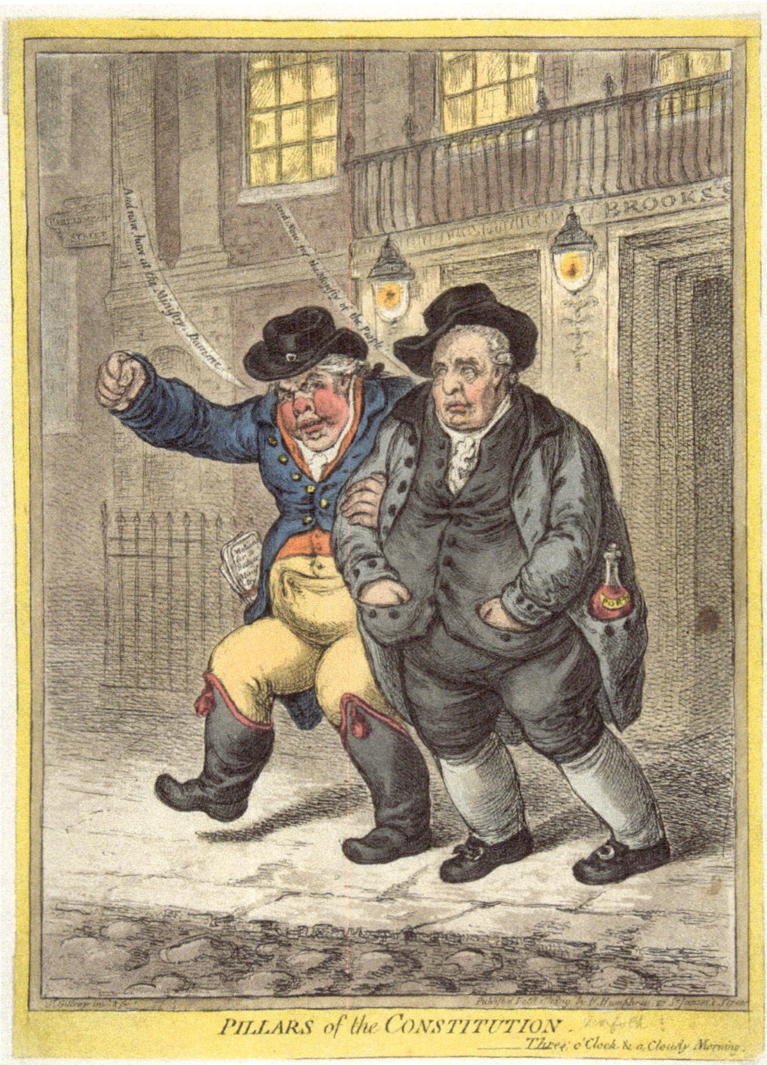
And now have at the Ministry. Damme
BROOKS'S
PILLARS of the CONSTITUTION.
Three o'Clock & a Cloudy Morning.

Figure 1.4 James Gillray, *Pillars of the Constitution*. Published by Hannah Humphrey, 1 February 1809, hand-coloured etching.

Notes

1 Hugh Stokes, *The Devonshire House Circle* (Smith, Elder & Co, 1917), p. 218.

2 Callum D. Smith, 'Radical socialites or sociable radicals?: The Foxite Whigs in caricature, 1780–1810' (PhD thesis, University of Bristol [SWW DTP], 2022).

3 See Christopher Clayton, 'The Political Career of Richard Brinsley Sheridan', in James Morwood and David Crane (eds), *Sheridan Studies* (Cambridge University Press, 1995), pp. 131–50; David Francis Taylor, 'Caricaturing Sheridan', in Jack DeRochi and Daniel Ellis (eds), *Richard Brinsley Sheridan: The Impresario in Political Cultural Context* (Pennsylvania State University Press, 2012), p. 214.

4 Louis Fagan, *The Reform Club: Its Founders and Architect* (B. Quaritch, 1887), pp. 16–17.

5 Stokes, *Devonshire House Circle*, p. 132; Anon., *SHERIDANIANA* (W. Simpkin and R. Marshall, 1826), p. 283.

6 See James Kelly, '"Bleeding, vomiting and purging": The medical response to ill-health in eighteenth-century Ireland', in Catherine Cox and Maria Luddy (eds), *Cultures of Care in Irish Medical History, 1750–1970* (Routledge, 2010), pp. 13–36; Marek H. Dominiczak, 'Cartoons: Another long-standing bridge between science and the arts', *Clinical Chemistry* 63:4 (2017), 934–5.

7 Elaine Chalus, 'Elite women, social politics, and the political world of late eighteenth-century England', *The Historical Journal* 43:3 (2000), 675–6; Judith S. Lewis, *Sacred to Female Patriotism: Gender, Class, and Politics in Late Georgian Britain* (Routledge, 2003).

8 See Peter Clark, *The English Alehouse* (Longman, 1983); Christina Parolin, *Radical Spaces* (ANU Press, 2010), p. 111; Peter Brett, 'Political dinners in early nineteenth-century Britain: Platform, meeting place and battleground', *History* (1996), 527–52; Stokes, *Devonshire House Circle*; Lloyd Charles Sanders, *The Holland House Circle* (Smith, Elder & Co, 1908).

9 Ian Newman, *The Romantic Tavern: Literature and Conviviality in the Age of Revolution* (Cambridge University Press, 2019), pp. 69–70.

10 Martyn J. Powell, 'Political toasting in eighteenth-century Ireland', *History: The Journal of the Historical Association* 91:304 (2006), 508–29; Rémy Duthille, 'Political toasting in the age of revolutions: Britain, America and France, 1765–1800', in Gordon Pentland and

Michael T. Davis (eds), *Liberty, Property and Popular Politics. England and Scotland 1688–1815* (Edinburgh University Press, 2016).

11 For Sheridan's heavy drinking in 1777, see his tavern bills in Charles C. Ludington, 'Drinking for Approval: Wine and the British Court from George III to Victoria and Albert', in Daniëlle De Vooght, *Royal Taste: Food, Power and Status at the European Courts after 1789* (Berg Publishers, 2016), p. 72; BL, Add. MS 44401, ff. 30–32. R.B. Sheridan's tavern bills from L. Reilly, 1777.

12 Anon., *The Tipling Dutchess Returning From Canvassing*, Pub. Aitken, A. (29 April 1784) BM Satires 6560, MN: J,3.10; Amelia Rauser, 'The butcher-kissing Duchess of Devonshire: Between caricature and allegory', *Eighteenth Century Studies* 36:1 (2002), 23–46.

13 See Mark Hailwood, *Alehouses and Good Fellowship in Early Modern England* (Boydell Press, 2014), pp. 113–71.

14 Roy Porter, 'The drinking man's disease: The "Pre-History" of alcoholism in Georgian Britain', *British Journal of Addiction* 80:4a (1985), 390.

15 Julia Skelly, 'The politics of drunkenness: John Henry Walker, John A. Macdonald, and Graphic Satire', *Canadian Art Review* 40:1 (2015), 74.

16 Sigmund Freud, *Jokes and Their Relation to the Unconscious* (W.W. Norton & Company, 1960), pp. 90–117; Skelly, 'The politics of drunkenness', 74.

17 Freud, *Jokes and Their Relation*, pp. 90–117.

18 Thomas Hobbes, *The Elements of Law, Natural and Politic* (Oxford University Press, 1999), pp. 54–5.

19 Hobbes, *The Elements of Law*, pp. 54–5.

20 Diana Donald, *The Age of Caricature: Satirical Prints in the Reign of George III* (Yale University Press, 1996), p. 51.

21 Vic Gatrell, *The First Bohemians* (Penguin Books, 2013), p. 43.

22 James Gillray, *Very Slippy-Weather*, Pub. Humphrey, Hannah (10 February 1808) BM Satires 11100, Museum Number: 1851,0901. 1248.

23 Tamara Hunt, *Defining John Bull: Political Caricature and National Identity in Late Georgian England* (Routledge, 2003), p. 15.

24 H.T. Dickinson, *Caricatures and the Constitution 1760–1832* (Cambridge University Press, 1986), p. 13.

25 Roy Porter, 'Seeing the past', *Past and Present Society* 118 (1988), 189.

26 Robert D. Hume, 'The value of money in eighteenth-century England: Incomes, prices, buying power – and some problems in cultural economics', *Huntington Library Quarterly* 77:4 (2014), 377.

27 M. Dorothy George, *English Political Caricature: A Study of Opinion and Propaganda, Volume 1* (Oxford University Press, 1959), p. 176.
28 Dickinson, *Caricatures and the Constitution*, p. 13; Donald, *The Age of Caricature*, p. 2; Eirwen Nicholson, 'Consumers and spectators: The public of the political print in eighteenth-century England', *The Journal of The Historical Association* 81:261 (1996), 10–11.
29 Donald, *The Age of Caricature*, p. 2; Nicholson, 'Consumers and spectators', 12–13.
30 Marc Baer, 'The Ruin of the Public Man: The Rise and Fall of Richard Brinsley Sheridan', in Morwood and Crane (eds), *Sheridan Studies*, p. 157.
31 Leslie Mitchell, *The Whig World* (Hambledon Continuum, 2005), p. 34.
32 James Sambrook, 'Club [Literary Club, Johnson's Literary Club] (act. 1764–1784)', *ODNB* (Oxford, 2006).
33 Martyn Powell, *The Politics of Consumption in Eighteenth-Century Ireland* (Palgrave Macmillan, 2005), p. 225.
34 Karen Harvey, 'Ritual encounter: Punch parties and masculinity in the eighteenth century', *Past & Present* 214 (2012), 165–203. For Irish Whiskey punch see James Gillray, *The Union Club*, Pub. Hannah Humphrey (21 January 1801), BM Satires 9699, MN: 1868,0808.6922.
35 John Cannon, *The Fox-North Coalition* (Cambridge University Press, 1969), pp. 82–106.
36 Iain Hampsher-Monk, 'Civic Humanism and parliamentary reform: The case of the society of the friends of the people', *Journal of British Studies* 18:2 (1979), 70–89.
37 A.D. Harvey, 'The Ministry of All the Talents: The Whigs in office, February 1806 to March 1807', *Historical Journal* 15:4 (1972), 619–48; Richard A. Gaunt, 'Ministry of All the Talents (act.1806–1807)', *ODNB* (Oxford, 2008).
38 Henry Stooks Smith, *The Register of Parliamentary Contested Elections. Containing the Uncontested Elections Since 1830*, 2nd edition (Simpkin, Marshall & Co, 1842), p. 166.
39 Norman Jeffares, 'Sheridan, Richard Brinsley (1751–1816)', *ODNB* (Oxford, 2004).
40 See James Kelly, 'The consumption and sociable use of alcohol in eighteenth-century Ireland', *Proceedings of the Royal Irish Academy*, 115C (2015), pp. 234–6.
41 Harald T. Gorgulla et al., 'Rhinophyma in literature and the arts', *Facial Plastic Surgery* 14:4 (1998), 229.
42 Porter, 'The drinking man's disease', 385–6.

43 Julia Skelly, *Addiction and British Visual Culture, 1751–1919: Wasted Looks* (Ashgate 2014), p. 2.
44 Peter Shaw, *The Juice Of The Grape* (T. Warner, 1733), pp. 33, 49; Porter, 'The drinking man's disease', 387.
45 Porter, 'The drinking man's disease', 389; Erasmus Darwin, *Zoonomia, Vol. I* (J. Johnson, 1794), p. 368.
46 Porter, 'The drinking man's disease', 394; Robert Willan, *Extract from an Account of the dreadful effects of Dram-drinking* (C. Dilly, 1803), pp. 7, 4–14.
47 See Figure 1.1.
48 W. O'Keeffe's prints were frontispieces; see Eaton Stannard Barrett, *The Rising Sun: A Serio-comic Satiric Romance, by Cervantes Hogg. In Three Volumes* (T. Tegg, 1809).
49 Baer, 'The Ruin of a Public Man', 166.
50 Willan, *Extract from an Account*, pp. 7, 4–14.
51 Willan, *Extract from an Account*, pp. 7, 4–14.
52 'Portland' is William Cavendish-Bentinck, 3rd Duke of Portland, who succeeded Grenville as Prime Minister. See Michael Roberts, *The Whig Party, 1807–1812* (Routledge, 1965), pp. 303–30.
53 See Skelly, *Addiction and Visual Culture*, pp. 1–19.
54 Porter, 'The drinking man's disease', 390–2.
55 Porter, 'The drinking man's disease', 390; T. Trotter, *An Essay, Medical, Philosophical and Chemical on Drunkenness* (T. Cadell and W. Davies, 1804), pp. 1–8, 179.
56 Porter, 'The drinking man's disease', 390.
57 Porter, 'The drinking man's disease', 391; William Buchan, *Domestic Medicine* (W. Strahan and T. Cadell, 1776), p. 101.
58 Porter, 'The drinking man's disease', 391.
59 Porter, 'The drinking man's disease', 391.
60 Porter, 'The drinking man's disease', 394–95.
61 Dana Rabin, 'Drunkenness and responsibility for crime in the eighteenth century', *Journal of British Studies* 44:3 (2005), 457.
62 Rabin, 'Drunkenness', 457; Richard Younger, *A Sovereign antidote, or, A Precious Mirthridate* (J. Hayes, 1664), p. 7.
63 Leslie Mitchell, *Charles James Fox* (Oxford University Press, 1992), p. 94.
64 Women suffered far worse in this new context. Rauser, 'The butcher-kissing duchess', 25; John Dinwiddy, *Radicalism and Reform in Britain, 1780–1850* (Hambledon Press, 1992), p. 1; Marilyn Morris, *Sex, Money and Personal Character in Eighteenth-Century British Politics* (Yale University Press, 2015).

65 Sambrook, 'Club [Johnson's Literary Club]', *ODNB*.
66 Fiona Haslam, *From Hogarth To Rowlandson: Medicine in Art in Eighteenth Century Britain* (Liverpool University Press, 1996), p. 87; Corinna Wagner, *Pathological Bodies: Medicine and Political Culture* (University of California Press, 2013), p. 232.
67 Wagner, *Pathological Bodies*, p. 232.
68 Haslam, *From Hogarth To Rowlandson*, p. 2.
69 Noelle Gallagher, 'Satire as medicine in the Restoration and early eighteenth century: The history of a metaphor', *Literature and Medicine* 31 (2013), 1; Roy Porter and Dorothy Porter, *In Sickness and In Health* (Penguin Books, 1988), pp. 21–42.
70 Gallagher, 'Satire as medicine', 2; Roy Porter, *Disease, Medicine and Society in England, 1550–1860* (Cambridge University Press, 1995), pp. 24–6.
71 Gallagher, 'Satire as Medicine', 3.
72 Anon., *SHERIDANIANA*, p. 216.
73 Skelly, *Addiction and Visual Culture*, p. 7; Julia Skelly, 'The Paradox of Excess: Oscar Wilde, Caricature, and Consumption', in Julia Skelly (ed.), *The Uses of Excess in Visual and Material Culture, 1600–2010* (Ashgate, 2014), p. 137.
74 Skelly, *Addiction and Visual Culture*, p. 9.
75 Skelly, *Addiction and Visual Culture*, p. 2.
76 Richard Brinsley Sheridan, *Authentic Memoirs of the Life and Death of the Right Honourable R.B. Sheridan* (T. Warner, 1816), p. 11.
77 Wenting Deng et al., 'Alcohol consumption and risk of stomach cancer: A meta-analysis', *Chemico-Biological Interactions* 336 (2021), 1–9.
78 Skelly, 'The politics of drunkenness', 74.
79 Skelly, 'The politics of drunkenness', 74.
80 Skelly, 'The politics of drunkenness', 79.
81 Robert R. Clewis, *The Origins of Kant's Aesthetics* (Cambridge University Press, 2023), p. 215.
82 John Morreal, *Humor Works* (HRD Press, Inc., 1997), pp. 26–30. Immanuel Kant is often cited as the father of the 'Incongruity Theory', Clewis, *The Origins of Kant's Aesthetics*, pp. 213–15.
83 Mike Goode, 'The Public and the Limits of Persuasion in the Age of Caricature', in Todd Porterfield (ed.), *The Efflorescence of Caricature, 1759–1838* (Ashgate, 2011), pp. 118, 122–5.
84 Dickinson, *Caricatures and the Constitution*, p. 11.
85 Goode, 'The Public and the LIMITS', 129.
86 See Johann Kaspar Lavater, *Physiognomy* (S. Gosnell, 1826).

87 Goode, 'The Public and the Limits', 132.
88 Skelly, 'The Politics of Drunkenness', 71.
89 Vic Gatrell, *City of Laughter: Sex and Satire in Eighteenth-Century London* (Atlantic Books, 2006), p. 230.
90 Mabell, Countess of Airlie, *In Whig Society 1775–1818* (Hodder & Stoughton, 1921), pp. 25, 120, 153.
91 Anon., *SHERIDANIANA*, p. 206.
92 Thomas Moore (ed.), *The Works of Lord Byron with His Letters and Journals, In Seventeen Volumes, Vol. IV* (John Murray, 1833), p. 85.
93 James Parton, *Caricature and Other Comic Art* (Harper & Brothers, 1877), p. 272.

References

Primary sources

Anon. *SHERIDANIANA*. W. Simpkin and R. Marshall, 1826.
Anon. *The Tipling Dutchess Returning From Canvassing*. Published by A. Aitken, 29 April 1784. BM Satires 6560. MN: J,3.10.
Barrett, Eaton Stannard. *The Rising Sun: A Serio-comic Satiric Romance, by Cervantes Hogg*. T. Tegg, 1809.
Buchan, William. *Domestic Medicine*. W. Strahan and T. Cadell, 1776.
Cochrane, Thomas, 10th Earl of Dundonald, Marquess of Maranhão. *The Register of Parliamentary Contested Elections. Containing the Uncontested Elections Since 1830*. 2nd edition. William Clowes and Sons, 1842.
Darwin, Erasmus. *Zoonomia, Vol. I*. J. Johnson, 1794.
Gillray, James, *The Union Club*. Published by Hannah Humphrey, 21 January 1801. BM Satires 9699. MN: 1868,0808.6922.
Gillray, James. *Very Slippy-Weather*. Published by Hannah Humphrey, 10 February 1808. BM Satires 11100. MN: 1851,0901.1248.
Lavater, Johann Kaspar. *Physiognomy*. S. Gosnell, 1826.
Sanders, Lloyd Charles. *The Holland House Circle*. Smith, Elder & Co, 1908.
Shaw, Peter. *The Juice Of The Grape*. T. Warner, 1733.
Sheridan, Richard Brinsley. *Authentic Memoirs of the Life and Death of the Right Honourable R. B. Sheridan*. T. Warner, 1816.
Stokes, Hugh. *The Devonshire House Circle*. Smith, Elder & Co., 1917.
Trotter, Thomas. *An Essay, Medical, Philosophical and Chemical on Drunkenness*. T. Cadell and W. Davies, 1804.

Willan, Robert. *Extract from an Account of the Dreadful Effects of Dram-drinking*. C. Dilly, 1803.

Secondary sources

Baer, Marc. 'The Ruin of the Public Man: The Rise and Fall of Richard Brinsley Sheridan'. In James Morwood and David Crane (eds), *Sheridan Studies*. Cambridge University Press, 2012.

Brett, Peter. 'Political dinners in early nineteenth-century Britain: Platform, meeting place and battleground'. *History* 81 (1996), 527–52.

Cannon, John. *The Fox-North Coalition*. Cambridge University Press, 1969.

Chalus, Elaine. 'Elite women, social politics, and the political world of late eighteenth-century England'. *The Historical Journal* 43:3 (2000), 675–6.

Chalus, Elaine. *Elite Women, Social Politics, and the Political World of Late Eighteenth-Century England*. Palgrave Macmillan, 2003.

Clark, Peter. *The English Alehouse*. Longman, 1983.

Clayton, Christopher. 'The Political Career of Richard Brinsley Sheridan'. In James Morwood and David Crane (eds), *Sheridan Studies*. Cambridge University Press, 1995.

Deng, Wenting, et al. 'Alcohol consumption and risk of stomach cancer: A meta-analysis'. *Chemico-Biological Interactions* 336 (2021), 1–10.

Dickinson, H.T. *Caricatures and the Constitution 1760–1832*. Cambridge University Press, 1986.

Dinwiddy, John. *Radicalism and Reform in Britain, 1780–1850*. Hambledon Press, 1992.

Donald, Diana. *The Age of Caricature: Satirical Prints in the Reign of George III*. Yale University Press, 1996.

Dominiczak, Marek H. 'Cartoons: Another long-standing bridge between science and the arts'. *Clinical Chemistry* 63:4 (2017), 934–5.

Duthille, Rémy. 'Political Toasting in the Age of Revolutions: Britain, America and France, 1765–1800'. In Gordon Pentland and Michael T. Davis (eds), *Liberty, Property and Popular Politics. England and Scotland 1688–1815*. Edinburgh University Press, 2016.

Freud, Sigmund. *Jokes and Their Relation to the Unconscious*. W.W. Norton & Company, 1960.

Gallagher, Noelle. 'Satire as medicine in the Restoration and early eighteenth century: The history of a metaphor'. *Literature and Medicine* 31 (2013), 1–25.

Gallagher, Noelle. 'The Paradox of Excess: Oscar Wilde, Caricature, and Consumption'. In Julia Skelly (ed.), *The Uses of Excess in Visual and Material Culture, 1600–2010*. Ashgate, 2014.

Gatrell, Vic. *City of Laughter: Sex and Satire in Eighteenth-Century London*. Atlantic Books, 2006.
Gatrell, Vic. *The First Bohemians*. Penguin Books, 2013.
Gaunt, Richard A. 'Ministry of All the Talents (act. 1806–1807)'. *Oxford Dictionary of National Biography*. Oxford University Press, 2008.
George, M. Dorothy. *English Political Caricature: A Study of Opinion and Propaganda, Volume 1*. Oxford University Press, 1959.
Gorgulla, Harald T., et al. 'Rhinophyma in literature and the arts'. *Facial Plastic Surgery*, 14:4 (1998), 229–33.
Goode, Mike. 'The Public and the Limits of Persuasion in the Age of Caricature'. In Todd Porterfield (ed.), *The Efflorescence of Caricature, 1759–1838*. Ashgate, 2011.
Hailwood, Mark, *Alehouses and Good Fellowship in Early Modern England*. Boydell Press, 2014.
Hampsher-Monk, Iain. 'Civic humanism and parliamentary reform: The case of the society of the friends of the people'. *Journal of British Studies* 18:2 (1979), 70–89.
Harvey, A.D. 'The Ministry of All the Talents: The Whigs in office, February 1806 to March 1807'. *Historical Journal* 15:4 (1972), 619–48.
Harvey, Karen. 'Ritual encounter: Punch parties and masculinity in the eighteenth century'. *Past & Present* 214 (2012): 165–203.
Haslam, Fiona. *From Hogarth to Rowlandson: Medicine in Art in Eighteenth Century Britain*. Liverpool University Press, 1996.
Hobbes, Thomas. *The Elements of Law, Natural and Politic*. Oxford University Press, 1999.
Hunt, Tamara. *Defining John Bull: Political Caricature and National Identity in Late Georgian England*. Ashgate, 2003.
Hume, Robert D. 'The value of money in eighteenth-century England: Incomes, Prices, buying power – and some problems in cultural economics'. *Huntington Library Quarterly* 77:4 (2014), 377–94.
Jeffares, Norman. 'Sheridan, Richard Brinsley (1751–1816)'. *Oxford Dictionary of National Biography*. Oxford University Press, 2004.
Kelly, James. 'The medical response to ill-health in eighteenth-century Ireland'. In Catherine Cox and Maria Luddy (eds), *Cultures of Care in Irish Medical History, 1750–1970*. Routledge, 2010.
Kelly, James. 'The consumption and sociable use of alcohol in eighteenth-century Ireland'. *Proceedings of the Royal Irish Academy*, 115C (2015), 234–6.
Kelly, James, and Martyn Powell (eds). *Clubs and Societies in Eighteenth-Century Ireland*. Four Courts Press, 2010.
Lewis, Judith S. *Sacred to Female Patriotism: Gender, Class, and Politics in Late Georgian Britain*. Routledge, 2003.

Ludington, Charles C. 'Drinking for approval: wine and the British Court from George III to Victoria and Albert'. In Daniëlle De Vooght (ed.), *Royal Taste: Food, Power and Status at the European Courts after 1789*. Berg Publishers, 2016.
Mabell, Countess of Airlie. *In Whig Society 1775–1818*. Hodder & Stoughton, 1921.
Mitchell, Leslie. *Charles James Fox*. Oxford University Press, 1992.
Mitchell, Leslie. *The Whig World*. Hambledon Continuum, 2005.
Moore, Thomas. *The Works of Lord Byron with His Letters and Journals. In Seventeen Volumes, Vol. IV*. John Murray, 1833.
Newman, Ian. *The Romantic Tavern: Literature and Conviviality in the Age of Revolution*. Cambridge University Press, 2019.
Nicholson, Eirwen. 'Consumers and spectators: The public of the political print in eighteenth-century England'. *The Journal of The Historical Association* 81:261 (1996), 10–13.
Parolin, Christina. *Radical Spaces*. ANU Press, 2010.
Parton, James. *Caricature and Other Comic Art*. Harper & Brothers, 1877.
Porter, Roy. 'The drinking man's disease: The "Pre-History" of alcoholism in Georgian Britain'. *British Journal of Addiction* 80:4a (1985), 385–95.
Porter, Roy. 'Seeing the past'. *Past and Present Society* 118 (1988), 186–205.
Porter, Roy. *Disease, Medicine and Society in England, 1550–1860*. Cambridge University Press, 1995.
Porter, Roy, and Dorothy Porter. *In Sickness and In Health*. Penguin Books, 1988.
Powell, Martyn. *The Politics of Consumption in Eighteenth-Century Ireland*. Palgrave Macmillan, 2005.
Powell, Martyn J. 'Political toasting in eighteenth-century Ireland'. *History: The Journal of the Historical Association* 91:304 (2006), 508–29.
Rabin, Dana. 'Drunkenness and responsibility for crime in the eighteenth century'. *Journal of British Studies* 44:3 (2005), 457–79.
Rauser, Amelia. 'The butcher-kissing Duchess of Devonshire: Between caricature and allegory'. *Eighteenth-Century Studies* 36:1 (2002), 23–46.
Roberts, Michael. *The Whig Party, 1807–1812*. Routledge, 1965.
Sambrook, James. 'Club [Literary Club, Johnson's Literary Club] (act. 1764–1784)'. *Oxford Dictionary of National Biography*. Oxford University Press, 2006.
Skelly, Julia. *Addiction and British Visual Culture, 1751–1919: Wasted Looks*. Ashgate, 2014.
Skelly, Julia. 'The paradox of excess: Oscar Wilde, caricature, and consumption'. In Julia Skelly (ed.), *The Uses of Excess in Visual and Material Culture, 1600–2010*. Ashgate, 2006.

Skelly, Julia. 'The politics of drunkenness: John Henry Walker, John A. Macdonald, and graphic satire'. *Canadian Art Review* 40:1 (2015), 74–9.

Smith, Callum D. 'Radical socialites or sociable radicals?: The Foxite Whigs in caricature, 1780–1810'. PhD thesis, University of Bristol, SWW DTP, 2022.

Smith, Henry Stooks. *The Register of Parliamentary Contested Elections. Containing the Uncontested Elections Since 1830.* Second Edition. William Clowes and Sons, 1842.

Taylor, David Francis. 'Caricaturing Sheridan'. In Jack DeRochi and Daniel Ellis (eds), *Richard Brinsley Sheridan: The Impresario in Political Cultural Context*. Pennsylvania State University Press, 2012.

Wagner, Corinna. *Pathological Bodies: Medicine and Political Culture.* University of California Press, 2013.

Wardrop, James. *The Works of Matthew Baillie, M.D., Vol. I.* Longman, Rees, Orme, Brown, and Green, 1825.

2

Bedroom eyes as bedside manner: Humorous expressions of medical impropriety in mid-nineteenth-century visual culture

Rebecca Whiteley

Who was the doctor in mid-nineteenth-century Britain? He was certainly a complicated and important figure.[1] On the one hand, he was becoming one of the core bourgeois professionals: an exemplum of the educated, self-contained, authoritative Victorian masculine ideal. On the other, this same doctor was always *potentially* a probing, touching, insinuating, swindling, seducing, murderous and deeply problematic character. How these two personas coexisted and conflicted in the Victorian popular consciousness, and how their contradictory aspects sparked humour in Victorian print culture, is the focus of this chapter.

There is a growing literature on the medical persona in the nineteenth century, addressing sources from legal records to novels to fine art.[2] Yet little has been done with the profusion of printed images produced in this period. From medical illustrations to 'popular' prints to pornography, there is a distinct body of images in which the doctor is presented as a sexual actor. In all of these, confusion about the doctor's identity – somewhere between professional and seducer – was intended to produce laughter. What can this material tell us about mid-Victorian perceptions of the doctor and the medical encounter? I argue that this problematic, morally dubious and potentially dangerous subject matter was so often expressed comically because this mode allowed for the speaking of the secret, the sublimated and the taboo.[3] Print culture, because of its ephemeral nature and broad reach, was especially suited to expressing these ideas. Indeed, through comic print, the problematics of the medical persona were not just spoken, they were defused and made safe.

Finding the material addressed in this chapter posed serious challenges. I set out to look for visual expressions of what I term 'medical impropriety' – of doctors seducing, coercing or engaging in sexual activity with patients. At the time of writing, there are no particular collections, journals or archives dedicated to this theme, and indeed, because of the illicit and often implicit nature of the material, even keyword searches are of limited use. I trawled digitised medical visual archives, print collections and illustrated journals, limiting searches by medium, date and certain keywords but discerning topic and content largely by eye. My sample is, therefore, far from comprehensive – not only was much of this sort of material surely lost, but what remains is very difficult to find in the archive. That, despite these difficulties, a distinct body of material dealing with the topic was to be found suggests that it was of enduring and quite general interest in the nineteenth century.

The images under discussion here were produced as single-sheet prints, as advertisements and as illustrations from the new popular periodical press. Some have essentially no metadata and their original context can only be guessed. But what links these images is their contribution to the explosion in printed visual culture in the mid-nineteenth century. Printing images became much cheaper in this period, and so they were produced for much wider audiences. This image culture was also newly ambitious, aiming to record all the great variety and rapid change of nineteenth-century life.[4] The ambition and reach of this new kind of 'picture world', to borrow Rachel Teukolsky's phrase, is significant.[5] It provides a useful array of attitudes to medicine and the doctor, from admiring, to ridiculing, to fearful. And because in aggregate it was produced by many kinds of people, and addressed to many more, it can give a wider view of cultural attitudes to medicine than more exclusively middle- and upper-class visual culture does.

The images addressed here originate mostly from Britain and France, though cultures of medicine across Western Europe and the United States were increasingly conversant with one another and the images, too, travelled both through export and copying. They originate in the mid-century, which is sometimes seen as a lull period in anti-doctor feeling, between earlier satires of the doctor as unregulated, self-involved and ineffective, and late-century depictions of the villainous, undetectable, unstoppable medical murderer.[6] But if this was the period when the doctor was legitimised as an upstanding bourgeois professional, these images suggest that not all doubts were quieted. I approach the printed images produced in this period as working in a deeply unstable medical culture, with a chimeric potential to both support and attack the ideal medical persona.

The problematic medical persona

In 1864 Heinrich Hasselhorst produced a chalk drawing and an oil painting depicting an earnest and respectably dressed doctor contemplating a naked female corpse (Figure 2.1). The image depicts an actual event: the anatomist Johann Christian Gustave Lucae studying the corpse of an 18-year-old who had died by suicide to establish the ideal proportions for the female body.[7] The doctor looks at the body with a mixture of detached professionalism and erotic appreciation. This image is part of a broader trend of erotically charged dissection paintings in the latter half of the century, turning on a new elision of power in the male medical professional: the physical and sexual dominance of the patient body.[8] To the modern eye, the wavering between medical and sexual penetration is disturbing. The two approaches to the body are so different that to substitute one with another is to break deep social taboos. In the context of the nineteenth century, however, and particularly given the elite male gaze that such images catered to, the slippage was natural, two expressions of the same dominance that such men exerted over other bodies. This image neatly encompasses the power dynamics at the heart of the medical persona that was forming in the mid-century, and of which we are the beneficiaries.

In the nineteenth century, the social identity and professional position of the doctor changed radically in Britain, Europe, North America and their colonies. Training lengthened, specialisms developed and medical and surgical interventions proliferated. The older system of relatively few elite university-trained physicians and many much lower-status surgeons and apothecaries shifted. A vast

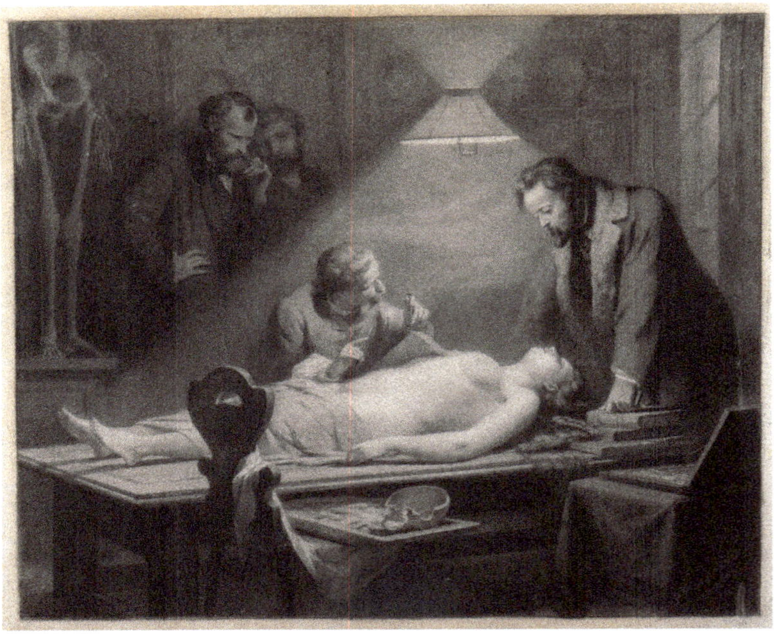

Figure 2.1 Heinrich Hasselhorst, *The dissection of a young, beautiful woman directed by J. Ch. G. Lucae (1814–85) in order to determine the ideal female proportions*, 1864, black chalk on paper.

middle class of 'general practitioners', who combined surgery, dispensing and medicine sought a new level of respectability and new pools of patients, especially among women and children.[9] Some medical discoveries, including anaesthesia and antiseptic practice, improved medicine's reputation for efficacy, with increased training and professional regulation cementing it as a respectable bourgeois profession. It is to the nineteenth century that we owe the ideal of the doctor as a committed, benevolent and highly trained professional.[10]

However, this identity emerged amidst much wider and more ambivalent public attitudes. Doctors had long struggled with reputational issues to do with their mercenary outlooks and the effectiveness of their remedies.[11] Although increased training and regulation from the mid-century challenged these ideas, fears arose that new modes of medical instruction were producing cold, unsympathetic, amoral and potentially maniacal practitioners.[12] Thus, the construction of the new medical persona as respectable bourgeois professional brought with it its own shadow, its dark side. Some scholars, including Tabitha Sparks and Alannah Tomkins, have demonstrated how middle-class culture in this period was heavily invested in making the doctor appear safe, respectable and marriageable.[13] Other areas of culture, as Anna Gasperini's work on penny bloods and Coral Lansbury's on anti-vivisection campaigns show, were committed to exposing the problematic, predatory, abusive nature of the doctor and particularly of his power over patients.[14] In all of these expressions of medical culture, a medico-sexual power dynamic is at the root of what makes the doctor dangerous and fascinating. His ability to expose and overpower the body, intellectually but also, always potentially, physically, is an expression of the bourgeois masculine ideal, and of the problems with that ideal.[15] As Michael Sappol observes (of American culture, but of relevance to European as well):

> physicians defined themselves professionally and socially in opposition not just to lower-class healers and anatomy rioters, but also to the body. In the rituals of the anatomical theater and the anatomy room, ambitious young men learned to dissect, and to regard that operation as a paradigm for the broader mastery of instrumental reason over the body, the lower class, the savage races, the material world, women, animals. Such mastery was not just an isolated part of professional identity, but (at least potentially) part of two larger projects: the making of the bourgeois self and the making of bourgeois society.[16]

This dynamic of power founded on professional authority was, therefore, both an inherent part of ideal bourgeois masculinity and bourgeois patriarchal society, and the tool with which its possessors engaged in all kinds of exploitation. This was the root of the problem for the Victorians: their ideal doctor had the capacity and indeed the inclination to sexually abuse patients, and while it was widely agreed that such inclinations should not be acted upon, when they were, public reactions were complex. The line to tread was one that could condemn the misbehaviour without attacking the system that facilitated it. While dissection portraits such as Hasselhorst's did tread this line studiously and earnestly, comic print culture did so with more unsteadiness, playfulness and criticality.

Considering my sources together, several themes emerge as flashpoints for discussions of medical impropriety. I briefly explore: physical closeness; women doctors; seduction; secrecy and voyeurism; and violence, before considering how the visual humour in these cases functioned for Victorian audiences.

Visualising medical impropriety

The image of the physician taking the patient's pulse had long been a shorthand for intimacy, visualising the potential for medico-sexual ambiguity. Taking the pulse was physically similar to gestures of courtship, such as touching and kissing the hand, and the pulse traditionally was understood to betray feelings of love and lovesickness.[17] This, surely, is the visual context of Figure 2.2, an anonymous and untitled print dating probably, judging by the fashions and medium, to the 1830s or 1840s and depicting a dentist inspecting the mouth of a young woman.

In this lithograph, the intimacy and the innuendo are stepped up. Instead of standing beside the seated patient and feeling the wrist, as was common in seventeenth- and eighteenth-century depictions, this dentist straddles the legs of his patient and touches her open mouth. The allusion to sexual touching and genital orifices is obvious, underscored by the dentist's half-lidded eyes, emphasised eyelashes and amused smile – he looks at her not openly and professionally, but with outrageous 'bedroom eyes'. The image points out what was always dangerous about a medical encounter – its intimacy. In this period, men and women who were not married were rarely physically close, and rarely alone, yet the medical encounter offered opportunities for both. Even among courting couples, unchaperoned encounters and physical closeness were bywords for impropriety and sexual misconduct.[18] What the comic and satirical images here examined do is render explicit what was *implicit* in any unchaperoned encounter between a man and a woman, medical or not.

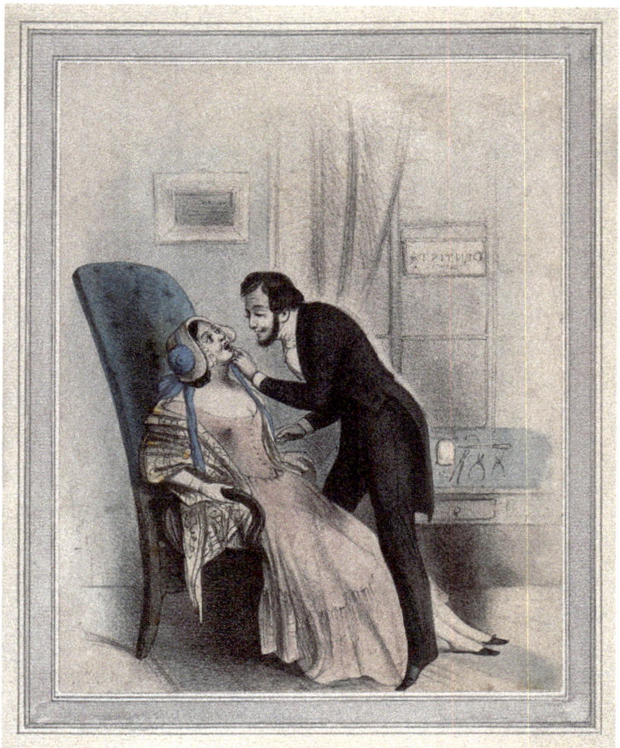

Figure 2.2 Anon., [A dentist examining a patient], [*c*.1830–50], hand-coloured lithograph.

While the dentist is fully and formally clothed in the black suit associated with the medical profession, the patient is in a vulnerable state of, if not undress, then of more intimate and penetrable dress. Her neckline is low, the shawl around her shoulders risks slipping off, her bodice is partially unbuttoned and both feet and ankles are on display. The dress also exposes the shape of breast, stomach and leg, and in colour alludes to the skin beneath. The two sets of clothing indicate, therefore, masculine self-contained power and feminine vulnerability and penetrability – his medical touch, it would seem, leaves her 'undone'. While the medical framing provides plausible deniability, the image clearly indicates seduction.

But medical theming wasn't just an excuse to depict physical closeness and (sometimes forced) sexual intimacy between men and women. The nature of medicine was in itself intriguing and exciting to Victorian audiences. The array of tools, including several sets of pliers, undermines the gentleness of the dentist's touch, particularly because this image predates the widespread use of anaesthetic. Images such as this suggest that, for contemporary audiences, the practitioner's power over the patient, combined with the interplay of sexual pleasure and the threat of pain and fear, was both troubling and attractive. Contemporary pornography indicates that power imbalance, from masculine dominance to sadistic violence, featured heavily in the sexual imagination of the period.[19] The doctor, as an inherently powerful, increasingly unquestionable and idealised masculine figure with inbuilt access to the body, was a natural location for the expression of sexual desire for dominance.[20]

The sexual dynamic expressed in these medico-comic images was resolutely heterosexual and patriarchal. It was because the doctor was a man, with a man's basic sexual urges, that the veneer of rational professionalism was always at risk of collapse. The rise of qualified women doctors, first in the United States from 1849, and across Europe from the 1860s, was presented by some as an answer to this problem.[21] If women could be trained to treat other women's intimate illnesses, the danger of the medical encounter would disappear – 'sapphic' interactions remaining essentially unexpressed in the visual sources I have found. But this did not make the woman doctor an unproblematic figure. Those opposed to women's practice saw the exposure to sickness, the exhausting work outside the home and engagement with dissection, as ruining the morals, modesty and femininity of the female medical student. If becoming a doctor hypersexualised the man, then it essentially desexed the woman.

This is reflected in widespread caricatures of the woman doctor as elderly, ugly and unfeminine. A *Punch* cartoon from 1856 accompanying an article titled 'Physicians in Muslin' contrasts an idealised and beautiful young woman with a caricature of a woman physician (Figure 2.3). Here the artist borrows several existing tropes from caricatures of physicians, including glasses, protruding nose and lower lip and a gold-headed cane held to the mouth.[22]

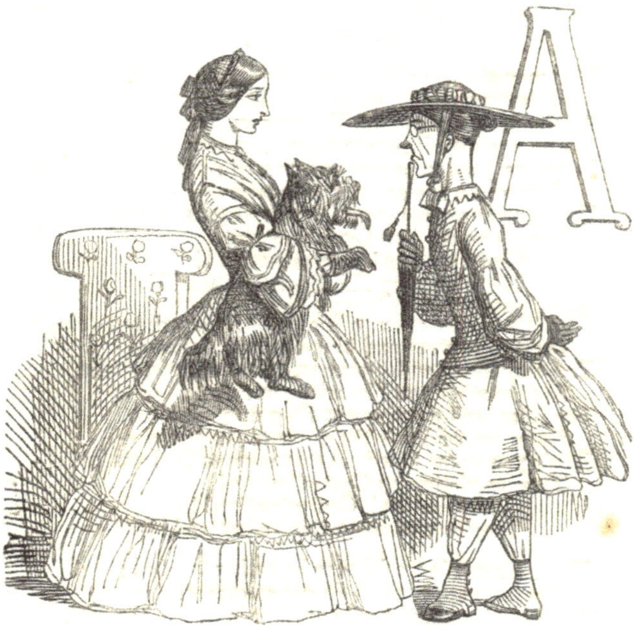

Figure 2.3 Anon., [Illustrated Initial], wood engraving. In Anon., 'Physicians in Muslin', *Punch* (5 April 1856), p. 133.

These elements, along with the large hat, severe hairstyle and short skirt, suggest that the woman physician is the antithesis of womanly ideals. However, not all images of the woman doctor represented her as 'desexed'; others emphasised her femininity in order to underscore the comic incongruity of her medical practice. Another *Punch* cartoon, this from 1865 (Figure 2.4), plays on the incongruity of effecting a professional, but not a sexual, role reversal. While in this image it is the woman who stands, and who takes the pulse, it is still the man who is the sexual aggressor. The incongruity between the professional and personal dynamics in this image are the source of its humour: the supposedly invalid patient looks with an active, predatory gaze while the supposedly authoritative doctor looks modestly down and away. When a woman becomes a doctor, therefore, it is still she who is made vulnerable by the intimacy of

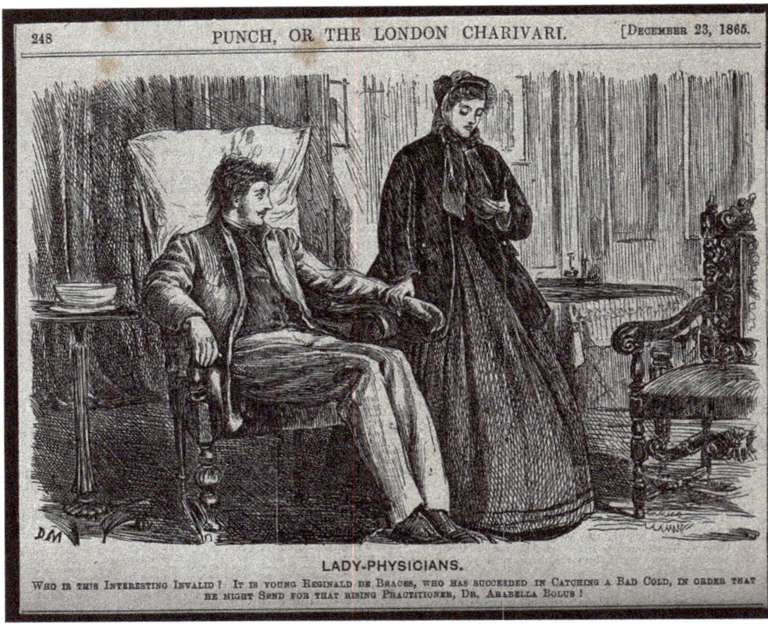
248 PUNCH, OR THE LONDON CHARIVARI. [DECEMBER 23, 1865.
DM
LADY-PHYSICIANS.
WHO IS THIS INTERESTING INVALID? IT IS YOUNG REGINALD DE BRACES, WHO HAS SUCCEEDED IN CATCHING A BAD COLD, IN ORDER THAT HE MIGHT SEND FOR THAT RISING PRACTITIONER, DR. ARABELLA BOLUS!

Figure 2.4 George du Maurier, 'Lady-Physicians', wood engraving. In *Punch* (23 December 1865), p. 248.

the medical interaction. Where women were not seen as desexed by medical practice, therefore, they were seen as vulnerable to sexual violation – by patients, by doctors and by the work itself.[23] These twin dangers: of becoming desexed and becoming hypersexualised, were oppressively obvious to early women practitioners. Curating the perfect level of femininity to be accepted both as women and as doctors was a large part of their professional labour.[24]

The comic image allowed for the artist to highlight the slippage between the medical and the sexual touch in an allusive, sidelong way. *Punch* and other mid-Victorian entertainment periodicals often balanced acknowledgement of problematic aspects of culture with a cloaking of safe, family friendly humour.[25] However, more explicitly critical material was produced, often by those with a grudge against normative middle-class culture. One example can be found in a set of four prints produced as advertisements and propaganda for the famous alternative practitioner and 'hygeist' James Morison.[26] These prints, collected under the title *The Morality of Modern Medicine Mongers*, depicted four aspects of the dark side of the doctor: the Family MD, who forces a patient to answer intimate questions; the Obscene MD, who publishes pornography under the guise of medical literature; the Mesmeric MD, who uses mesmerism to control and seduce patients; and the Obstetric MD, who persuades a reluctant patient to undergo a pelvic examination (Figure 2.5).[27] A later edition in which all four plates are reproduced on one sheet is dated 1852, but the original colour plates were likely printed between 1828 and 1840.[28]

Alternative practitioners abounded in the nineteenth century, much to the chagrin of the regulars. These 'irregulars' were not limited by any professional demands on education or training, and could offer treatments and medications that catered to people's anxieties and dissatisfactions with regular practice. Some irregulars were obviously frauds and sold ineffective panaceas through a combination of expansive promises and effective advertising. Other irregulars had more comprehensive theories of medicine, often addressing legitimate concerns with regular practice, including: over-use of complex medications, interventionist and even experimental attitudes to patient care and the protectionism of medical knowledge.[29] This last was of particular relevance to those anxious about medical seduction, indeed the two issues are linked in three of the four Morison prints. As medical knowledge became ever more specialised and professionalised, patients' authority over their bodies and their treatment fell away and they became subject to their doctors'. Patients were expected to trust in their doctors' knowledge and judgement, but also their professional integrity. Much of this debate in the mid-century was focused on the speculum. This tool allowed a practitioner to visually examine the cervix and to more easily treat gynaecological diseases. However, it also involved penetrating the vagina of the patient with a distinctly phallic object. Critics argued that not only was this, in itself, morally wrong, tantamount to sexual assault, but that women were all too likely to become addicted to the procedure, to have their modesty and their morals degraded by it.[30]

These anxieties are expressed in Morison's print 'The Obstetric M.D.' (Figure 2.5): the doctor's professionalism as a cover for

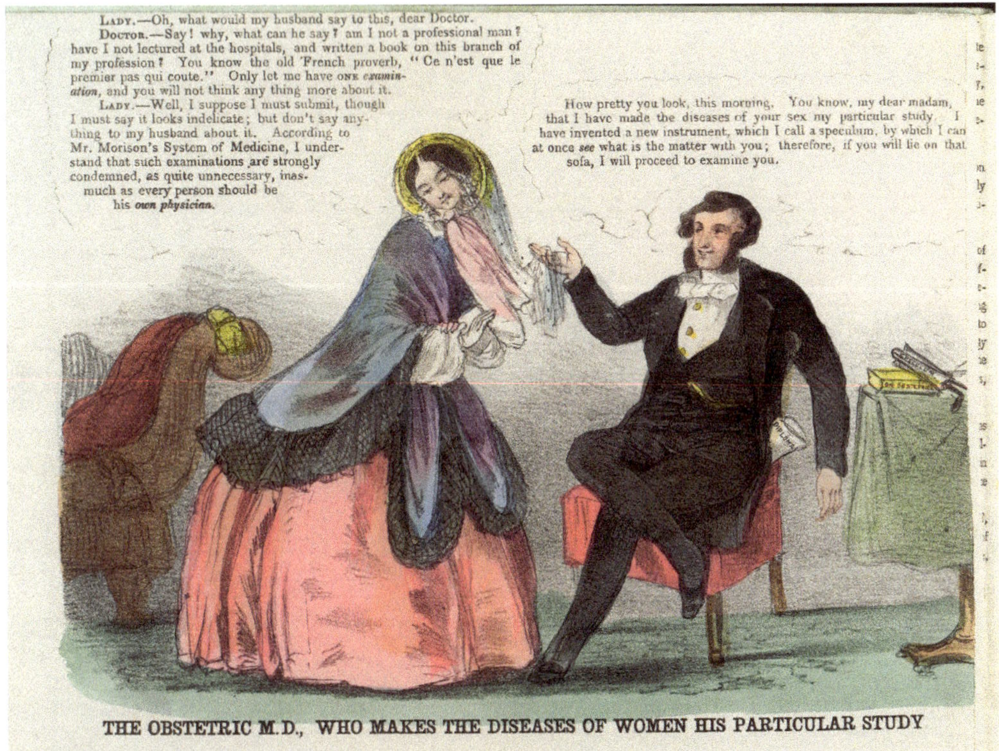

Figure 2.5 Anon., 'The Obstetric M.D.', hand-coloured lithograph. In James Morison, *Morality of Modern Medicine-Mongers* ([London]: [British College of Health], [1852?]).

seduction, the misleading and manipulation of patients and the use of the speculum as a medicalised tool for sexual penetration. Of course, this image is selling something and denigrates regular medicine in order to do so, but the image could only work if such fears already existed or had the potential to exist for viewers. Text is used to make these points explicit where other comedic prints leave them ambiguous, but this image underscores the extent to which even a relatively 'mild' image of medical seduction could have explosive implications for Victorian viewers. It is worth noting that in this image, and that of the dentist (Figure 2.2), the two practitioners have similar expressions of amused enjoyment. In both, the doctor reaches to touch the headwear of the patient, indicating not a professional touch, but a flirtatious one. To touch the headdress – an element of clothing specific to women and associated with modesty and propriety – emphasises the gender dynamic between the two figures, highlighting the femininity of the patient. It also acts as an obvious visual precursor to other forms of touching, and to acts of exposure and undress.

It is also significant that in both images, the lithographic medium is used to draw attention to the 'bedroom eyes' of the practitioner. Where elsewhere the lithographic capacity for shading and diffuse line is employed, in rendering the eyes both artists have used a deep, inky black line: the gaze is dark, sly, suggestive. Indeed, looking itself is a feature in all of these works, and plays on the medium in which they were produced. Following the work of Foucault, much attention has been paid to the clinical gaze and the way it objectified and dehumanised the patient.[31] For Victorian audiences, the manner of the medical look was clearly of interest, as patients found they lost control over their own bodies and medical narratives as they exposed themselves to the probing and knowledge-making gazes of their doctors. This, indeed, was part of the problem with the speculum. While a digital pelvic examination was often legitimised by the use of drapery to protect the patient body from sight if not touch, the speculum exam involved not only looking, but looking within the body. Highly intimate, it also further disempowered the patient by giving the doctor knowledge of their body that the person could not have. All these prints feature looking as a precursor to, and key aspect of, medical seduction. Indeed, by looking at these prints we become implicated in the doctor's invasion of the private, the feminine and the domestic. We observe the private consultation, and in identifying the sexual beneath the medical we also become a voyeur. In all three images, the direction of gaze between patient and doctor is crucial, and in all three the viewer of the print becomes the third in a triangle of illicit looking.

It is worth remembering that the very existence of these kinds of images: affordable prints depicting scenes and themes of interest from daily life and aimed at a general viewership, were very new. Of course, there were still wealth, class, literacy and geographic barriers to access, but this kind of visual media was much more available than, for example, the political satirical prints of the Georgian period.[32] As such, the dynamics of sight comments not just on this issue of medical culture, but much more widely on the pleasures and risks of looking and visually representing. The proliferation of print culture in this period was seen as something of a problem. It was appealing to people of all classes and was understood to have a powerful influence over less educated viewers, and especially women. Unregulated images could corrupt or influence vulnerable minds in serious ways, and so women are doubly in danger here: as both the subject of the image and its viewer.[33] These particular images were dangerous not only because they pointed out problems with medical culture, but because they encouraged erotic looking and general interest in improper subjects. Indeed, they might even inspire both doctors and patients to engage in such behaviour. As these images indicate, part of the problem with the medical encounter was that it gave women patients, as well as doctors, opportunities to initiate clandestine sexual encounters. While the public were mostly worried about predatory doctors, doctors themselves were deeply concerned with the risks posed to their careers by sexually deviant patients.[34]

The viewer of the print occupies an uncertain space, therefore, both separate from and also engaged in the scene represented. The fact that medical consultations happened in private and domestic or semi-domestic spaces was part of what made them problematic. The danger of the private interaction, and the constant risk of exposure or discovery is always implicit and would have been much more obvious for a Victorian viewer, embedded in a culture obsessed with the ideal of the domestic and the risk that extramarital sex posed to that ideal.[35] In some images, this danger is explicit: the text in Figure 2.5 indicates that both doctor and patient are conscious that their interaction must be hidden from the patient's husband. Indeed, it is this secrecy that most clearly indicates to the viewer that the examination is improper. While not in itself obscene, this image makes obvious allusions to the contemporary visual culture of pornography: the secret liaison, the extramarital affair and risk of discovery were all common tropes in written and visual pornography of the period. Indeed, the medical encounter itself was to be found represented in this genre.

While a less common theme than the sexual misdemeanours of other professional men – most usually clergy – doctors do feature in pornography. The series of flap prints *Grand theâtre des petites passions de société* exposed a whole variety of sexual misdemeanours engaged in by French society, each hidden behind a door that the viewer can open. One, 'Le docteur est bien long' (Figure 2.6) depicts a man waiting impatiently outside a doctor's room. Opening the door, we find the doctor masturbating and fingering the vulva of his patient. The caption can be translated as 'Rest assured, Madame, I always choose my remedies from the animal kingdom.' The pun plays on the contemporary anxieties around medicines taken not from the natural world but from synthesised chemicals, while his actual remedy is animal in the sexual sense. While not all pornography was meant to be comic, this series was clearly intended both to titillate and amuse. The flap mechanism gives power to the viewer to be a voyeur, to enjoy peeking at sexual interactions that were intended to be private. It also gives a much broader power to the viewer to expose the hypocrisies and corruptions of society, and indeed to laugh at and criticise its upper echelons.

Looking at Figures 2.5 and 2.6 together elucidates the broad visual contexts in which print in this period worked. The same medium – hand-coloured lithograph – the startlingly similar domestic contexts and even colour palettes show how easily the sexually suggestive popular image blended with and referenced the sexually explicit pornographic one. Of course, not all viewers would have seen these exact two prints, but the medium, style and themes were part of a much larger cross-genre visual language.

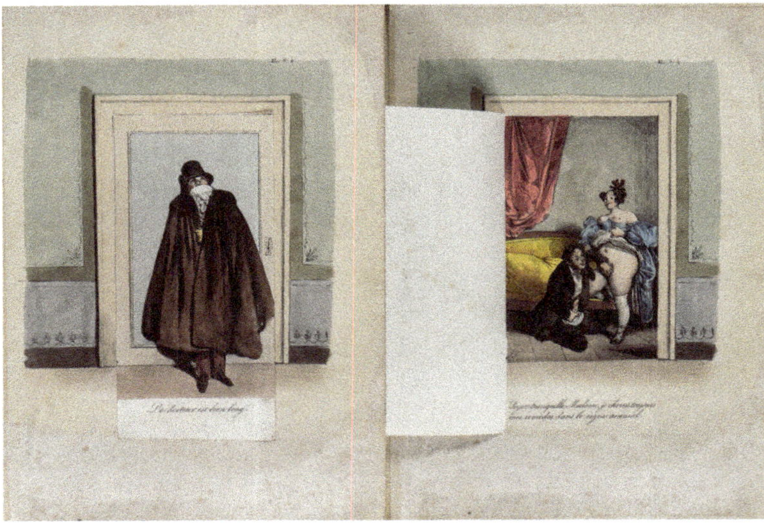

Figure 2.6 Anon., 'Le docteur est bien long', hand-coloured lithograph. In Anon., *Grand theâtre des petites passions de société* ([Paris?]: [s.n.], [*c*.1830s]).

The explicit voyeurism and exposure of the pornographic print, as well as the medical theming, allow us to see the contexts in which a viewer would have approached the less explicit 'Obstetric M.D.' It is significant, too, that humour is an element of both images. Laughter is produced by the disconnect between the expectation of professional medical behaviour, and the actual highly improper sexual behaviour displayed by the doctors. Each image provides an erotic pleasure cloaked in a critical comedic one, allowing the viewer to enjoy being at once a voyeuristic actor in the sexual scene, and a detached critic of such misbehaviour.

Nervous laughter

John Morreall has described the incongruity theory of humour as 'some thing or event we perceive or think about [that] violates our normal mental patterns and normal expectations'.[36] In these images we expect to see a medical consultation and our expectation is violated when instead we find a seduction. But this, I argue, is not a complete account of the humour in these images. After we are shocked by the incongruity, the emotion subsides, and congruity is re-established because it wasn't ridiculous or impossible for a doctor to seduce a patient. It was entirely possible: cases were prosecuted in court and reported in the press.[37] By making use of the visual language of seduction, an already familiar aspect of sexual politics, the interaction is presented as entirely expectable. The response these images script, I argue, is a jolt and a laugh, followed by an eye roll, a tut, an 'I'm not surprised'. This isn't surreal humour or extreme humour, it's somewhere between jaded and indulgent.

To look at this interpretation more closely, let us first take the surprise. These images might be seen as satire, as attacks on the way that medicine as it was developing in this period seemed to facilitate, even to invite, sexual impropriety. Roy Porter, in his foundational article 'The Rise of Physical Examination', argues that doctors in this period were enabled to examine and touch bodies in ways that broke barriers of bodily privacy and sexual propriety through a process of ritualisation. The creation of 'reassuring ritualized, consensual sanctions' made safe actions that in other contexts would be highly inappropriate, tantamount to sexual abuse.[38] The mid-nineteenth century was the period when these rituals were being established, but before they were completely secure, it was 'the threat of the surreptitious slippage from one code into another that leaves clinical practice so subject to the anarchy of *double entendre*'.[39] The commitment of the medical establishment to these rituals may have seemed, to critical observers, astonishing. Indeed, polemicists repeatedly expressed incredulity at how society had fallen, seemingly unconsciously, into the nefarious grip of the improper medical encounter.[40] Images like those discussed here pointed to the risks of slippage, the social anarchy, that the rituals were trying to do away with.

However, these images are not simply satires aimed at disrupting the ritualisation of the medical encounter. After the initial surprise of identifying seduction in place of consultation, the images settle back into Morreall's 'normal mental patterns and normal expectations'. This is because the misogyny and sexual violence at the heart of these images was extensively used in visual humour. Nineteenth-century theories of masculinity embraced dominion over women, the capacity for violence and strong sexual urges. The ideal middle-class educated man, whose superiority brought him all kinds of privileges over other classes of people, was supposed, in theory, to control the more basic of these urges. These expectations strengthened over the course of the century, but occasional lapses of control, which included extra-marital sex and sexual violence, continued to be widely, if tacitly, accepted.[41] Indeed sexual violence against women formed a central and enduring part of humour, including in visual satires. Such images were funny to both men and women because the power dynamic was legitimated by notions of sexual difference and hierarchy.[42] The misuse of masculine power was funny because people could see the incongruity between ideal behaviour and that represented, but were not outright appalled by it.

This is best exemplified in a final visual example, a lithographic illustration from the French comic periodical *Le Charivari*. In the images examined so far, the predatory nature of the doctor is implied. While he does not sexually touch or force the patient, his control of the interaction, based on a potent mix of masculine, professional, intellectual and physical authority, make no explicit exertion of force necessary. But in Charles Jacques's 'Le Médecin de théâtre', one of a series of cartoons on the theme of medical culture, the doctor bribes *and* physically coerces an actress (Figure 2.7). The caption can be translated as:

> Because you absolutely insist, my beautiful one, I find that you have a fever ... a terrible fever ... and I will sign the certificate that will excuse you from having to perform tomorrow ... but I urge you to look after yourself and not to eat anything more at supper tonight than a simple macaroni, a stuffed chicken and a light lobster salad. [Translation Dr Katherine Goodson Walker]

The text is mild, hinting at seduction – a sick note in exchange for a dinner. Indeed, by itself, it could even be read to simply mock the disparity between doctors' prescriptions and what was actually within the means of their more impoverished patients. That such a

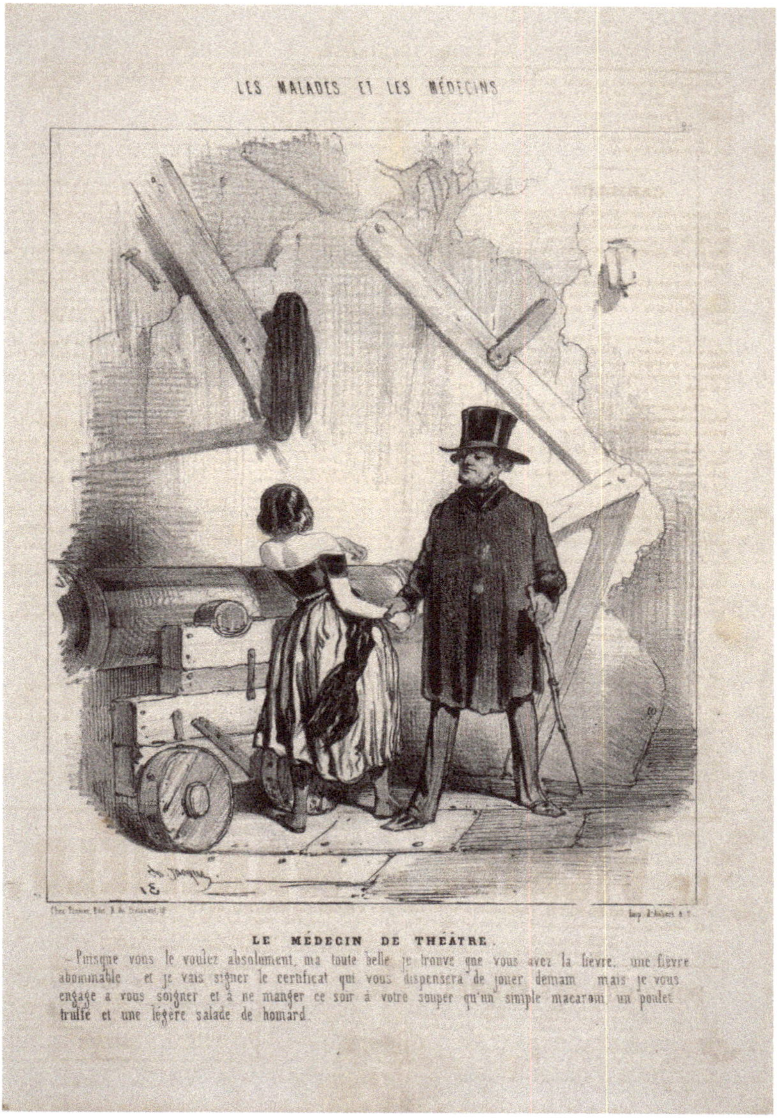
LES MALADES ET LES MÉDECINS
LE MÉDECIN DE THÉATRE.
– Puisque vous le voulez absolument, ma toute belle je trouve que vous avez la fièvre. une fièvre abominable et je vais signer le certificat qui vous dispensera de jouer demain mais je vous engage à vous soigner et à ne manger ce soir à votre souper qu'un simple macaroni un poulet truffé et une légère salade de homard.

Figure 2.7 Charles Jacque, 'Le Médecin de théâtre', lithograph. In *Le Charivari* (1843), p. 25.

meal would be followed by seduction, and a sexual encounter, is a potential left unspoken, but implied in the doctor's shifting of the relationship from professional to personal. But combined with the image, the meaning of the text changes. Here the familiar gesture of pulse-taking is shifted and darkened, the grasp becomes controlling. The actress expresses helpless fear and repulsion in her posture and the doctor is presented as nothing less than a Gothic villain. It is interesting to note that once again the doctor's eyes are dark, lidded, predatory – bedroom eyes of a more sinister sort. But unlike in the other images, where the gazes of both parties are in interplay, suggesting some level of complicity, here the actress has no gaze, and no agency, the interaction and the power is entirely one-sided.

To a modern audience, this is an image of sexual violence with a vague medical theming; there is no balance between proper and improper, no levity to produce humour. But for a nineteenth-century audience, as already discussed, masculine power, sexual violence and particularly the sexual exploitation of working-class women by middle-class men, were practically accepted, if morally dubious.[43] Indeed, it is certainly the class differential that allows for the representation of physical violence here. This is not a middle-class patient who must be secretly seduced, but a working-class woman and an actress, only one step away from a prostitute, who can be compelled without consequence.[44] Holmstrom has noted that the beautiful corpses in the dissection paintings with which we began were understood to deserve their medico-sexual punishment because they embodied the threat of both the elite New Woman and the disease-carrying prostitute to patriarchal power.[45] Here, too, the doctor brings order and control to the potential chaos of the woman outside the home through medical and sexual dominance.

These images of medical impropriety were both interesting and amusing to a nineteenth-century audience because they spoke to the dangerous problematics of medical culture, indeed often raising issues that were otherwise ignored or suppressed. But then they reconcile the danger within conventional comic frameworks of seduction imagery, even when the seduction is coercive and one-sided, as in Figure 2.7. In these popular images, the actual medical edifice is kept safe. This follows Mary Douglas's analysis of the joke as something that 'offers alternative patterns, one apparent, one hidden: the latter, by being brought to the surface impugns the validity of the first'.[46] However, the excitement of the joke, Douglas argues, 'lies in the suggestion that any particular ordering of experience may be arbitrary and subjective. It is frivolous in that it produces no real alternative, only an exhilarating sense of freedom from form in general'.[47] Jokes, in this system, can be understood as 'anti-rites': similar to rites in that they connect different systems, but different in that their point is to challenge, not to strengthen, that which is dominant. This they do safely, offering a psychological relief without effecting a material social or cultural revolution.[48] While I doubt this (or any one) theory's ability to encompass all instances of humour across time, place, media and context, Douglas's theory does help in understanding the role of medical impropriety jokes for mid-Victorian audiences. This is particularly so when we return to Porter's theory about the ritualising of the medical encounter in this period: while the dominant culture was committed to these new rituals confirming the right of the doctor to examine the body, medical impropriety jokes disordered, challenged and criticised them, but only within the world of the joke.[49] Indeed, it is arguably this eventual non-productivity that makes them funny, and that distinguishes them from the large body of earnest polemics and campaign materials produced by middle-class Victorians for their various social causes.

This recognition and then dismissal of great social evils caused by patriarchal systems characterises mid-nineteenth-century British culture. It is identified with regard to sexual violence by Carolyn Conley, prostitution by Judith R. Walkowitz and medical misadventure by Alannah Tomkins.[50] Both Conley and Tomkins note that in court and in community, men accused of sexual assault usually received every possible assistance towards acquittal, especially if they were respectable middle- or upper-class members of the community. Where the crime could not be denied, sentencing often reflected a general feeling that the issue was neither serious, nor one to cause permanent damage to the perpetrator's reputation. Extreme cases were separated as exceptional and comparisons between these and lesser crimes were avoided.

How humour came to feature in this rather depressing endeavour can be explained by examining a strange phenomenon noted by

Tomkins. Around the mid-century, newspaper reports began to describe spontaneous applause from the gallery when doctors were acquitted of crimes. She argues that 'In the 1860s, applause was a way to defend the medical persona against the reallocation of their role from expert witness to attacker in a decade when medical status was still quite friable.'[51] While not exactly comic, this intriguing public response indicates the same underlying need for performativity, for an overt confirmation of the patriarchal and class protections afforded to doctors. As Tomkins points out, 'A profession that is more confident of its status does not require the reassurance of such applause.'[52] We can see the comic images addressed in this chapter in a similar light: as a performative, perhaps slightly hysterical, public response to the dangers of the medical encounter. Applause in the courtroom and laughter at the print both acknowledge the problematic and then dismiss it.

To some degree, whether these prints attack or support institutionalised medicine depends on the individual viewer. Some were certainly committed campaigners against new gynaecological and obstetric practice and maintained genuine anger and fear towards doctors. However, I argue that there is something inherent in the representational style of the images that encourages the continued support of regular medicine. It has been widely noted that the graphic humour of the mid-century was gentler, less satirical and more supportive of the status quo.[53] Indeed, in the images addressed here, the suggestions of medical impropriety are made gently, often allusively. This was particularly the case when we remember that certain levels of masculine dominance and sexual violence were accepted, especially where the perpetrator was 'respectable' and middle-class. If we compare these images to the much more grotesque and bawdy Georgian satires by the likes of James Gillray, Thomas Rowlandson and Isaac Cruikshank, or the radical and explicit late-century imagery of Félicien Rops and Jules Abel Faivre, we can see how the mid-century cartoons work as apologies for, as well as criticisms of, the problem. The naturalistic style, the often middle-class and elegant theming, the use of allusion and a visual language of flirtation make the images safe to circulate widely, but they also downplay the seriousness of the issue. Even in the

Morison print (Figure 2.5), the cut is really in the text, not the image, and is thus less obvious. These images allow us to recognise medical impropriety, but they also encourage us to laugh it off.

If historians of graphic comedy are often rather dismissive of both the style of humour and the social and political toothlessness of mid-nineteenth-century imagery, this does not mean that the images are simple or ineffectual. In fact, they were effective and powerful tools for supporting medical culture while avoiding didacticism, pomposity or hypocrisy. Indeed, exploring how they engaged with mid-century anxieties around the newly forming medical culture, and particularly how they defused them, is crucial to understanding how medicine came to command such widespread social respect, even reverence, from then until now. As other chapters in this volume so neatly show, medical culture is rather good at laughing at itself, at making jokes out of things that are frightening, serious, destructive. Very often, this humour poses no threat to the institution of medicine or its workings, even where the point of the joke is to criticise. Rather, the humour works because of the disconnect (or incongruity) between the ideal and the reality of a highly idealised profession. While we might like to think we are both more socially progressive and more able to criticise powerful institutions than the Victorians, when it comes to the medical edifice, we in the twenty-first century might do well to recognise our own tendency to nervous laughter at medical impropriety.

Acknowledgements

My thanks to Dr Katherine Goodson Walker for her invaluable assistance in interpreting the nuances and double entendres of some French sources.

Notes

1 I approach the nineteenth-century medical persona as inherently male. While women practised medicine in many forms and were registered as doctors in increasing numbers in the latter half of the century, the

ideal of the doctor, and most discourse around it, assumed maleness. As discussed later in this chapter, the female medical persona was constructed largely in response to the 'default' male.

2 See, for example, Alannah Tomkins, *Medical Misadventure in an Age of Professionalisation, 1780–1890* (Manchester University Press, 2017); Tabitha Sparks, *The Doctor in the Victorian Novel: Family Practices* (Ashgate, 2009); Anna Gasperini, *Nineteenth Century Popular Fiction, Medicine and Anatomy: The Victorian Penny Blood and the 1832 Anatomy Act* (Springer, 2019); Mary Hunter, *The Face of Medicine: Visualising Medical Masculinities in Late Nineteenth-Century Paris* (Manchester University Press, 2016); Melissa Dickson, 'Hats, Cloaks, and Stethoscopes: The Symbolic Fashions of the Nineteenth-Century Medical Practitioner', in Janine Hatter and Nickianne Moody (eds), *Fashion and Material Culture in Victorian Fiction and Periodicals* (Edward Everett Root, 2019), pp. 103–18.

3 Mary Douglas, *Implicit Meanings: Selected Essays in Anthropology*, 2nd edition (Routledge, 1999), pp. 146–64.

4 Patricia Mainardi, *Another World: Nineteenth-Century Illustrated Print Culture* (Yale University Press, 2017), p. 235.

5 Rachel Teukolsky, *Picture World: Image, Aesthetics, and Victorian New Media* (Oxford University Press, 2020).

6 For earlier, see Fiona Haslam, *From Hogarth to Rowlandson: Medicine in Art in Eighteenth Century Britain* (Liverpool University Press, 1996). For later, see Angus McLaren, '"Not a Stranger, a Doctor": Medical Men and Sexual Matters in the Late Nineteenth Century', in Roy Porter and Mikuláš Teich (eds), *Sexual Knowledge, Sexual Science: The History of Attitudes to Sexuality* (Cambridge University Press, 1994), pp. 267–83; Coral Lansbury, 'Gynaecology, Pornography, and the anti-vivisection movement', *Victorian Studies* 28:3 (1985), 413–37; Andrew Smith, *Victorian Demons: Medicine, Masculinity and the Gothic at the Fin de Siècle* (Manchester University Press, 2004); Sparks, *The Doctor in the Victorian Novel*, pp. 111–31.

7 See Wellcome catalogue record https://wellcomecollection.org/works/hahd7nuh

8 See Natasha Ruiz-Gómez, 'The Model Patient: Observation and Illustration at the Musée Charcot', in Andrew Graciano (ed.), *Visualizing the Body in Art, Anatomy, and Medicine since 1800: Models and Modeling* (Routledge, 2019), pp. 203–32; Mary Hunter, 'The waiting time of prostitution: Gynaecology and temporality in Henri de Toulouse-Lautrec's *Rue Des Moulins*, 1894', *Art History* 42:1 (2019), 68–93; Neil Graham Holmstrom, 'Beautiful, Dead, Dissected:

The Dismembered Female Body in Artistic Representation' (PhD thesis, University of Tasmania, 2017); Elisabeth Bronfen, *Over Her Dead Body: Death, Femininity and the Aesthetic* (Manchester University Press, 1992), pp. 3–14.

9 Irvine Loudon, *Medical Care and the General Practitioner 1750–1850* (Clarendon Press, 1986).

10 See Anne Digby, *Making a Medical Living: Doctors and Patients in the English Market for Medicine, 1720–1911* (Cambridge University Press, 1994); Michael Brown, *Performing Medicine: Medical Culture and Identity in Provincial England, c.1760–1850* (Manchester University Press, 2011), pp. 113–49.

11 Digby, *Making a Medical Living*, pp. 37–64; Sparks, *The Doctor in the Victorian Novel*, pp. 12–15; Tomkins, *Medical Misadventure*, pp. 7–10.

12 See, for example, Ornella Moscucci, 'Clitoridectomy, circumcision, and the politics of sexual pleasure in mid-Victorian Britain', in Andrew H. Miller and James Eli Adams (eds), *Sexualities in Victorian Britain* (Indiana University Press, 1996), pp. 60–78; Cheryl Blake Price, 'Medical Bluebeards: The Domestic Threat of the Poisoning Doctor in the Popular Fiction of Ellen Wood', in Louise Penner and Tabitha Sparks (eds), *Victorian Medicine and Popular Culture* (University of Pittsburgh Press, 2016), pp. 81–93; McLaren, '"Not a Stranger, a Doctor"'; Tomkins, *Medical Misadventure*.

13 Sparks, *The Doctor in the Victorian Novel*, pp. 23–45; Tomkins, *Medical Misadventure*, p. 173.

14 Gasperini, *Nineteenth Century Popular Fiction, Medicine and Anatomy*; Lansbury, 'Gynaecology, pornography, and the antivivisection movement'.

15 For general works on masculinity in this period, see John Tosh, *A Man's Place: Masculinity and the Middle-Class Home in Victorian England* (Yale University Press, 2007); Joanne Begiato, *Manliness in Britain, 1760–1900: Bodies, Emotion, and Material Culture* (Manchester University Press, 2020).

16 Michael Sappol, *A Traffic of Dead Bodies: Anatomy and Embodied Social Identity in Nineteenth-Century America* (Princeton University Press, 2002), pp. 168–9.

17 Laurinda S. Dixon, *Perilous Chastity: Women and Illness in Pre-Enlightenment Art and Medicine* (Cornell University Press, 1995), pp. 85–91; Sally Holloway, *The Game of Love in Georgian England: Courtship, Emotions, and Material Culture* (Oxford University Press, 2019), pp. 31–4.

18 Jennifer Phegley, *Courtship and Marriage in Victorian England* (Praeger, 2012), pp. 31–67.

19 Lisa Z. Sigel, *Governing Pleasures: Pornography and Social Change in England, 1815–1914* (Rutgers University Press, 2002), pp. 50–80; Steven Marcus, *The Other Victorians: A Study of Sexuality and Pornography in Mid-Nineteenth Century England* (Weidenfeld & Nicolson, 1966), pp. 197–251.

20 Hunter, *The Face of Medicine*, pp. 127–8; Elizabeth Stephens, 'Touching Bodies: Tact/Ility in Nineteenth-Century Medical Photographs and Models', in Kate Fisher and Sarah Toulalan (eds), *Bodies, Sex and Desire from the Renaissance to the Present* (Palgrave Macmillan, 2011), pp. 87–101; Sappol, *A Traffic of Dead Bodies*, p. 207.

21 For general histories of women's battle for professional training and recognition see Alison Bashford, *Purity and Pollution: Gender, Embodiment and Victorian Medicine* (Macmillan, 1998), pp. 85–108; Susan Wells, *Out of the Dead House: Nineteenth-Century Women Physicians and the Writing of Medicine* (The University of Wisconsin Press, 2001); Claire Brock, *British Women Surgeons and Their Patients, 1860–1918* (Cambridge University Press, 2017); Steven J. Peitzman, *New and Untried Course: Woman's Medical College and Medical College of Pennsylvania, 1850–1998* (Rutgers University Press, 2000).

22 See, for example, the caricatures of Thomas Rowlandson: *A Medical Inspection, or Miracles Will Never Cease* (1814); *The Anatomist* (1811); *Medical Dispatch, or, Doctor Doubledose Killing Two Birds with One Stone* (1810). Or, in a more naturalistic mode, Louis-Léopold Boilly's *La Malade* (1827).

23 Bashford, *Purity and Pollution*, p. 58.

24 Teja Varma Pusapati, 'Claiming Medicine as a Profession for Women: The English Woman's Journal's Campaign for Female Doctors', in Beth Rodgers, Alexis Easley and Clare Gill (eds), *Women, Periodicals and Print Culture in Britain, 1830s–1900s: The Victorian Period* (Edinburgh University Press, 2022), pp. 122–4; Jessica Dandona, '"The Lady Anatomist": Fragmented Bodies, Photographic Assemblage and the "Art" of Dissection at Woman's Medical College of Pennsylvania, 1895–98', in John Nott and Anna Harris (eds), *Making Sense of Medicine: Material Culture and the Reproduction of Medical Knowledge* (Intellect, 2022), pp. 106–24; Peitzman, *New and Untried Course*.

25 Vic Gatrell, *City of Laughter: Sex and Satire in Eighteenth-Century London* (Atlantic Books, 2006), pp. 417–34; Frank Palmeri,

'Cruikshank, Thackeray, and the Victorian eclipse of satire', *Studies in English Literature, 1500–1900* 44:4 (2004), 753–77; Robert Bernard Martin, *The Triumph of Wit: A Study of Victorian Comic Theory* (Clarendon Press, 1974), pp. 25–46.

26 Brown, *Performing Medicine*, pp. 206–9.

27 See Sarah Bull, 'Managing the "Obscene M.D.": Medical publishing, the medical profession, and the changing definition of obscenity in mid-Victorian England', *Bulletin of the History of Medicine* 91 (2017), 713–43.

28 That is, between the date mentioned on the wrapper as when Morison founded his college, and when he died.

29 See, for example, John S. Haller, *Medical Protestants: The Eclectics in American Medicine, 1825–1939* (Southern Illinois University Press, 1994); Kevin A. Morrison, 'Dr Locock and His Quack: Professionalizing Medicine, Textualizing Identity in the 1840s', in Louise Penner and Tabitha Sparks (eds), *Victorian Medicine and Popular Culture* (University of Pittsburgh Press, 2016), pp. 9–25; Bull, 'Managing the "Obscene M.D."'; Tomkins, *Medical Misadventure.*

30 Ornella Moscucci, *The Science of Woman: Gynaecology and Gender in England, 1800–1929* (Cambridge University Press, 1990), pp. 112–26; Kathryn Yeniyurt, 'When it hurts to look: Interpreting the interior of the Victorian woman', *Social History of Medicine* 27:1 (2014), 22–40; George Morant, *Hints to Husbands: A Revelation of the Man-Midwife's Mysteries*, 3rd edition (Simpkin, Marshall & Co, 1857).

31 Michel Foucault, *The Birth of the Clinic: An Archaeology of Medical Perception*, trans. A.M. Sheridan (Routledge, 2003).

32 Brian Maidment, 'The gallery of comicalities: Graphic humour, wood-engraving, and the development of the comic magazine, 1820–1841', *Victorian Periodicals Review* 50:1 (2017), 214–27.

33 Lynda Nead, *Victorian Babylon: People, Streets, and Images in Nineteenth-Century London* (Yale University Press, 2000), pp. 150–60; Brian Maidment, *Comedy, Caricature and the Social Order, 1820–50* (Manchester University Press, 2013), pp. 113–43.

34 Tomkins, *Medical Misadventure*, p. 162.

35 Lynda Nead, *Myths of Sexuality: Representations of Women in Victorian Britain* (Basil Blackwell, 1988), pp. 48–90; see also Tosh, *A Man's Place*, pp. 53–78; Jeffrey Weeks, *Sex, Politics and Society: The Regulations of Sexuality Since 1800* (Routledge, 2014), pp. 27–46.

36 John Morreall, *Comic Relief: A Comprehensive Philosophy of Humor* (Wiley-Blackwell, 2009), p. 11.

37 Martin J. Wiener, *Men of Blood: Violence, Manliness and Criminal Justice in Victorian England* (Cambridge University Press, 2004), pp. 115–6.
38 Roy Porter, 'The Rise of Physical Examination', in W.F. Bynum and Roy Porter (eds), *Medicine and the Five Senses* (Cambridge University Press, 1993), p. 180.
39 Porter, 'The Rise of Physical Examination', p. 197.
40 See, for example, Morant, *Hints to Husbands*; George Gregory, *Medical Morals, Illustrated with Plates and Extracts from Medical Works; Designed to Show the Pernicious Social and Moral Influence of the Present System of Medical Practice, and the Importance of Establishing Female Medical Colleges, and Educating and Employing Female Physicians for Their Own Sex* (The Author, 1852).
41 Carolyn A. Conley, *The Unwritten Law: Criminal Justice in Victorian Kent* (Oxford University Press, 1991), pp. 68–95; Tomkins, *Medical Misadventure*, pp. 157–9; Wiener, *Men of Blood*, pp. 76–122.
42 Gatrell, *City of Laughter*, pp. 345–87.
43 Judith R. Walkowitz, *Prostitution and Victorian Society: Women, Class and the State* (Cambridge University Press, 1980), pp. 32–47; Marcus, *The Other Victorians*, pp. 128–46.
44 See Conley, *The Unwritten Law*, pp. 68–95; Hunter, 'The waiting time of prostitution'; Maria Luddy, 'Prostitution from 1800', in Sarah Toulalan and Kate Fisher (eds), *The Routledge History of Sex and the Body: 1500 to the Present* (Routledge, 2013), pp. 409–26; Abigail Solomon-Godeau, 'The legs of the countess', *October* 39 (Winter 1986), 83–94.
45 Holmstrom, 'Beautiful, Dead, Dissected', pp. 58–68.
46 Douglas, *Implicit Meanings*, pp. 149–50.
47 Douglas, *Implicit Meanings*, pp. 150–1.
48 Douglas, *Implicit Meanings*, p. 155.
49 See also Peter L. Berger, *Redeeming Laughter: The Comic Dimension of Human Experience*, 2nd edition (De Gruyter, 2014), p. 67.
50 Conley, *The Unwritten Law*, pp. 68–95; Walkowitz, *Prostitution and Victorian Society*, pp. 32–47; Tomkins, *Medical Misadventure*, pp. 157–98.
51 Tomkins, *Medical Misadventure*, p. 173.
52 Tomkins, *Medical Misadventure*, p. 174.
53 Gatrell, *City of Laughter*, pp. 417–34; Palmeri, 'Cruikshank, Thackeray, and the Victorian Eclipse of Satire'; Martin, *The Triumph of Wit*, pp. 25–46.

References

Bashford, Alison. *Purity and Pollution: Gender, Embodiment and Victorian Medicine*. Palgrave Macmillan, 1998.

Begiato, Joanne. *Manliness in Britain, 1760–1900: Bodies, Emotion, and Material Culture*. Manchester University Press, 2020.

Berger, Peter L. *Redeeming Laughter: The Comic Dimension of Human Experience*. 2nd edition. De Gruyter, 2014.

Brock, Claire. *British Women Surgeons and Their Patients, 1860–1918*. Cambridge University Press, 2017.

Bronfen, Elisabeth. *Over Her Dead Body: Death, Femininity and the Aesthetic*. Manchester University Press, 1992.

Brown, Michael. *Performing Medicine: Medical Culture and Identity in Provincial England, c.1760–1850*. Manchester University Press, 2011.

Bull, Sarah. 'Managing the "Obscene M.D.": Medical publishing, the medical profession, and the changing definition of obscenity in mid-Victorian England'. *Bulletin of the History of Medicine* 91 (2017), 713–43.

Conley, Carolyn A. *The Unwritten Law: Criminal Justice in Victorian Kent*. Oxford University Press, 1991.

Dandona, Jessica. '"The Lady Anatomist": Fragmented Bodies, Photographic Assemblage and the "Art" of Dissection at Woman's Medical College of Pennsylvania, 1895–98'. In John Nott and Anna Harris (eds), *Making Sense of Medicine: Material Culture and the Reproduction of Medical Knowledge*, pp. 106–24. Intellect, 2022.

Dickson, Melissa. 'Hats, Cloaks, and Stethoscopes: The Symbolic Fashions of the Nineteenth-Century Medical Practitioner'. In Janine Hatter and Nickianne Moody (eds), *Fashion and Material Culture in Victorian Fiction and Periodicals*, pp. 103–18. Edward Everett Root, 2019.

Digby, Anne. *Making a Medical Living: Doctors and Patients in the English Market for Medicine, 1720–1911*. Cambridge University Press, 1994.

Dixon, Laurinda S. *Perilous Chastity: Women and Illness in Pre-Enlightenment Art and Medicine*. Cornell University Press, 1995.

Douglas, Mary. *Implicit Meanings: Selected Essays in Anthropology*. 2nd edition. Routledge, 1999.

Foucault, Michel. *The Birth of the Clinic: An Archaeology of Medical Perception*. Translated by A.M. Sheridan. Routledge, 2003.

Gasperini, Anna. *Nineteenth Century Popular Fiction, Medicine and Anatomy: The Victorian Penny Blood and the 1832 Anatomy Act*. Springer, 2019.

Gatrell, Vic. *City of Laughter: Sex and Satire in Eighteenth-Century London*. Atlantic Books, 2006.

Gregory, George. *Medical Morals, Illustrated with Plates and Extracts from Medical Works; Designed to Show the Pernicious Social and Moral Influence of the Present System of Medical Practice, and the Importance of Establishing Female Medical Colleges, and Educating and Employing Female Physicians for Their Own Sex*. The Author, 1852.

Haller, John S. *Medical Protestants: The Eclectics in American Medicine, 1825–1939*. Southern Illinois University Press, 1994.

Haslam, Fiona. *From Hogarth to Rowlandson: Medicine in Art in Eighteenth Century Britain*. Liverpool University Press, 1996.

Holloway, Sally. *The Game of Love in Georgian England: Courtship, Emotions, and Material Culture*. Oxford University Press, 2019.

Holmstrom, Neil Graham. 'Beautiful, Dead, Dissected: The Dismembered Female Body in Artistic Representation'. PhD thesis, University of Tasmania, 2017.

Hunter, Mary. *The Face of Medicine: Visualising Medical Masculinities in Late Nineteenth-Century Paris*. Manchester University Press, 2016.

Hunter, Mary. 'The waiting time of prostitution: Gynaecology and temporality in Henri de Toulouse-Lautrec's *Rue Des Moulins*, 1894'. *Art History* 42:1 (2019), 68–93.

Lansbury, Coral. 'Gynaecology, pornography, and the antivivisection movement'. *Victorian Studies* 28:3 (1985), 413–37.

Loudon, Irvine. *Medical Care and the General Practitioner 1750–1850*. Clarendon Press, 1986.

Luddy, Maria. 'Prostitution from 1800'. In Sarah Toulalan and Kate Fisher (eds), *The Routledge History of Sex and the Body: 1500 to the Present*, pp. 409–26. Routledge, 2013.

Maidment, Brian. *Comedy, Caricature and the Social Order, 1820–50*. Manchester University Press, 2013.

Maidment, Brian. 'The gallery of comicalities: Graphic humour, wood-engraving, and the development of the comic magazine, 1820–1841'. *Victorian Periodicals Review* 50:1 (2017), 214–27.

Mainardi, Patricia. *Another World: Nineteenth-Century Illustrated Print Culture*. Yale University Press, 2017.

Marcus, Steven. *The Other Victorians: A Study of Sexuality and Pornography in Mid-Nineteenth Century England*. Weidenfeld & Nicolson, 1966.

Martin, Robert Bernard. *The Triumph of Wit: A Study of Victorian Comic Theory*. Clarendon Press, 1974.

McLaren, Angus. '"Not a Stranger, a Doctor": Medical Men and Sexual Matters in the Late Nineteenth Century'. In Roy Porter and Mikuláš Teich (eds), *Sexual Knowledge, Sexual Science: The History of Attitudes to Sexuality*, pp. 267–83. Cambridge University Press, 1994.

Morant, George. *Hints to Husbands: A Revelation of the Man-Midwife's Mysteries*. 3rd edition. Simpkin, Marshall & Co., 1857.

Morreall, John. *Comic Relief: A Comprehensive Philosophy of Humor*. Wiley-Blackwell, 2009.

Morrison, Kevin A. 'Dr Locock and His Quack: Professionalizing Medicine, Textualizing Identity in the 1840s'. In Louise Penner and Tabitha Sparks (eds), *Victorian Medicine and Popular Culture*. University of Pittsburgh Press, 2016.

Moscucci, Ornella. 'Clitoridectomy, Circumcision, and the Politics of Sexual Pleasure in Mid-Victorian Britain'. In Andrew H. Miller and James Eli Adams (eds), *Sexualities in Victorian Britain*, pp. 60–78. Indiana University Press, 1996.

Moscucci, Ornella. *The Science of Woman: Gynaecology and Gender in England, 1800–1929*. Cambridge University Press, 1990.

Nead, Lynda. *Myths of Sexuality: Representations of Women in Victorian Britain*. Basil Blackwell, 1988.

Nead, Lynda. *Victorian Babylon: People, Streets, and Images in Nineteenth-Century London*. Yale University Press, 2000.

Palmeri, Frank. 'Cruikshank, Thackeray, and the Victorian eclipse of satire'. *Studies in English Literature, 1500–1900* 44:4 (2004), 753–77.

Peitzman, Steven J. *New and Untried Course: Woman's Medical College and Medical College of Pennsylvania, 1850–1998*. Rutgers University Press, 2000.

Phegley, Jennifer. *Courtship and Marriage in Victorian England*. Praeger, 2012.

Porter, Roy. 'The Rise of Physical Examination'. In W.F. Bynum and Roy Porter (eds), *Medicine and the Five Senses*, pp. 179–97. Cambridge University Press, 1993.

Price, Cheryl Blake. 'Medical Bluebeards: The Domestic Threat of the Poisoning Doctor in the Popular Fiction of Ellen Wood'. In Louise Penner and Tabitha Sparks (eds), *Victorian Medicine and Popular Culture*, pp. 81–93. University of Pittsburgh Press, 2016.

Pusapati, Teja Varma. 'Claiming Medicine as a Profession for Women: The English Woman's Journal's Campaign for Female Doctors'. In Beth Rodgers, Alexis Easley and Clare Gill (eds), *Women, Periodicals and Print Culture in Britain, 1830s–1900s: The Victorian Period*, pp. 120–39. Edinburgh University Press, 2022.

Ruiz-Gómez, Natasha. 'The Model Patient: Observation and Illustration at the Musée Charcot'. In Andrew Graciano (ed.), *Visualizing the Body in Art, Anatomy, and Medicine since 1800: Models and Modeling*, pp. 203–32. Routledge, 2019.

Sappol, Michael. *A Traffic of Dead Bodies: Anatomy and Embodied Social Identity in Nineteenth-Century America*. Princeton University Press, 2002.

Sigel, Lisa Z. *Governing Pleasures: Pornography and Social Change in England, 1815–1914*. Rutgers University Press, 2002.
Smith, Andrew. *Victorian Demons: Medicine, Masculinity and the Gothic at the Fin de Siècle*. Manchester University Press, 2004.
Solomon-Godeau, Abigail. 'The legs of the countess'. *October* 39 (Winter 1986), 65–108.
Sparks, Tabitha. *The Doctor in the Victorian Novel: Family Practices*. Ashgate, 2009.
Stephens, Elizabeth. 'Touching Bodies: Tact/Ility in Nineteenth-Century Medical Photographs and Models'. In Kate Fisher and Sarah Toulalan (eds), *Bodies, Sex and Desire from the Renaissance to the Present*, pp. 87–101. Palgrave Macmillan, 2011.
Teukolsky, Rachel. *Picture World: Image, Aesthetics, and Victorian New Media*. Oxford University Press, 2020.
Tomkins, Alannah. *Medical Misadventure in an Age of Professionalisation, 1780–1890*. Manchester University Press, 2017.
Tosh, John. *A Man's Place: Masculinity and the Middle-Class Home in Victorian England*. Yale University Press, 2007.
Walkowitz, Judith R. *Prostitution and Victorian Society: Women, Class and the State*. Cambridge University Press, 1980.
Weeks, Jeffrey. *Sex, Politics and Society: The Regulations of Sexuality Since 1800*. Routledge, 2014.
Wells, Susan. *Out of the Dead House: Nineteenth-Century Women Physicians and the Writing of Medicine*. The University of Wisconsin Press, 2001.
Wiener, Martin J. *Men of Blood: Violence, Manliness and Criminal Justice in Victorian England*. Cambridge University Press, 2004.
Yeniyurt, Kathryn. 'When it hurts to look: Interpreting the interior of the Victorian woman'. *Social History of Medicine* 27:1 (2014), 22–40.

3

'The top set's artificial, but the bottom's my own!': Comic representations of false teeth and denture users in mid-twentieth-century British seaside postcards

Georgia Haire

Behind closed doors in a 1950s dental office, a large woman with sizeable breasts and an exaggerated behind speaks with her dentist. Gesturing to her teeth, she exclaims: 'The top set's artificial, but the bottom's my own!'[1] With a raised eyebrow, the blushing dentist eyes her teeth, or perhaps his stare drifts further down her figure. The viewer's gaze, as the dentist's might be, is drawn to the woman's chest, and then further down, to her bottom, which interrupts the border of the image. In this seaside postcard (Figure 3.1), illustrated by the graphic artist Donald McGill (1875–1962), the comedic potential of dentures and dentistry, and the situations they facilitate, are realised. The postcard's innuendo pokes fun at the use of false teeth, the experiences of denture users and the lewd double meanings that can lend dental terminology comedic effect. Moreover, the invisibility of the dental prostheses is contrasted with other hyper visible parts of the body, such as the woman's rear. The humorous imagery evoked in this postcard, and others like it, can reveal the bodily norms constructed around the visibility – or invisibility – of dentures in mid-twentieth-century Britain, and the anxieties associated with their usage.

Seaside postcards were cheap, mass-produced and popular souvenirs for the working and lower-middle classes holidaying in British seaside resorts in the mid-twentieth century.[2] During this period, denture usage was a common experience for British audiences. By 1968, when the first Adult Dental Health Survey was carried out in England and Wales, 37 per cent of the adult population over the age of 16 wore a full set of dentures.[3] Unlike in public health campaigns and denture-care product advertisements with which this audience was familiar, these seaside postcards saw dentures comically portrayed, intended to incite laughter. Using seaside postcards, this chapter explores comic representations of dentures and denture users in mid-twentieth-century Britain, demonstrating the emotional, class-entrenched meanings derived from such prostheses.

In visual comedy, dentures were discernible, even if they were to be laughed at – or rather, it was exactly because of the subversion of the usual social taboos surrounding the detectability of false teeth that such opportunities for laughter arose. Dentures could be anxiety-inducing for their users, who might have experienced difficulties adapting to their use, such as when speaking or eating, and keeping them in, hidden and in place. As a prosthesis, dentures are designed to remain concealed within the mouth, undetectable to others. In comedic seaside postcards, stress-inducing scenarios involving loose or visible false teeth become a source of fun, laughter and light mockery.

The following analysis demonstrates how postcard artwork subverted the (in)visibility of false teeth to create humour. Going beyond medical and professional framings, this chapter offers a fresh perspective on the cultural and social meanings attached to false teeth. The first section examines the contextual relationship between dentures and British humour, as well as the availability of dental care in the National Health Service (NHS); the second section explores comedic seaside print culture in mid-twentieth-century Britain; and the final section analyses depictions of false teeth and denture users within comic postcards, making connections between comedy, bodily anxieties and denture stigma.

Dentures, humour and the NHS

The introduction of the NHS in 1948 offered British people access to free at the point of use comprehensive healthcare. This included dental care and the provision of dentures – albeit very briefly.[4] Just a few years later in 1951, charges were introduced that limited the accessibility of dentures and, subsequently, these charges were extended to more general dental treatment.[5] However, during that short period, huge numbers of British people were able to obtain dental prostheses; in the first year of the NHS alone, two million sets of dentures were issued.[6] While they were often hidden within the mouth, false teeth were a very commonly used and recognised prosthetic among the British population.

While its origin has been difficult to trace, the humorous stereotype of the bad British smile perhaps has some basis in the types of dental work carried out in this period (which focused on function, rather than cosmetics), as well as the limited kinds and standards of treatment readily available to the British public. When the NHS began service, orthodontics was still a developing specialism in terms of regulation, education, standardisation and professionalisation.[7] The machinations of the NHS and the Dental Estimates Board meant that orthodontic treatment was not routinely offered to patients, or required prior approval before treatment could begin, leading to discrepancies in how approval was obtained and who was eligible to receive treatment.[8] Cosmetic treatments for patients with natural teeth were not a priority for dentists during this time, and often were not even a possibility – if teeth were in a very bad state, which they frequently were, they had to be removed altogether.[9] It was not until later into the twentieth century that orthodontic treatment became more accessible on the NHS. However, decades later, the value of these cosmetic treatments was still being questioned by the state. In 1986, a Report of the Committee of Enquiry into Unnecessary Dental Treatment criticised the practice of orthodontics in the NHS, suggesting that it was of little benefit to patients, because it was often of a purely cosmetic nature.[10] For dental professionals throughout Britain in the mid-twentieth century, the maintenance of a healthy, crooked-toothed mouth, or the usage of dentures, was more medically urgent and feasible than carrying out cosmetic treatments. Therefore, dentures occupied a place of tension, as while they were a functional replacement for unhealthy teeth, they also offered aesthetic improvement for their users.

Because of the millions who benefited from the NHS's early years of free dentures, there were a significant number of denture users in Britain during the mid-twentieth century. The inclusion of dentures and denture-care within seaside postcards demonstrates the commonality of false teeth as a medical prosthesis within this period – they were not limited to the dentist's office or denture lab, but an everyday presence in the lives of British people. Although the situations shown within the postcard imagery are set up for laughs or play to innuendos, the inclusion of such a wide range of users, of different ages, sexes and social backgrounds within these postcards reflects the many and various types of individuals that received dentures during this period.

Dentures at the British seaside

Seaside postcards covered many different aspects of British life and carried a particularly prurient interest in the body, often depicting clinical scenarios within their artwork, as well as figures such as dentists, dentures and denture users. These postcards were typically humorous in nature and sometimes intentionally unsavoury, bordering on offensive, such as the bawdy example given at the beginning of this chapter. The production numbers for these postcards were significant; Donald McGill's (Figure 3.1) publisher, D. Constance Ltd, sold over four million cards in 1954 alone.[11] The average yearly output of cards from major British firms, such as the publishing and illustration company Bamforth & Co. Ltd, was around the 100 million mark in the middle of the twentieth century.[12] Despite their popularity and the breadth of the subjects they depict, there is a lack of critical discussion around medical themes within seaside postcards and in particular, dentistry and dentures.[13] While scholarship has explored print culture, cartoons and caricatures of medical professionals in the eighteenth and early nineteenth century, little attention has been paid to such depictions within the twentieth century.[14] Postcards are very different from caricature, cartoons and satirical prints in terms of circulation, style and, in some ways, purpose, but there are some commonalities between these types of media: for example their use of paper, their affordability and their wide viewership. The politically minded cartoons of the eighteenth century and beyond sought to underline, reflect and shift public opinion, while seaside postcards were more focused on the light-hearted scenarios and situations that British people faced in their everyday lives. They did not offer serious criticism of society or notable individuals, or make suggestions for

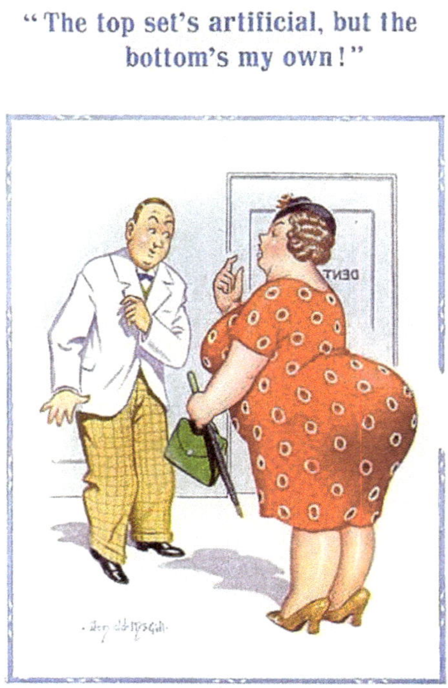

Figure 3.1 Donald McGill, 'The top set's artificial, but the bottom's my own!' *c.*1950s, postcard, Donald McGill Museum.

moral improvement. Fundamentally, however, both mediums were reflective of contemporary British life and sought to amuse their respective audiences, while also conveying prescient social issues.[15]

Like eighteenth- and nineteenth-century caricaturists, postcard artists such as McGill pushed the limits of good taste. For instance, McGill came up against the Obscene Publications Act of 1959 and moral sensibilities of contemporary authorities, such as the Home Office, who oversaw the policy on obscene publications, as well as local police forces.[16] In 1954, McGill was prosecuted under the Obscene Publications Act, having breached the rules with the publication of his more risqué designs, and was subsequently fined £50.[17] Those who transgressed the Act were scrutinised, prosecuted and punished with fines and/or the destruction and confiscation of goods – processes that saw vendors suffer too; many seaside shops were raided and their stocks confiscated.[18] In this prohibitory context, the double entendres often deployed in seaside postcards served an important purpose, as postcard producers sought to avoid censorship by the authorities.

Prints and postcards are alike in terms of the speed at which they were produced and disseminated, making them both highly reactive mediums that could quickly respond to different concerns, trends or audience interests. Like the humorous, socio-political caricatures of the eighteenth and nineteenth centuries, seaside postcards depicting dental scenarios demand close reading. For historians of medicine, these comedic depictions are useful for understanding contemporary bodily norms and how such norms were constructed and upheld within culture and society. As Andrew Stott has noted, comedy is not immune to ideology, but rather saturated in it, meaning that the body within comedic media is derived from normative culture concepts of the body and beauty.[19] Although comedy is informed by such norms, it also challenges them through parody, mockery and subversion.

Indeed, in a well-known 1941 essay on the art of McGill, for the literary journal *Horizon*, author and social critic George Orwell (1903–50) analysed conventions within the genre of seaside postcards, which he noted as specialising in 'very low humour'.[20] Although Orwell derided the content of these postcards, as well as the vulgar jokes they made, he concluded that their existence, and the 'worm's-eye view of life' they stood for, was 'symptomatically important'.[21] Orwell viewed these types of dirty jokes and comic depictions as a kind of rebellion within a society that demanded so much from its citizens: 'it has to demand faultless discipline and self-sacrifice, it must expect its subjects to work hard, pay their taxes, and be faithful to their wives, it must assume that men think it's glorious to die on the battlefield and women want to wear themselves out with child-bearing'.[22] In this way, as part of the seaside holiday, these postcards offered an outlet for thoughts and tendencies that, for many, could not be ordinarily articulated or expressed. This interpretation of comedic seaside postcards aligns with Mikhail Bakhtin's theory of the carnivalesque, ever-present in scholarship on comedy, which posits that the medieval carnival offered a temporary liberation of the social order and the suspension of the hierarchy and customs that dictated it.[23] The liminal space and laughter of the carnival temporarily liberated people from the imposed and restrictive etiquette of the 'real' world, offering opportunity for a form of cross-class and subversive communication that was otherwise impossible outside of carnival celebrations.[24] Seaside cartoons, as conceptualised by Orwell, provided a small, visual slice of this carnivalesque. Dentures also had a clear, strict and well-established etiquette around their usage and visibility within British society, meaning they had powerful comedic, carnivalesque, subversive potential within seaside postcard artwork.

As well as acknowledging these realities and offering an outlet for the inexpressible, postcards offered – and symbolised – escapism and relief from the everyday. The situations depicted were familiar to most people during this period, but transformed the banal into something lighter and more jovial than what was experienced in the 'real' world. As James Walvin has argued, the vulgarity of comic postcards reflected a more relaxed holidaying public, exuding fun, enjoyment and a certain level of permissiveness that was often sorely absent from the harsh realities of urban and industrial life.[25] The removal from everyday life that postcards embodied, both geographically and in their tone, afforded holiday-goers space for relaxation and amusement, distanced but not wholly untethered from the world of home. In relation to denture use and misuse, the fictional, outrageous, yet all-too-recognisable world of the postcard represented a more relaxed and permissive view on the visibility of these prostheses than was typically permitted in 'normal' society. Within this quasi-liberatory medium, dentures were reframed as humorous objects, rather than as simply sources of embarrassment and anxiety – although embarrassment is humorous to some, of course.

The jokes and images contained within seaside postcards were suggestive and full of light-hearted innuendos – told with a knowing wink and a nudge. This low-stakes, bawdy visual and textual language had a practical purpose in relation to sending postcards back home to friends and family. Benny Green, in his popular book on comic seaside postcards, posited that a certain euphemistic code of language was necessary 'for the successful smuggling across the frontiers of respectability of those disgraceful and disturbing messages to suburbia'.[26] Essentially, double entendre was required for the postcards to fulfil their primary function, marketability – and to avoid the censorship or fines associated with the Obscene Publications Act. In order for messages from the permissive and joyous world of the seaside to acceptably permeate the 'real' world, outright offensive or sexual language had to be disguised.

The mid-twentieth-century British seaside holiday offered a physical escape from the polite restrictions of society and created a space, if only liminal, of pleasure, hope and fun for working-class Britons.[27] The comic postcard capitalised on this escapism with risqué subject matter that was also liminal. The geographical, temporal and social marginality of the postcard made this possible: they were sold at the seaside, they were cheap, seemingly frivolous and purchased by predominantly working-class holidaymakers.[28] At home, in the 'real' world, the visibility of dentures was stigmatised, but by the seaside, these prostheses, in or out of the mouths of their users, were played and displayed for laughs.

Comedic postcards and the social stigma of dentures

Denture users experienced a variety of anxieties related to their false teeth, in terms of beauty and aesthetics, social interactions and practical everyday use. The postcards discussed here relate to these quotidian issues, showing dentures in use outside of the dental clinic. Taboo or anxiety-producing subjects were ripe for exploration in comic media, specifically because they were related to unmentionable topics and caused discomfort – both socially and, in the case of dentures, for the denture user.[29] While the denture user was set up as a comedic figure within seaside postcards, largely through their difficulties using their prostheses, dentures themselves were also presented as objects of fun; even – or especially – as disembodied objects, false teeth had the capacity to evoke humour. As an object, freed from the user's mouth, they represented something gone amiss or out of place, a body part without its corporeal context, rendered ridiculous by distance. It followed then, owing to their connections to discomfort and social taboo, that dentures and their users were frequently portrayed within seaside postcards in a comic light. This section explores the quotidian nature of dentures within this comic imagery; the prosthetic anxieties users contended with; disembodied dentures; and the class dynamics at work within the portrayals of false teeth and their users in seaside postcards.

Comic postcards featured many routine aspects of British life, such as marriage, work, leisure, sex, drunkenness and relationships. A familiar cast of caricatured characters were also seen throughout such designs: the hen-pecked husband, the bossy wife, the merry drunkard, newlyweds, bimbos, among others. Within this medium, the domestic and the dental often intersected. In these scenes, false teeth become a prop through which fictional couples expressed their grievances with one another or considered the inner workings of their relationship. In one 1960s postcard published by Bamforth & Co. Ltd and illustrated by Brian Fitzpatrick (1932–74), a woman is in bed with her husband. The woman is heavily made up, with her hair in rollers, and is wearing a revealing see-through negligee. With her arms crossed, but her breasts uncovered, she looks down at her husband next to her and complains that he never bites her ears any more like he did on their honeymoon. Her spouse has the duvet tucked right up to his chin, with only his small, balding head visible next to her imposing figure. With a wide-eyed, anxious look, he responds: 'How the hell can I – my teeth are in the bathroom!'[30] In this scenario, while the husband's dentures are in the correct place from a dental hygiene perspective, they are matter socially out of place – prohibiting him from performing affectionate husbandly duties. Another postcard shows a married couple on a trip; the husband is crouched over a suitcase with a toothbrush held aloft in his hand, exclaiming to his wife: 'Well, Ethel, I've remembered my toothbrush!' while she replies, 'Yes – but it's a pity you forgot your teeth!'[31]

Some scenes featuring married couples and dentures were repeated many times in different iterations. Another common postcard scenario depicted a married couple out for dinner. In these images, one individual within the couple refrains from eating while the other goes ahead, with a waiter standing tableside, eager to check that all was well with the meal.[32] Either the husband or wife would reassure the waiter that everything was okay, they were just waiting until their partner was finished with the false teeth so they could begin their own meal. The implication being, here, that the married couple shared a set of dentures and had to alternate their use in order to complete common actions that involved their teeth or mouth. Perhaps the need to share their prostheses was motivated by the increased scarcity of dentures after the introduction of NHS fees for false teeth in 1951. In these examples the captioned statement of the diners was written colloquially, identifying them as either Scottish or from the North. Their implied geographic background and the frugality of the couple suggests they are from a working-class background and thus can be read as another example of the class-entrenched humour at work within British seaside postcards, as well as how denture users were directly portrayed within mid-twentieth-century popular culture.

These scenarios would have been somewhat familiar to contemporary denture users, who would have had to contend with issues similar to, or exactly like, those depicted in these postcards: dentures hindering intimacy, the loss or forgetting of dentures or the expense of dentures. Many of them would also have had anxieties about denture slippage or about revealing and losing control of their prosthesis. In these examples, not only are these concerns made light of, but they are amplified to the point of ridiculousness, for comic effect. Writing about portrayals of prostheses used in nineteenth-century literature, Ryan Sweet has discussed how the slippage or exposure of prostheses impacts on the autonomy of the user.[33] Sweet states that such incidents underscored physical difference, despite the fact that the use of prostheses was meant to help users meet certain ideals of bodily normality, thus offering a critique of such standards.[34] Indeed, in the case of the mid-twentieth-century postcard, the lack of control a denture user exacted over their dentures – or their fear of lapses – is humorously portrayed. Dentures are depicted as, ironically, creating a barrier for engagement with certain 'normal' bodily behaviours – eating dinner, biting a lover's ear – but their ubiquity in this period infers a critique of social standards around their visibility, rather than one of bodily standards. Although the denture user is no doubt the subject of the joke, there is a sense of empathy or understanding in these portrayals that an observing user could relate to their own experience. As discussed, the aim of these comic postcards was not to influence or shift public opinion, but rather to reflect – and laugh at – everyday experiences to which holidaying Britons could relate.

In comic postcards, dentures often show up without their owners, or at least out of their mouths. In a postcard published by Bamforth & Co. Ltd, a red-faced woman stands over a set of dentures, which has presumably just fallen out of her own mouth, while playing a tennis match. Her equally embarrassed opponent exclaims: 'Your set!' – making a pun out of a set within a tennis match and a set of false teeth.[35] Whereas dentures as objects were portrayed as humorous objects with this medium, conversely, their absence is also framed as funny. Dentures that had gone missing, been misplaced, or had ended up out of the mouths of their users, were a frequent occurrence in postcards. In these postcards, their very absence from the mouth of the user is the basis for the whole joke. Sometimes they are not even visible within the image, but merely referred to within the caption. The matter out of place – the disembodied denture – does not have to be seen to evoke laughter.

Another comic theme including dentures revolves around their misuse – not as teeth, but as a tool. Out of their place within the mouth, these disembodied dentures are depicted in places and situations where the postcard consumer would not usually expect to see them, incongruous to their surroundings.[36] One postcard scenario, depicted in a few different ways, involved dentures being used as a decorative baking tool – particularly effective for the scalloped effect around a pie crust. These scenes involved another person expressing shock or surprise at the decorative uses for dentures in baking. Another Bamforth postcard published in the late 1960s depicts three workers in a bakery. In the foreground, a red-faced man adjusts some doughnuts on a baking tray. In front of him sit three golden, freshly baked pies. In the background, two uniformed women walk by the kitchen door, carrying a tray of baked goods. Both look shocked as they survey the scene. The caption reveals their conversation, as one woman says: 'I've heard he uses his false teeth to scallop the edges of his pies.'[37] In response, the other woman reveals a lewd rumour to the other, with a hand cupped to her ear states: 'You should see what he uses to put the holes in doughnuts.'[38] The incongruous associations between the baked goods, the baker's teeth and his genitals, prompt further opportunities for comedy within the imagery – and possible disgust.

Such portrayals had a class dynamic, in terms of how denture users were coded and perceived, particularly in terms of what such prostheses might say about the health of the working classes. Across twentieth-century popular culture, working-class people were frequently associated with excess. Portrayed within the media as excessive in their eating, smoking, drinking and spending habits, they were presented as unable to control either themselves or their impulses, behaviour which often led to obesity and disease.[39] Such excess was also framed as threatening or dangerous by the media, medical sources, the state and the upper classes. Beverley Skeggs has outlined the long tradition of associating dirt and pollution with the working classes, noting how such qualities were positioned as a threat that could readily 'spill over and contaminate the order of the nation'.[40] Such excesses were not only considered a threat to the working-class individual and family, but to all of society. In terms of twentieth-century public health, these connections are evident, particularly in terms of the type of audiences targeted for paternalistic public health messaging, as well as those who were deemed in most need of monitoring and educating and who were portrayed as most threatening. In this period, it was the working-class population of Britain that was portrayed by the state and upper-class commentators as endangering the overall health of the nation – including in terms of their poor dental health, which was also symptomatic of, and the root cause of, poor bodily health overall.[41]

Dentures as objects, rather than their wearer, similarly caused anxieties about contamination. Dentures themselves were evocative of unhygienic qualities through their connections to types of 'matter out of place' which Mary Douglas describes as 'marginal stuff'.[42] As an object that traverses the boundary of the body, like spittle, dentures represent something dirty, visceral and unnaturally out of place. Furthermore, as Elizabeth Grosz has demonstrated, saliva, and by extension, dentures and the mouth, reveal the perilous divisions between the body's inside and outside.[43] Dentures therefore expose a vulnerability in the body, through their ability to penetrate and inhabit the inside–outside status of the mouth. Moreover, dentures themselves represent a severed part of the body and are uncanny in this resemblance to the teeth and gums. William Ian Miller has highlighted how severance, no matter what is separated from the body, is unnerving because it disturbs the integrity of the body.[44] In this way, the uncannily separated body part (or approximation of that body part) is closely related to horror, fear and repulsion: uncanniness can unsettle us, producing disgust.

In the mouths of the working classes, then, dentures had a doubly repellent meaning: they were both the consequence of poor dental health, and a signifier of the supposedly uncontained nature of the working class body – threatening to spill beyond their proper, bounded site. Comic rendering of denture users were therefore symbolically loaded, capturing class-coded national anxieties about British health. In seaside postcards, denture users and their prosthetic issues were laughed at, or were the subject of the joke, and it appears as if a form of 'punching down' humour is utilised within them. However, these forms of media were largely aimed at, and consumed by, working-class audiences. In keeping with the carnivalesque nature of the seaside, I argue that working-class denture users were aware of societal perceptions about their mouths and prostheses use and chose to be in on the joke through the consumption of these ephemeral products.

The visible denture was stigmatised within everyday social situations that users encountered – they were a prosthesis that belonged, and preferably remained, in the mouth. When untethered, they were representative of the perceived excesses of the working class, an individual's attempts to maintain bodily normality and the threatening tendency of the body's interior to overspill. Their visibility transgressed social mores, creating feelings of disgust, shame or embarrassment for both the denture user and observer. However, mid-twentieth-century comic seaside postcards subverted these dental taboos. In this medium, the ubiquitous but usually invisible denture became a source of comedy, rather than anxiety. In doing so, the perceived concerns about the health of the working classes, bodily standards and difficulties with dental prosthetics invited laughter from postcard audiences.

Conclusion

Within the closing decades of the twentieth century, dentures had become a less ubiquitous object, both in comedy and among the British public: dental health had improved, and false teeth were not as frequently required by or prescribed to patients.[45] As they became less commonly worn, their visibility waned within the contemporary comedic offering. Simultaneously, there were shifts and changes within comic culture. Certain types of humour and styles of joke were no longer popular among the British population. Whereas once the anarchic, politically incorrect humour of the bawdy seaside postcard served a purpose within the repressive world of mid-twentieth-century Britain, its nudging jokes and unsavoury depictions of gender relations were set against the political landscape of the later century. Speaking to *The Independent* in 1996, Roy Clarke, the writer of the British sitcom *Last of the Summer Wine*, blames this decline on political correctness:

> False teeth, wooden legs and surgical trusses used to be a standard area for comics ... everything was fair game. People don't make jokes about such things nowadays because of body-consciousness. Before the 1960s, certainly here in the North, there was no consciousness of style. The attitude, in fact, was anti-style. People who dressed stylishly or took too much care of their bodies were regarded with suspicion. If you were 50 you were expected to look 50. There was nothing wrong with getting a bit old and fat and having a laugh about it. This terrible self-consciousness didn't appear until the 1960s.[46]

Clarke's statement highlights changes in comedy as well as broader societal changes in how the body was regarded and presented in the latter half of the twentieth century. As Nathalie Olah has argued, the physical body carries the burden of respectability and with it, the categories of 'tasteful' and 'distasteful' bodies that emerged within the consumerist, capitalist world of modern Britain in the latter half of the twentieth century.[47] In other words, in a world in which so much value was attributed to one's body and one's image, there was little to laugh at without crossing one or many lines. Alongside these changes, some of the spaces and places – like the seaside resort – previously associated with the working classes have diminished in popularity, and with them these types of comedic postcards waned in the latter part of the twentieth century. The world of the British seaside began to be abandoned in favour of holidays to Spain and the rest of Europe, with the rise of cheaper air travel and package holidays, and with this, a new, international postcard and souvenir culture developed.[48]

The inclusion of denture users and false teeth within seaside postcards demonstrates how culturally visible these prostheses were during this period, even if they were supposed to be theoretically invisible in the mouths of their users. This chapter has touched on how dentures could be anxiety-making for users, for example by having their teeth slip out and made visible to others. Although, in some cases, denture users were the butt of the joke in mid-twentieth-century comic material, such media was nevertheless an outlet for such anxieties, and a subversion of the stresses that false teeth could cause for the user. When faced with the many challenges of dental prostheses, one could only laugh, and such laughter allowed users to process and cope with prosthetic difficulties. More specifically, it was this anxiety surrounding the use and wearing of dentures that enabled their potent adoption within comedy. A study of seaside postcards also indicates the ways in which bodily norms surrounding the mouth, teeth and dentures were constructed within British culture.

Later into the twentieth century, dentures became artistically unseen once again, largely because of the decrease in their usage and their associations with old-fashioned forms of dentistry, as well as with older people.[49] Moreover, denture technology became more discreet with the development of new materials and other methods for tooth replacement, such as dental implants and veneers. These new medical developments have spurred a whole comic context of their own, with further opportunities for comedy and anxiety.[50] Dentures no longer represented a common medical experience and thus were no longer a recognisable object or a familiar prosthesis for many in late-twentieth-century Britain and beyond. This is not to say that dentures were no longer considered a comedic object, but the type of humour surrounding them shifted, as did the type of experience symbolised within such jokes. Over the course of the twentieth century, the comedic potential of dentures changed, but nevertheless endured.

Notes

1 Donald McGill, 'The top set's artificial, but the bottom's my own!', *c.*1950s, postcard, Donald McGill Museum.
2 Svetlin Stratiev, 'The Margin of the Printable: Seaside Postcards and Censorship', in Lara Feigel and Alexandra Harris (eds), *Modernism on Sea: Art and Culture at the British Seaside* (Peter Lang Ltd, 2009), p. 194. In mid-twentieth-century Britain, a souvenir seaside postcard would cost around three or four pence each; see Alan Wykes, *Saucy Seaside Postcards* (Bloomsbury Books, 1988), p. 108.
3 P.G. Gray, J.E. Todd, G.L. Slack and J.S. Bulman, *Adult Dental Health in England and Wales in 1968* (Her Majesty's Stationery Office, 1970), p. 120.
4 Charles Webster, *The National Health Service: A Political History* (Oxford University Press, 2002), p. 1.
5 John Eversley, 'The history of NHS charges', *Contemporary British History* 15 (2001), 56.
6 Richard Barnett, *The Smile Stealers: The Fine and Foul Art of Dentistry* (Thames & Hudson, 2017), p. 232.
7 This was not the case in other areas of the world; in the United States, orthodontics was a much more advanced specialism that had been established and organised as such much earlier. This may further account for the stereotype of bad British teeth, when compared to the American stereotype of the straight-toothed Hollywood smile. For more on the development of orthodontics in Britain, and the differences between North American and British orthodontics, see Geoffrey Stuart Taylor and Malcolm Nicolson, 'The emergence of orthodontics as a specialty in Britain: The role of the British Society for the Study of Orthodontics', *Medical History* 51 (2007), 379–98.
8 B.C. Leighton and J.P. Moss, 'Orthodontics in the National Health Service', *British Dental Journal* 24 (1998), 24–6.
9 J.D. Hooper, 'The pattern of orthodontics in the National Health Service', *Orthodontist* 1 (1969), 2–8.
10 Unknown author, *A History of the British Orthodontic Societies (1907–1940)* (British Orthodontic Society, 2002), pp. 103–4.
11 Stratiev, 'The Margin of the Printable', p. 193.

12 Marcus Hearn, *The Bamforth Collection: Saucy Postcards* (Constable & Robinson Ltd, 2013), p. 16.
13 On how humour can deepen our understandings of the contemporary history of healthcare, see: Julian M. Simpson and Stephanie J. Snow, 'Why we should try to get the joke: Humor, laughter, and the history of healthcare', *The Oral History Review* 44 (2017), 77–93.
14 See Diana Donald, *The Age of Caricature: Satirical Prints in the Reign of George III* (Yale University Press, 1996); Vic Gatrell, *City of Laughter: Sex and Satire in Eighteenth-Century London* (Atlantic Books, 2006); Fiona Haslam, *From Hogarth to Rowlandson: Medicine in Art in Eighteenth-century Britain* (Liverpool University Press, 1996); Temi Odumosu, *Africans in English Caricature 1769–1819: Black Jokes White Humour* (Harvey Miller, 2018); T.G.H. Drake, 'The Medical Caricatures of Thomas Rowlandson', *Bulletin for the History of Medicine* 12 (1942), 323–35; and John Trevers and Martin Orskey, *Open Wide!: A Series of Eighteenth & Nineteenth Century Caricatures on Dentistry* (Wynchwood Books, 2009).
15 Linus Abraham, 'Effectiveness of cartoons as a uniquely visual medium for orienting social issues', *Journalism & Communication Monographs* 11 (2009), p. 128.
16 Christopher Hilliard, *A Matter of Obscenity: The Politics of Censorship in Modern England* (Princeton University Press, 2021), p. 64.
17 Rebecca Jones, 'Postcard Censorship', *BBC*, 25 October 2005, https://www.bbc.co.uk/radio4/today/reports/arts/postcard_censorship_20040714.shtml; For examples of banned seaside art, see 'Banned Saucy Seaside Postcards by Donald McGill Go on Show', *The Telegraph*, 5 August 2010, https://www.telegraph.co.uk/news/picturegalleries/uknews/7928713/Banned-saucy-seaside-postcards-by-Donald-McGill-go-on-show.html.
18 'Saucy Seaside Postcards and Censorship', The Postal Museum, https://www.postalmuseum.org/blog/saucy-seaside-postcards-and-censorship/; Hilliard, *A Matter of Obscenity*, pp. 64–6.
19 Andrew Stott, *Comedy* (Routledge, 2005), p. 102.
20 George Orwell, *The Art of Donald McGill* (Greaves & Thomas, 2009), p. 1.
21 Orwell, *The Art of Donald McGill*, p. 12.
22 Orwell, *The Art of Donald McGill*, p. 11.
23 Mikhail Bakhtin, *Rabelais and His World* (Indiana University Press, 1984), p. 10.
24 Bakhtin, *Rabelais and His World*, p. 10.

25 James Walvin, *Beside the Seaside: A Social History of the Popular Seaside Holiday* (Allen Lane, 1978), p. 119.
26 Benny Green, *I've Lost my Little Willie!: A Celebration of Comic Postcards* (Elm Tree Books Ltd, 1976), p. 23.
27 Darren Webb, 'Bakhtin at the Seaside: Utopia, Modernity and the Carnivalesque', *Theory, Culture & Society* 22 (2005), 132.
28 Stratiev, 'The Margin of the Printable', p. 194.
29 Dave Huxley, 'VIZ: Gender, class and taboo', in Stephen Wagg (ed.), *Because I Tell a Joke or Two: Comedy, Politics and Social Difference* (Routledge, 1998), p. 280.
30 Author's Personal Collection, 'Why don't you bite my ears', Brian Fitzpatrick, no date. Viewable at University College Cork, Archival Collections. Humour Collection: Bamfoth and Co. Ltd. Postcards Collection Listing. IE BL/VC/H/B/5 27 No date. Couple in bed. 1 item.
31 Author's Personal Collection, 'I've remembered my toothbrush!', Donald McGill, no date, postcard.
32 Author's Personal Collection, 'The steak's a'richt laddie', Donald McGill, no date, postcard; Author's Personal Collection, 'Doesn't madam like her food?', Brian Fitzpatrick, no date, postcard.
33 Ryan Sweet, *Prosthetic Body Parts in Nineteenth-Century Literature and Culture* (Palgrave Macmillan, 2022), p. 85.
34 Sweet, *Prosthetic Body Parts*, p. 85.
35 Author's Personal Collection, 'All sorts of things come out on the courts!', artist unknown, no date, postcard.
36 For further discussion of incongruity theory and humour, see Stott, *Comedy*, pp. 131–8.
37 Author's Personal Collection, 'I've heard he uses false teeth', Brian Fitzpatrick, no date, postcard.
38 Author's Personal Collection, 'I've heard he uses false teeth', Brian Fitzpatrick, no date, postcard.
39 Owen Jones, *Chavs: The Demonization of the Working Class* (Verso Books, 2011), p. 126; Imogen Taylor, '"CHAV MUM CHAV SCUM": Class disgust in contemporary Britain', *Feminist Media Studies* 8 (2008), 27–34, 19.
40 Beverley Skeggs, *Class, Self, Culture* (Routledge, 2004), p. 104.
41 Speaking at the British Dental Association's (BDA) annual general meeting in 1907, the BDA president J.C. Oliver blamed the poor state of the nation's teeth on: 'The great ignorance of the great working populations respecting the teeth, their uses, and their effect on health': British Dental Association, 'Bad Teeth and Degeneracy, Inspection of Children's Teeth', *South Wales Daily News*, 20 May 1907, p. 6.

42 Mary Douglas, *Purity and Danger: An Analysis of Concepts of Pollution and Taboo* (Routledge, 2001), pp. 50, 122.

43 Elizabeth Grosz, *Volatile Bodies: Toward a Corporeal Feminism* (Indiana University Press, 1994), p. 193.

44 William Ian Miller, *The Anatomy of Disgust* (Harvard University Press, 1997), p. 27.

45 At the time of the 1998 Adult Dental Health Survey, 87% of all adults had some natural teeth, while up to the age of 45, that figure was almost 100%, meaning fewer people needed dentures than they did a few decades earlier: J.G. Steele et al., 'Total tooth loss in the United Kingdom in 1998 and implications for the future', *British Dental Journal* 189 (2000), 598–603, 598. In the twenty-first century, the number of denture users in the UK had dropped further. The 2021 Adult Oral Health Survey reported that the proportion of adults who used dentures was highest among adults aged 75 years and over at 39 per cent, and lowest among adults aged 16–24 years at one per cent: 'Adult Oral Health Survey 2021: Self-reported Health of Teeth and Gums', *Gov.uk*, 25 January 2024, https://www.gov.uk/government/statistics/adult-oral-health-survey-2021/adult-oral-health-survey-2021-self-reported-health-of-teeth-and-gums.

46 Tim Minogue, 'Smile a Perfect Smile, but don't Laugh ... we have Officially Lost our Dentures', *The Independent*, 8 June 1996, https://www.independent.co.uk/news/uk/home-news/smile-a-perfect-smile-but-don-t-laugh-we-have-officially-lost-our-dentures-1336158.html.

47 Nathalie Olah, *Bad Taste, Or the Politics of Ugliness* (Dialogue Books, 2023), p. 79.

48 John K. Walton, *The British Seaside: Holidays and Resorts in the Twentieth Century* (Manchester University Press, 2000), p. 45.

49 By 2009, 40% of adults aged 65–74 in the UK wore some form of dentures, increasing to 70% among those aged 75 or older: Adult Dental Health Survey 2009, 'Theme 4: Complexity Maintenance' (2011), p. 16.

50 See, for example, the jokes made online in response to the veneers of former Love Island contestant, Sam Gowland: Melody Fletcher, 'Love Island's Sam Gowland furiously hits back after being mocked for "horrendous" £6k veneers as he insists they're "the best you can get"', *Daily Mail*, 10 August 2024, https://www.dailymail.co.uk/tvshowbiz/article-13733351/Love-Islands-Sam-Gowland-furiously-hits-mocked-horrendous-6k-veneers-insists-theyre-best-get.html.

References

Abraham, Linus. 'Effectiveness of cartoons as a uniquely visual medium for orienting social issues'. *Journalism & Communication Monographs* 11 (2009), 117–65.

Adult Dental Health Survey 2009. 'Theme 4: Complexity Maintenance' (2011).

Author's Personal Collection. 'All sorts of things come out on the courts!' Artist unknown. No date. Postcard.

Author's Personal Collection. 'Doesn't madam like her food?' Brian Fitzpatrick. No date. Postcard.

Author's Personal Collection. 'I've heard he uses false teeth.' Brian Fitzpatrick. No date. Postcard.

Author's Personal Collection. 'I've remembered my toothbrush!' Donald McGill. No date. Postcard.

Author's Personal Collection. 'The steak's a'richt laddie.' Donald McGill. No date. Postcard.

Author's Personal Collection. 'Why don't you bite my ears.' Brian Fitzpatrick. No date. Postcard.

Bakhtin, Mikhail. *Rabelais and His World*. Indiana University Press, 1984.

Barnett, Richard. *The Smile Stealers: The Fine and Foul Art of Dentistry*. Thames & Hudson, 2017.

Donald, Diana. *The Age of Caricature: Satirical Prints in the Reign of George III*. Yale University Press, 1996.

Douglas, Mary. *Purity and Danger: An Analysis of the Concepts of Pollution and Taboo*. Routledge, 2000.

Drake, T.G.H. 'The medical caricatures of Thomas Rowlandson'. *Bulletin for the History of Medicine* 12 (1942), 323–35.

Eversley, John. 'The history of NHS charges'. *Contemporary British History* 15 (2001), 53–75.

Fletcher, Melody. 'Love Island's Sam Gowland furiously hits back after being mocked for "horrendous" £6k veneers as he insists they're "the best you can get"'. *Daily Mail*, 10 August 2024. https://www.dailymail.co.uk/tvshowbiz/article-13733351/Love-Islands-Sam-Gowland-furiously-hits-mocked-horrendous-6k-veneers-insists-theyre-best-get.html.

Gatrell, Vic. *City of Laughter: Sex and Satire in Eighteenth-Century London*. Atlantic Books, 2006.

Gray, P.G., J.E. Todd, G.L. Slack and J.S. Bulman, *Adult Dental Health in England and Wales in 1968*. Her Majesty's Stationery Office, 1970.

Green, Benny. *I've Lost my Little Willie!: A Celebration of Comic Postcards*. Elm Tree Books Ltd, 1976.

Grosz, Elizabeth. *Volatile Bodies: Toward a Corporeal Feminism*. Indiana University Press, 1994.

Haslam, Fiona. *From Hogarth to Rowlandson: Medicine in Art in Eighteenth-century Britain*. Liverpool University Press, 1996.

Hearn, Marcus. *The Bamforth Collection: Saucy Postcards*. Constable & Robinson Ltd, 2013.

Hilliard, Christopher. *A Matter of Obscenity: The Politics of Censorship in Modern England*. Princeton University Press, 2021.

Hooper, J.D. 'The pattern of orthodontics in the National Health Service', *Orthodontist* 1 (1969), 2–8.

Huxley, Dave. 'VIZ: Gender, Class and Taboo'. In Stephen Wagg (ed.), *Because I Tell a Joke or Two: Comedy, Politics and Social Difference*, 271–88. Routledge, 1998.

Jones, Owen. *Chavs: The Demonization of the Working Class*. Verso Books, 2011.

Jones, Rebecca. 'Postcard Censorship', BBC, 25 October 2005. https://www.bbc.co.uk/radio4/today/reports/arts/postcard_censorship_20040714.shtml.

Leighton, B.C., and J.P. Moss. 'Orthodontics in the National Health Service'. *British Dental Journal* 24 (1998), 24–6.

Miller, William Ian. *The Anatomy of Disgust*. Harvard University Press, 1997.

Minogue, Tim. 'Smile a Perfect Smile, but don't Laugh ... We Have Officially Lost Our Dentures'. *The Independent*, 8 June 1996. https://www.independent.co.uk/news/uk/home-news/smile-a-perfect-smile-but-don-t-laugh-we-have-officially-lost-our-dentures-1336158.html.

No author. 'Adult Oral Health Survey 2021: Self-reported Health of Teeth and Gums'. *Gov.uk*, 25 January 2024. https://www.gov.uk/government/statistics/adult-oral-health-survey-2021/adult-oral-health-survey-2021-self-reported-health-of-teeth-and-gums.

No author, *A History of the British Orthodontic Societies (1907–1940)*. British Orthodontic Society, 2002.

No author. 'Banned Saucy Seaside Postcards by Donald McGill go on Show'. *The Telegraph*, 5 August 2010. https://www.telegraph.co.uk/news/picturegalleries/uknews/7928713/Banned-saucy-seaside-postcards-by-Donald-McGill-go-on-show.html.

No author. 'British Dental Association, Bad Teeth and Degeneracy, Inspection of Children's Teeth'. *South Wales Daily News*, 20 May 1907.

No author. 'Saucy Seaside Postcards and Censorship', *The Postal Museum*. https://www.postalmuseum.org/blog/saucy-seaside-postcards-and-censorship/.

Odumosu, Temi. *Africans in English Caricature 1769–1819: Black Jokes White Humour*. Harvey Miller, 2018.
Olah, Nathalie. *Bad Taste, Or the Politics of Ugliness*. Dialogue Books, 2023.
O'Reilly, Sally. 'Bawdy Beautiful'. In Martin Myrone (ed.), *Rude Britannia: British Comic Art*, pp. 110–13. Tate Publishing, 2010.
Orwell, George. *The Art of Donald McGill*. Greaves & Thomas, 2009.
Simpson, Julian M., and Stephanie J. Snow. 'Why we should try to get the joke: Humor, laughter, and the history of healthcare', *The Oral History Review* 44 (2017), 77–93.
Skeggs, Beverley. *Class, Self, Culture*. Routledge, 2004.
Steele, J.G., et al. 'Total tooth loss in the United Kingdom in 1998 and implications for the future', *British Dental Journal* 189 (2000), 598–603.
Stott, Andrew. *Comedy*. Routledge, 2005.
Stratiev, Svetlin. 'The Margin of the Printable: Seaside Postcards and Censorship'. In Lara Feigel and Alexandra Harris (eds), *Modernism on Sea: Art and Culture at the British Seaside*, pp. 191–200. Peter Lang, 2009.
Sweet, Ryan. *Prosthetic Body Parts in Nineteenth-Century Literature and Culture*. Palgrave Macmillan, 2022.
Taylor, Imogen. '"CHAV MUM CHAV SCUM": Class disgust in contemporary Britain', *Feminist Media Studies* 8 (2008), 27–34.
Taylor, Geoffrey Stuart, and Malcolm Nicolson. 'The emergence of orthodontics as a specialty in Britain: The role of the British Society for the Study of Orthodontics', *Medical History* 51 (2007), 379–98.
Trevers, John, and Martin Orskey. *Open Wide!: A Series of Eighteenth & Nineteenth Century Caricatures on Dentistry*. Wynchwood Books, 2009.
Walton, John K. *The British Seaside: Holidays and Resorts in the Twentieth Century*. Manchester University Press, 2000.
Walvin, James. *Beside the Seaside: A Social History of the Popular Seaside Holiday*. Allen Lane, 1978.
Webb, Darren. 'Bakhtin at the Seaside: Utopia, Modernity and the Carnivalesque'. *Theory, Culture & Society* 22 (2005), 121–38.
Webster, Charles. *The National Health Service: A Political History*. Oxford University Press, 2002.
Wykes, Alan. *Saucy Seaside Postcards*. Bloomsbury Books, 1988.

Part II

Dying laughing: Death, disfigurement, disease and disability

4

Dancing, laughing and sexing (with) death: Edvard Munch's gendered medical humour

Allison Morehead

Edvard Munch's lithograph *Dance of Death* (1915) is a self-portrait of the ageing Norwegian artist cuddling up to, and perhaps inappropriately touching, a skeleton.[1] Munch depicts himself in profile, with naked torso, muscular arm bent at the elbow and hand resting possessively on the skeleton's rib cage while the artist's nose nuzzles the side of the skeleton's face and his lips approach its jaw (Figure 4.1). The skeleton, meanwhile, appears inanimate, more of an anatomical preparation than the vitalised skeletons that typify dance of death imagery. A long rectangular frame squashes the two figures into tight relation, cutting the composition below the artist's bent elbow and at the skeleton's pelvis. In a subsequent state of the lithograph, the frame has been squared to bisect the artist's upper arm and the skeleton's mid-section (Figure 4.2). This altered composition edits out the artist's musculature and allows space for the schematic rendering of a disembodied forearm holding some kind of circular offering.[2]

Combining the closely related iconographies of the dance of death, self-portraiture with death and death and the maiden, Munch's lithograph courts a grotesque form of humour theorised by the French poet and critic Charles Baudelaire. The potential for this grotesque humour to be medical, gendered and sexualised is inferred by an earlier work by Munch, a drypoint entitled *The Women and the Skeleton* from 1896 (Figure 4.3). In this print, two naked women contemplate a skeleton mounted on a stand, an anatomical preparation evidently for use in an anatomy lesson.[3]

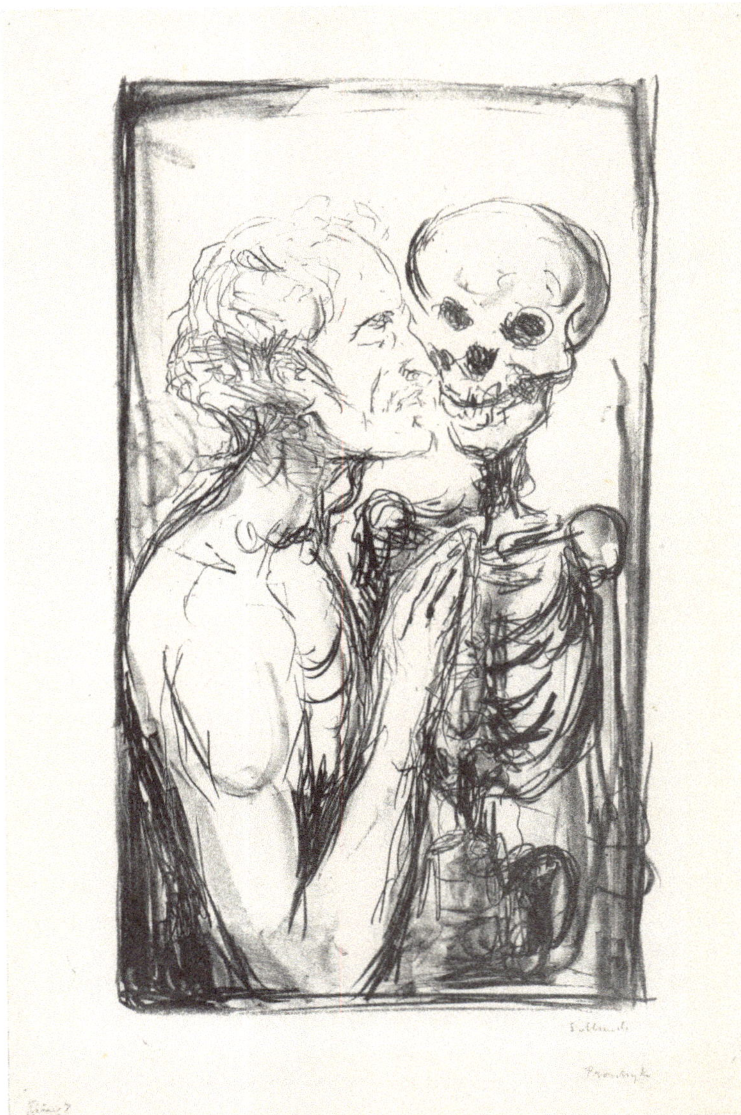

Figure 4.1 Edvard Munch, *Dance of Death*, 1915, lithographic crayon on paper, further worked on the stone, 500 × 285 mm (image), 596 × 400 mm (sheet), Woll 509, II/III.

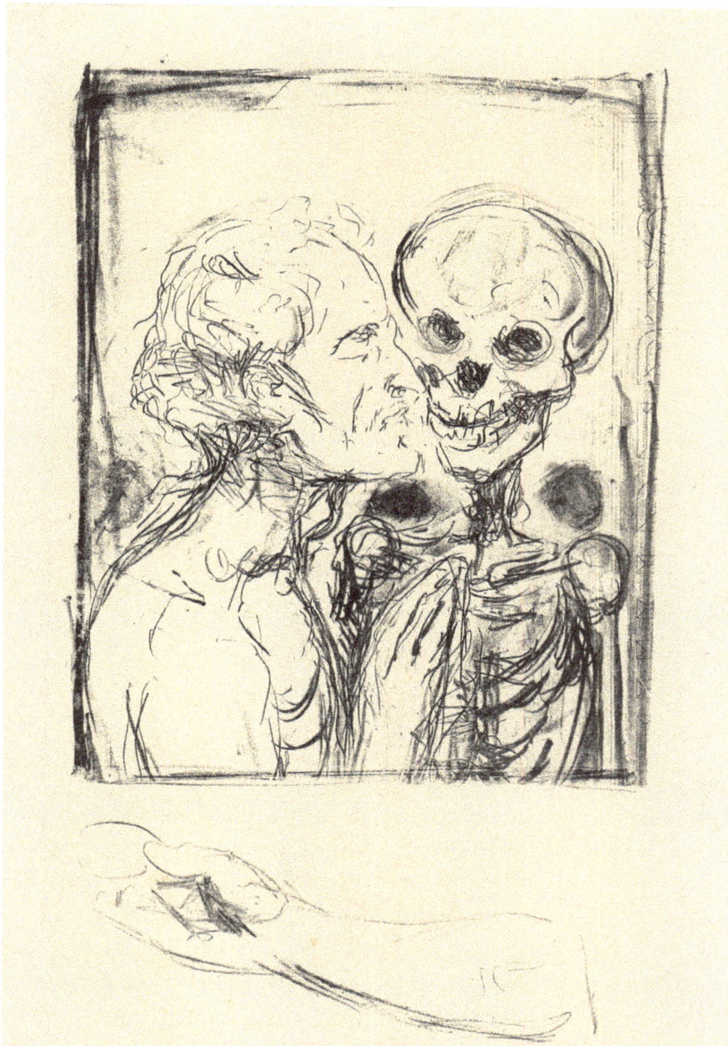

Figure 4.2 Edvard Munch, *Dance of Death*, 1915, lithographic crayon on paper, further worked on the stone, 480 × 292 mm (image), 556 × 366 mm (sheet), Woll 509, III/III.

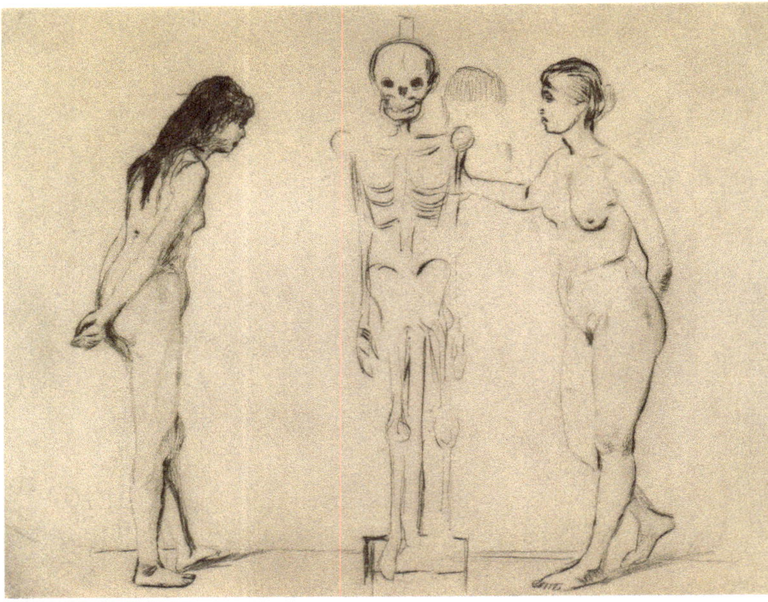

Figure 4.3 Edvard Munch, *The Women and the Skeleton*, 1896, drypoint on copper plate, 315 × 421 mm (image), 440 × 598 mm (sheet), 315 × 429 mm (plate), Woll 51, II/III.

On first glance, the print might not seem to include any element of humour, but entertaining the possibility of humour draws attention to the subtle gesture of the woman on the right, who places her hand behind or inside the ribcage of the skeleton. This grotesque, mischievous and perhaps even erotic act of penetration recalls both X-ray photographs and dissection. It lays claim to a transparency of knowledge at the heart of both medical and artistic studies of anatomy, and does so not long after women had begun studying medicine in Norway.[4] The act is rendered more curious by the faint shadow cast between the skeleton and the woman on the right, and by the incongruity of two *naked* women, perhaps artist's models, contemplating an even more 'naked', stripped-to-the-bone anatomical preparation.[5] The print might be considered an extremely distant cousin of a contemporaneous photograph of women medical students in the United States who are

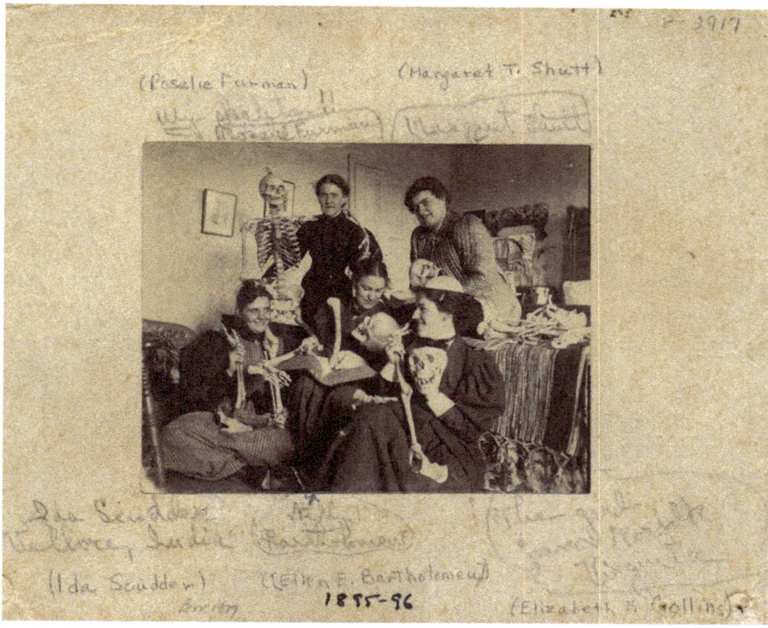

Figure 4.4 Anonymous photographer, Students at the Woman's Medical College of Pennsylvania, Philadelphia, 1895–96, black and white photograph.

shown amorously cradling and joking around with skeletons and skeleton parts (Figure 4.4).[6]

The possibility of medical humour in Munch's *oeuvre* is strengthened by the artist's status as a medical insider.[7] The son and brother of doctors who accompanied his father on house calls and on long stints in army hospitals from a young age, Munch grew up within, and was very much part of, a medical fraternity in his home country of Norway. Throughout his life, homosocial medical communities throughout Europe enabled him to gain access to vulnerable subjects for his art practice, brought him enthused medical friends and patrons and allowed him to secure the latest in medical treatments. In the larger project that houses this research, I argue that Munch's deep and lifelong embeddedness in medical contexts, his privileged status and connections within medical communities, affords his work a unique and critical perspective on the medicalisation of modern life.[8]

*

The dance of death is an exceptionally flexible and highly mobile iconography with an extensive and complex history in Europe, stretching back to the medieval period and arguably proliferating in the wake of the Black Death.[9] Originating in both visual and literary traditions, the dance of death commonly represents a procession of living individuals of different classes, walks of life and types accompanied by, dancing with or otherwise interacting with animated skeletons. The imagery signals both the inevitability of death, functioning as *memento mori*, as well as death's democratisation; everyone, from king to pauper, faces death as an equal. In tracing the dance of death's transition from public wall paintings in the late medieval period to more intimate spheres of printmaking cultivated during the Renaissance, historians have tended, as Sofie Oosterwijk and Stefanie Knöll have argued, to emphasise the dance of death's moralising function. Literary scholars, on the other hand, have long recognised its potential for humour and specifically for political satire.[10] In its grotesque and carnivalesque juxtapositions, the dance of death represents the putative equalising of death in order to highlight a *lack* of equality in life.

Munch's lithograph intertwines the iconography of the dance of death with the iconographies of self-portraiture with death, and death and the maiden, which also have their own trajectories. The former dates to early Renaissance dance of death murals, in which the artist's self-portrait intensified uncertainty over whether the death figures were separate entities or future representations of once-living selves.[11] In the late nineteenth century, the Swiss artist Arnold Böcklin gave new impetus to this iconography.[12] In his *Self-Portrait with Death Playing the Fiddle* (1872), Böcklin depicted himself in the midst of painting, palette and rag in his left hand, brush held poised to paint in his right, while just over his left shoulder a skeletal figure draws a bow across a fiddle with bony fingers. The artist looks directly out of the image, head turned slightly to his left and pulled back, as if, in scrutinising himself in a mirror, he has been startled by his own reflection and by the figure of death behind him. This disquieting painting introduces an extra note of ambiguity into the genre of self-portraiture, in which the artist often depicts themselves triumphantly, even defiantly, creating the 'great' work that the viewer now contemplates.[13] That ambiguity is heightened by the fact that, although interrupted at some point in his work by death, the artist has nevertheless survived to complete the artwork now before the viewer through which the artist achieves a certain immortality.

The iconography of death and the maiden has a slightly different genealogy that merged with and elaborated the dance of death after about 1500.[14] Emerging from *vanitas* traditions, death and the maiden is also part of a much larger class of Western cultural texts that address alterity and disorder within patriarchal structures via what Sarah Webster Goodwin and Elisabeth Bronfen call the 'multiply coded feminine body'. 'Our culture', Goodwin and Bronfen argue, 'posits death and the feminine as what is radically other to the norm, the living or surviving masculine subject; they represent the disruption and difference that ground a narcissistic sense of self and stability in a cultural system. But the system must also eliminate them or posit them as limit in order to survive.'[15] Or, as Bronfen succinctly states elsewhere, 'both femininity and death cause a disorder to stability, mark moments of ambivalence, disruption or duplicity and their eradication produces a recuperation of order, a return to stability'.[16] Representations of death and femininity, therefore, tend towards managing disorder, which is ultimately a fear of collapsing boundaries between self and other. Such fears arguably intensified in the midst of, and through, the modern processes of medicalisation that coincided with Munch's life and career.

In Munch's drypoint *Death and the Woman* (1894), a woman and an animated skeleton embrace passionately as a prelude, it seems, to impossibly reproductive intercourse implied by the phallic femur jutting out from between the woman's fleshy legs and by the spermatozoa and foetuses surrounding the dancing couple (Figure 4.5).[17] The print revels in the disruption of death and the feminine, which is implied to be managed, incompletely perhaps, only by the heroic (pro)creative act of the artist himself. *Death and*

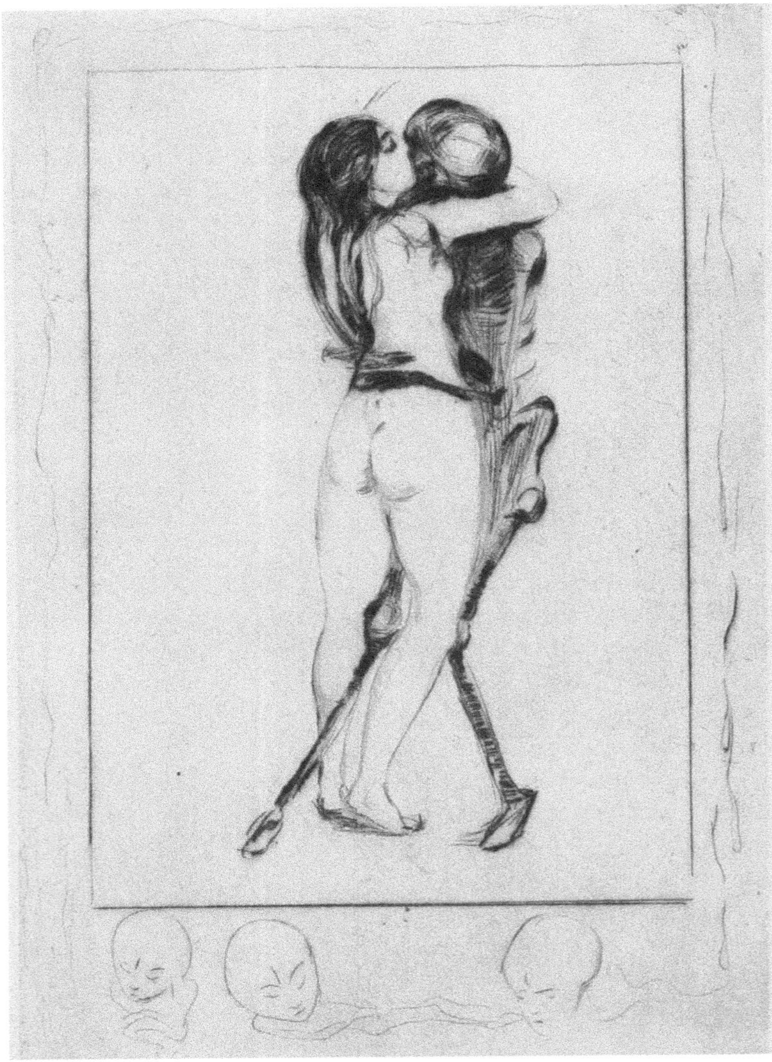

Figure 4.5 Edvard Munch, *Death and the Woman*, 1894, drypoint, 291 × 208 mm (image), 510 × 352 mm (paper), 310 × 221 mm (plate).

the Woman is among the many emotionally laden, shocking and seemingly ponderous works that contribute to the artist's reputation of having little to no interest in or capacity for humour.[18] But is there not some dark humour in that phallic femur, the idea of reproductive sex between a vital and voluptuous woman and a decidedly unfleshy skeleton?[19]

In the early twentieth century, the German-Austrian artist Ivo Saliger produced some distinctly unfunny death and the maiden imagery that throws into relief both the possibilities for a new medical context for the dance of death and the critical potential for humour in Munch's *Dance of Death* lithograph.[20] Beginning around 1920, Saliger made a number of prints, including *The Physician* (*c.* 1920), in which a doctor physically repels the skeletal figure of death, in this case to save a young naked woman. In a 1973 letter to a student at Case Western Reserve University in the United States, Saliger claimed that he began these prints to honour the Swiss physician who had worked in vain to save his young sister's life after she received a diagnosis of lymphomatoid granulomatosis in 1918.[21] Dedicating his prints to 'physicians world-wide', Saliger refused to limit the print runs, thereby ensuring the widest circulation possible. In another print work by Saliger, entitled *The Physician of the X-Rays* (*c.* 1920–40), a radiologist, eerily lit from the console of his X-ray machine and sporting round protective glasses that add to the disquieting atmosphere, manipulates the rays over the nubile body of a female patient. In doing so, he heroically repels a death figure clothed as the Grim Reaper, who is depicted cowering before the physician's modern diagnostic technology. The studied seriousness of these works, which approach kitsch, their thoroughly uncritical lionisation of the male physician's powers, translates into horror when one recognises Saliger as among the Nazi party's favoured artists, especially for his depictions of idealised white German womanhood.[22] Saliger's images were meant to heroicise the male doctor's efforts in overcoming death, effectively managing the threat to patriarchy that is both death and femininity. But they also stand as horrendous reminders of medical professionals' active roles in the Holocaust.[23]

Munch's *Dance of Death* is of a very different order from Saliger's self-serious images of physicians repelling death to save sexualised young women. Instead, Munch manipulates and transforms the three iconographies – the dance of death, the self-portrait with death and death and the maiden – to humorous, critical, sad and disturbing effect. First and perhaps most dramatically, Munch in some sense occupies the role of the maiden in amorous relation to death, but as a vulnerable ageing man who was 52 in 1915. The artist's age is emphasised in the final state of the print (Figure 4.2), in which Munch squared the frame to edit out the musculature of his arm so that his naked torso appears more sunken and pathetic, his body more atrophied and abject. At the same time, he depicts himself as usurping death's role as sexual aggressor, cosying up to the skeleton with a ribald, 'pucker-up' style of humour, ridiculed by the skeleton's perpetual grin, by its apparent lack of engagement with its suitor or assailant and by its ambiguous sex. Anxieties about the uncertain sex of skeletons is often negotiated, in both dance of death imagery and anatomical illustration, by hyperbolic signs of femininity, such as long flowing hair and remnants of rounded breasts, implying that a more conventional skeleton should be assumed male.[24] In Munch's print, there is no such sexing of the skeleton; it remains resolutely and queerly ambiguous, the viewer and perhaps the artist himself uncertain, unaware, maybe even uncaring of the sex of the bodily remains he accosts.

Self-portraiture with death involves figuring death as a future self, or more precisely future remains of the self. Böcklin depicted himself as taken aback at seeing himself accompanied by and doubled as death. Part of the sad joke in Munch's *Dance of Death* is that the figure of death is also the self, and a self that, like an anatomical preparation, does not pursue the artist-self, return his embrace or take up the invitation to dance, only remaining perpetually and enigmatically grinning. The death-self's lack of response to the artist-self's advances, the skeleton's insistence on its anatomical function rather than its role as living allegory, thus points out that no one, neither artist nor physician, can really know death. Munch's lithograph thus underscores the narcissistic and overdetermined construction of deathly remains as retaining some putatively essential connection to the self.[25]

Much of what I have described so far in Munch's *Dance of Death* hews to what Charles Baudelaire called the 'significative comic', a satirical mode that, in Baudelaire's words, 'derives from one's sense of superiority over others ... and is grasped by reason and analysis'.[26] The age, role and gender reversals that Munch introduced can be read as a knowing kind of self-satire of the ageing artist, and more broadly a satire of the knowing male subject, including artists and physicians who study anatomy, penetrating and even violating a dead body in order to become a professional artist or doctor. Both are envisioned and subtly mocked here as heroic figures with the power to overcome death. The 'significative comic' is what Christiane Hertel calls 'laughter at the object of the caricature', in the case of Munch's *Dance of Death* a knowing kind of laughter at the artist/physician himself.[27] But Baudelaire also describes a mode of humour he calls both the 'absolute comic' and the grotesque. This mode, he insists, still involves superiority, but man's superiority over nature rather than over others. The 'absolute comic', Baudelaire argues, is 'grasped synthetically by intuition and excites a spontaneous, excessive, violent laughter'.[28]

Munch was clearly familiar with Baudelaire's ideas on the 'absolute comic', although probably not directly through the Frenchman's essay 'On the Essence of Laughter' (1855). Rather, Munch gained intimate knowledge of Baudelaire's grotesque through a commission he received in 1896 to illustrate two poems from Baudelaire's *Les Fleurs du mal* (*The Flowers of Evil*, 1857), 'Une Charogne' ('A Carcass') and 'Le Mort Joyeux' ('The Joyful Corpse').[29] In the most elaborated versions of these illustrations, which were never completed, Munch produced surprisingly literal illustrations of the two poems, whose titles would otherwise indicate the potential for allegory and grotesque humour.[30] Munch's illustration for 'A Carcass' shows flowers and plants above, or emerging from, the head and chest of the rotting corpse, surrounded on two sides by a border of flies all spectacularly evoked in the poem (Figure 4.6). But Munch focuses his illustration on the poet's passionate embrace of his idealised beloved to whom the poem is addressed. In Munch's most developed composition for 'The Joyful Corpse', a skeleton leisurely lounges in a bucolic landscape, contemplating the flowering plants and basking in the light of a rising or setting sun (Figure 4.7). 'The Joyful Corpse'

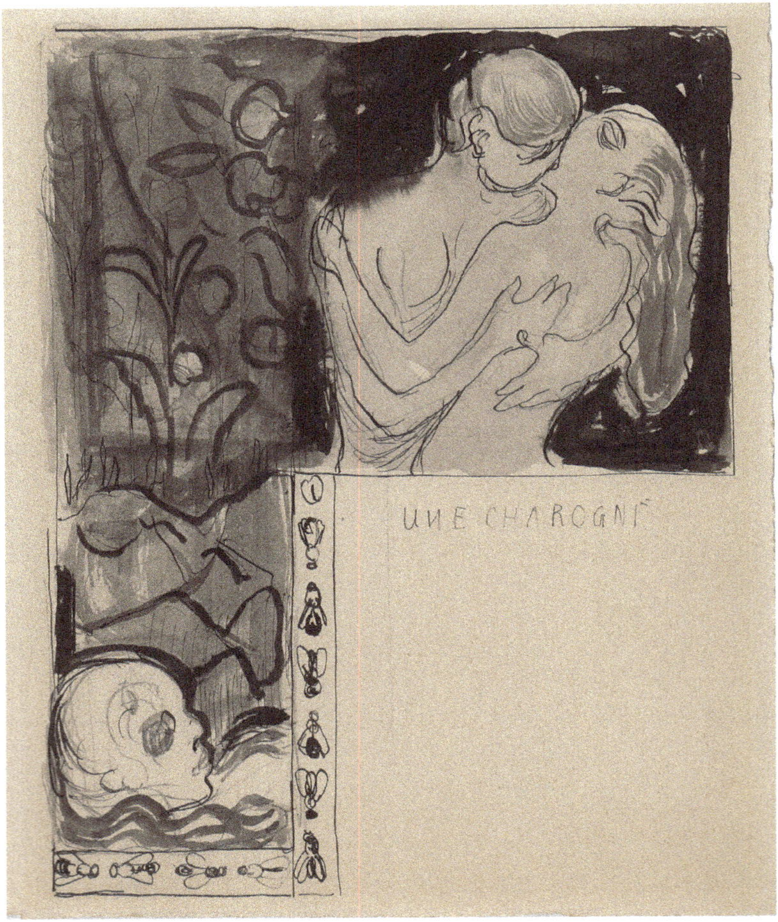

Figure 4.6 Edvard Munch, *Une Charogne. Illustration for 'Les Fleurs du Mal'*, 1896, pen, brush, wash, pencil, 260 × 226 mm.

is a short paean to the joys of death as 'oblivion', a rejection of death rituals, and an invitation to the 'ravens' and the 'worms' to 'burrow through' the poet's bodily 'ruins'.[31] In his image of a reclining skeleton in an idyllic landscape, however, Munch eschewed the poem's grotesque imagery for a more elegiac, contemplative tone.

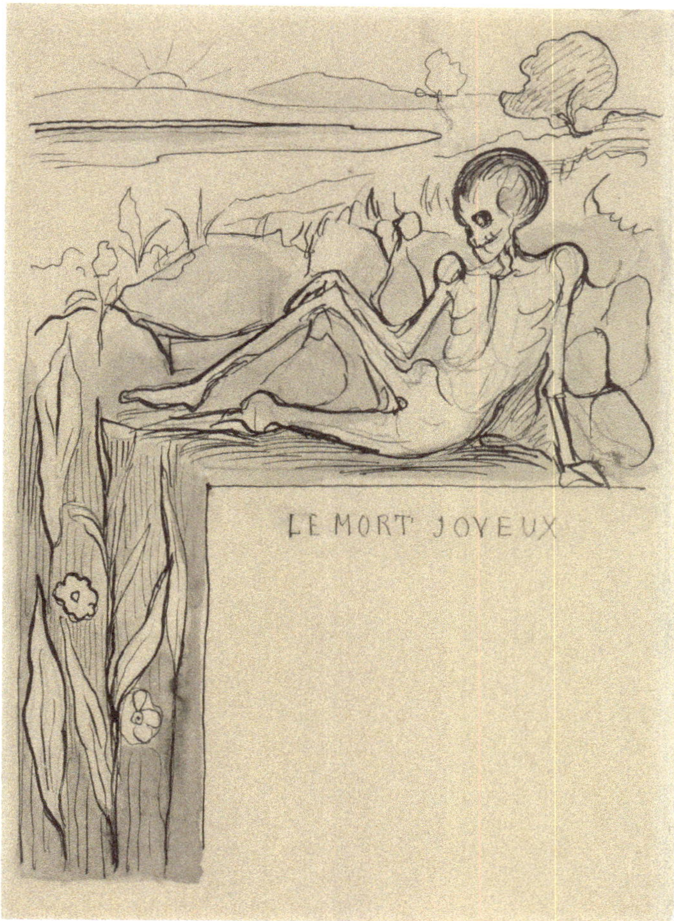

Figure 4.7 Edvard Munch, *Le Mort Joyeux. Illustration for 'Les Fleurs du Mal'*, 1896, Indian ink (pen and wash), pencil, 280 × 205 mm.

In other drawings connected to the project, however, Munch entertained the possibility of a more grotesquely humorous mode.[32] At the top of one ink drawing, very likely a study for 'A Carcass', a skeleton appears in extreme, comical foreshortening, with a puny bony arm, almost clown-like face, and enormous feet beyond which a giant fly, made plausible by the exaggerated perspective, exits the

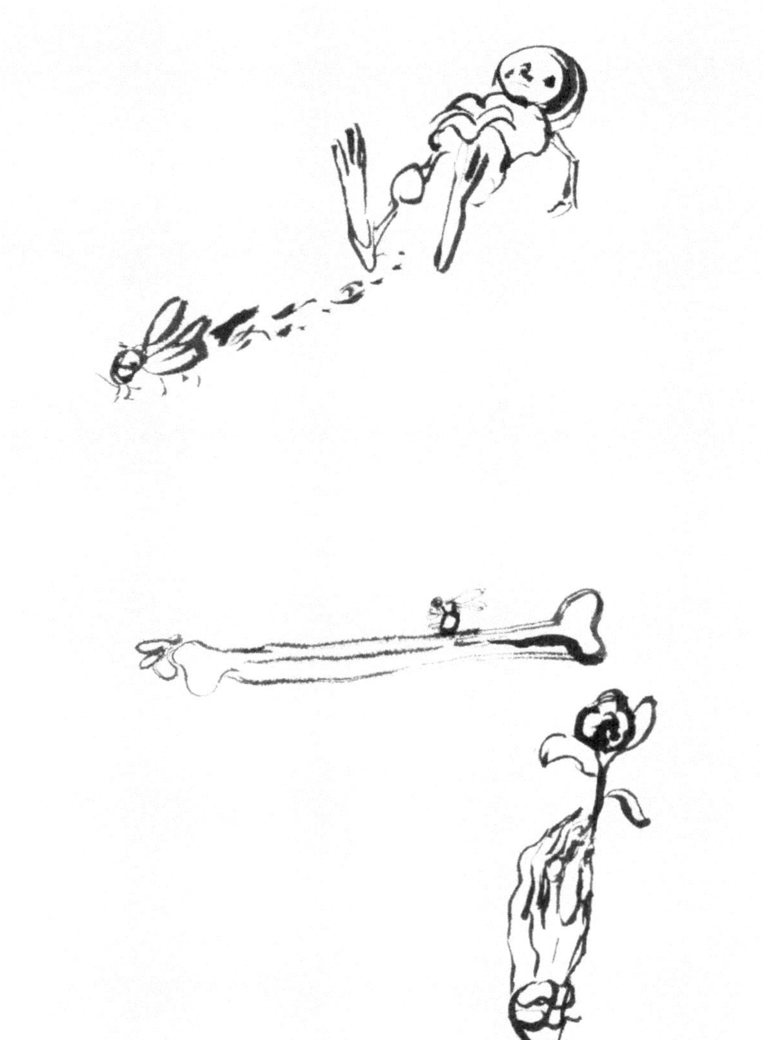

Figure 4.8 Edvard Munch, *Skeleton and Fly; Two Flies on a Bone; Hand Holding a Flower*, 1896, Indian ink (brush), 230 × 380 mm.

body from between the skeleton's legs (Figure 4.8). Below this, two flies take a break on a long bone, below which a bony hand delicately holds a single flower. The flies confined to the border in the more finalised illustration for 'A Carcass' are the main characters in this drawing, sending up the seriousness of death and highlighting the more grotesque lines of the poem, including the flies 'buzzing round that putrid belly', revelling in the corpse's putrescence and decay.[33]

A third poem by Baudelaire from *The Flowers of Evil*, the especially humorous and ironic 'Danse macabre' ('Dance of Death'), is obviously relevant to this discussion. In this lengthy poem, Baudelaire addresses death in the skeletal form of a 'noseless' woman, the slimmest at the ball who charms her potential suitors with the 'eternal smile' of her 'thirty-two teeth' and 'the curved trellis of [her] ribs', through which all can see the 'wandering' form of 'the insatiable asp'. Countering 'some lovers drunken with flesh' who 'will call you/ A caricature', the poet beseeches: 'who has not clasped a skeleton in his arms/ Who has not fed upon what belongs to the grave?' The last three and a half stanzas of the poem are in the voice of feminised death. She reminds the 'dancing couples' that they all 'smell of death!' and assures them, speaking of herself in the third person, that 'Death admires you / At your antics, ridiculous Humanity, / And frequently, like you, scenting herself with myrrh, / Mingles her irony with your insanity!'[34] While Munch was not commissioned to illustrate this poem, Baudelaire's sexualised imagery of the feminised, transparent, perpetually smiling skeleton resonates with both Munch's lithograph *Dance of Death* (Figures 4.1 and 4.2) and his drypoint *The Women and the Skeleton* (Figure 4.3).

In his programmatic essay 'On the Essence of Laughter', Baudelaire asserts humour as 'satanic' and therefore both 'profoundly human' and 'essentially contradictory'. Humour, he argues, is 'a token of an infinite grandeur and an infinite misery – the latter in relation to the absolute Being of whom man has an inkling, the former in relation to the beasts'. In distinguishing between the 'significative' and the 'absolute comic', or the grotesque, Baudelaire asserts a difference between humour that expresses superiority over other people and what he implies is a more profound and meaningful humour that expresses the superiority of man over nature. The former he aligns with 'imitation' and the latter with 'creation'. He writes: 'the laughter caused by the grotesque has about it something profound, primitive and axiomatic ... [it] emerges as a unity which calls for the intuition to grasp it'. The grotesque, in Baudelaire's formulation, is thus the purview not of any artist, but of the genius: the 'absolute comic turns out to be the prerogative of those superior artists whose minds are sufficiently open to receive any absolute ideas at all'. Ultimately, he concludes, the grotesque is the risky domain of that rare artist who is deeply aware of, and able to mobilise, 'a permanent dualism in the human being – that is, the power of being oneself and someone else at one and the same time'. '[A]n artist is only an artist', he continues, 'on condition that he is a double man and that there is not one single phenomenon of his double nature of which he is ignorant'.[35]

This doubling, the 'absolute comic' that Baudelaire asserts as a mark of the 'superior' artist, is at the heart of the Baudelairean grotesque in Munch's *Dance of Death*. In his lithograph Munch depicts himself as multiply multiple, including as gender fluid. He is the artist pawing his own future remains in a narcissistic act of necrophilia, the artist/physician with intimate knowledge of anatomy, the maiden dancing with an ironically immobile anatomical preparation and death accosting death itself, who nevertheless rebuffs its own advances with an 'eternal smile of ... thirty-two teeth'. But there is further irony and ambiguity in an ongoing oscillation between who is superior to whom.[36] As the artist/physician, Munch asserts his superiority over both man and nature, using both 'significative' and 'absolute' modes of humour. But with Munch in the guise of the maiden and death's accoster whose advances are ignored, skeletal death takes the upper hand over its fleshy double. This questioning of superiority and power highlights the profound irony in Baudelairean humour, which, in Michèle Hanoosh's terms, can be summarised as, 'the nature to which we feel superior is also that in which we must live'.[37] Ultimately, Munch's lithograph presents the viewer with the conundrum of who has the last laugh – artist/physician or death/maiden?

Munch's *Dance of Death* lithograph includes one further humorous aspect, which escapes Baudelaire's theory of the grotesque while both prolonging and interrupting the superiority theory of humour. In the lithograph (see Figures 4.1 and 4.2) an odd element is just visible along the right-hand side of the image: distinct traces of industrially produced lettering that contrast with the artist's signature expressionist idiom. In the first, very preliminary state of the lithograph (Figure 4.9), printed only as trial proofs, this lettering is revealed in full as 'DAMENUNDERTØI', which translates as 'ladies' underwear'. Evidently, the artist worked with lithographic crayon on a piece of advertising, the top parts of which were, along with the image, transferred to the lithographic stone before the image was further worked directly on the matrix for subsequent states.[38] This irreverent conserving of traces of the industrial lettering, redolent of Pop Art before its time, is a small but significant part of the 'joke' of this chapter's concern, a joke initially only available to insiders, specifically Munch's circle of collectors and now scholars, including myself, who have come to know his work intimately.[39]

On one hand, the words 'ladies' underwear' are in keeping with the 'absolute comic', words that, once revealed, elicit more of an immediate belly laugh than the rational, satirical humour also at play. And, because that laughter is primarily available to 'insiders', the artist, as well as the collector, patron or scholar of the work, those who, in other words, were part of a largely homosocial male community with the privilege of 'reading' the text, that superiority is further asserted. The act of appropriating a piece of advertising for a commodity often marketed to women but arguably prioritising men's pleasure deploys a humour that perhaps more fully excludes women from the inside jokes of both art and medicine.

But the formal incongruity of 'ladies' underwear', the industrially produced text layered with the artist's signature expressionism, introduces another possibility for print's humour.[40] This humour likely escaped Munch's intentions and his aristocratic Baudelairean sensibility that makes the superiority theory most plausible for an artist who laboured to mythically construct his own genius.[41] The lettering is funny because it seems so incidental, even accidental and alien to the artist's intentions, his gestural style and the viewer's expectations of the artist's moody, expressionist work. And yet, it is fortuitous, the remnants of 'ladies' underwear' in engineered lettering highlighting the nakedness of fleshy women *and* skeletons

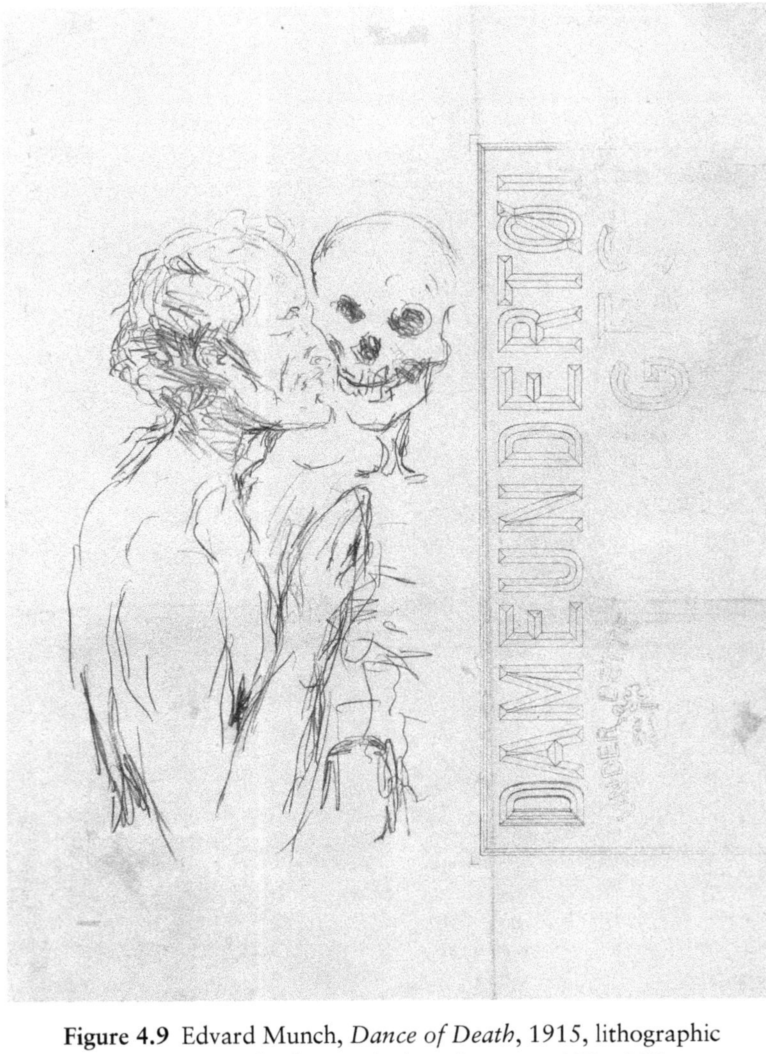

Figure 4.9 Edvard Munch, *Dance of Death*, 1915, lithographic crayon on paper, further worked on the stone, 420 × 250 mm (image), 650 × 477 mm (sheet), Woll 509, I/III.

and undergirding the privileged gender play of the print as well as the exclusion of women from most of the joke. But perhaps it is the exclusion of women that is being highlighted as incongruous. In this reading, the lettering becomes a literal sign of 'woman' reasserted where the maiden has otherwise been replaced by an artist/physician feeling up death. From this perspective, it is as if the artist's models in *The Women and the Skeleton* (Figure 4.3), depicted as so casually and naturally naked, have come to take their revenge, inserting themselves into Munch's self-portrait not unlike how one woman sticks her hand inside the ribcage of a skeleton to physically lay claim to an otherwise masculine domain of knowledge.

'Ladies' underwear' is funny because it transgresses Munch's form, imposing itself, in Henri Bergson's words, as 'something mechanical encrusted upon the living'.[42] Or maybe 'ladies' underwear' is funny because the transgression questions what *is* mechanical and what is alive, what is natural and what is not, the industrially produced lettering or the expressionist gesture, the anatomical preparation, the animated lecherous artist or the missing maiden? The grotesque humour of Munch's print both vaunts and undercuts the male artist's and the male physician's ability to cheat death and overcome femininity through modern technology, through modern printmaking and through modern medicine. But as a different kind of joke, 'ladies' underwear' threatens to carry the day.

Notes

1 Gerd Woll, *Edvard Munch: The Complete Graphic Works*, 2nd edition (Philip Wilson, 2012), cat. 509, p. 334. In a brief discussion of this lithograph, Eric Forssmann characterises the artist's approach to the skeleton as seeking a hug from a friend. See Eric Forssmann, 'Tanz und Tod im Werk Edvard Munchs', in Franz Link (ed.), *Tanz und Tod in Kunst und Literatur* (Duncker & Humblot, 1993), pp. 310–11.

2 The composition recalls the artist's 1895 lithograph, *Self-Portrait with Skeleton Arm*. See Woll, *Munch: Complete Graphic Works* cat. 37, pp. 62–3.

3 Woll, *Munch: Complete Graphic Works* cat. 51, pp. 82–3.

4 Women were granted the right to study medicine in Norway in 1884, but the first woman did not graduate until 1893.

5 This analysis is indebted to Alison Chang, 'The Art and Science of Observation: *The Women and the Skeleton*', in Heidi Bale Amundsen and Allison Morehead (eds), *Lifeblood – Edvard Munch* (MUNCH, 2025), pp. 131–5. On the power of the 'naked' dancing skeleton as a kind of impossible ideal, see Ashby Kinch, 'The *danse macabre* and the medieval community of death', *Mediaevalia* 23 (2002), 194–7.

6 John Harley Warner, 'Witnessing Dissection: Photography, Medicine, and American Culture', in John Harley Warner and James M. Edmonson, *Dissection: Photographs of a Rite of Passage in American Medicine: 1880–1930* (Blast Books, 2009), pp. 13, 23, 119, 133, 153. Warner notes that women medical students often posed humorously with skeletons, but were rarely, if ever, pictured joking around with a cadaver. I have not yet encountered literature that closely examines continuities between modern dissection photography and dance of death iconography. On the continuities between the dance of death and earlier anatomical illustrations, see Maike Christadler, 'From Allegory to Anatomy: Femininity and the Danse Macabre', in Sophie Oosterwijk and Stefanie Knöll (eds), *Mixed Metaphors: The Danse Macabre in Early Modern Europe* (Cambridge Scholars Publishing, 2011), pp. 101–29.

7 On the homosocial humour of medical training, see Lela Kerley, 'Merriment, medical humor, and masculinity at the Bal de l'Internat, 1897–1911', *Nineteenth-Century Art Worldwide* 13:2 (Autumn 2014), https://www.19thc-artworldwide.org/autumn14/kerley-on-merriment-medical-humor-and-masculinity-at-the-bal-de-l-internat (accessed 27 September 2023).

8 Amundsen and Morehead (eds), *Lifeblood – Edvard Munch*.

9 There is an extensive literature on the iconography of the dance of death, largely focused on the medieval and Renaissance periods, and especially the woodcuts of Hans Holbein the Younger (1523–5). For starting points, see Franz Link (ed.), *Tanz und Tod in Kunst und Literatur* (Duncker & Humblot, 1993); Wolfgang Neumann (ed.), *Tanz der Toten – Todestanz: Der monumentale Totentanz im deutschsprachigen Raum* (J.H. Röll, 1998); Kinch, 'The *danse macabre*'; Dagmar Eichberger, 'Close encounters with death: changing representations of women in Renaissance art and literature', in Bernard J. Muir (ed.), *Reading Texts and Images: Essays on Medieval and Renaissance Art and Patronage in Honour of Margaret M. Manion* (University of Exeter Press, 2002), pp. 273–96; Sophie Oosterwijk, 'Of corpses, constables and kings: the Danse Macabre in late-medieval and Renaissance culture', *The Journal of the British Archaeological Association* 157

(2004), 61–90; Elina Gertsman, *The Dance of Death in the Middle Ages: Image, Text, Performance* (Brepols, 2010); Oosterwijk and Knöll (eds), *Mixed Metaphors*. On the flexibility, adaptability and mobility of the iconography, see Sophie Oosterwijk, 'Dance, Dialogue and Duality: Fatal Encounters in the Medieval *Danse Macabre*', in Oosterwijk and Knöll (eds), *Mixed Metaphors*, p. 10. For a brief discussion of the dance of death, Black Death and epidemics, see Luisa Rittershuis and Kathrin Eschenberg, 'Black Death, plagues, and the Danse Macabre: Depictions of epidemics in art', *Historical Social Research* 22 (2021), 330–41. The argument that the imagery of the dance of death proliferated in the wake of the Black Death has been challenged. See Gertsman, *Dance of Death in the Middle Ages*, pp. 42–3.

10 Sophie Oosterwijk and Stefanie Knöll, 'Introduction', in Oosterwijk and Knöll (eds), *Mixed Metaphors*, p. 2.

11 One of the earliest self-portraits of an artist included in a dance of death is the no longer extant wall painting by Niklaus Manuel Deutsch in Bern, 1516–19, copied by Albert Kauw, 1649, Bernisches Historisches Museums, Inv. 822.23. See Gertsman, *The Dance of Death in the Middle Ages*, pp. 166–7.

12 Sharon Latchaw Hirsh, 'Arnold Böcklin: Death Talks to the Painter', *Arts Magazine* 55:6 (February 1981), 84–9. Subsequent examples, cited by Hirsh, include Hans Thoma, *Self-Portrait*, 1875 (Städtische Kunstsammlungen, Karlsruhe) and James Ensor, *The Skeleton Painter*, *c.*1896 (Koninklijk Museum voor Schone Kunsten, Antwerp).

13 Anthony Bond and Joanna Woodall, *Self-Portrait: Renaissance to Contemporary* (National Portrait Gallery, 2006).

14 Stefanie Knöll, 'Death and the Maiden', in Helen Fronius and Anna Linton (eds), *Women in Death: Representations of Female Victims and Perpetrators in German Culture 1500–2000* (Camden House, 2008), pp. 9–27. See also Jean Wirth, *La Jeune fille et la mort: Recherches sur les thèmes macabres dans l'art germanique de la Renaissance* (Droz, 1979); Eichberger, 'Close encounters with death'; Christadler, 'From Allegory to Anatomy', p. 106.

15 Sarah Webster Goodwin and Elisabeth Bronfen, 'Introduction', in Sarah Webster Goodwin and Elisabeth Bronfen (eds), *Death and Representation* (The Johns Hopkins University Press, 1993), pp. 13–14. See also Elisabeth Bronfen, *Over Her Dead Body: Death, Femininity and the Aesthetic* (Manchester University Press, 1992) and Karl S. Guthke, *The Gender of Death: A Cultural History in Art and Literature* (Cambridge University Press, 1999).

16 Bronfen, *Over Her Dead Body*, p. xii. See also Janet Wolff, 'Death and the Maiden: Does Semiotics Justify Murder?', in *Resident Alien: Feminist Cultural Criticism* (Yale University Press, 1995), pp. 59–67.
17 Woll, *Edvard Munch: The Complete Graphic Works*, cat. 3, p. 39. For the related painting, *Death and Life*, see Gerd Woll, *Edvard Munch: Complete Paintings*, vol. 1 (Thames & Hudson, 2009), cat. 345, p. 329. See also the lithograph, *The Kiss of Death* (1899) in Woll, *Edvard Munch: The Complete Graphic Works*, cat. 144, p. 163.
18 The seemingly endless possibilities for humour in appropriations of Munch's *The Scream* might also belie this assumption.
19 With thanks to Christine Slobogin for pointing out the potential for dark humour in this work.
20 There is very little scholarly work on Saliger. For a biography, see *Benezit Dictionnaire des peintres, sculpteurs, dessinateurs et graveurs*, vol. 7 (Librairie Grund, 1966), p. 483. Arguably, another death and the maiden image by Saliger does contain an element of humour, specifically the 'knees-up' poses of the print's two protagonists. See www.sepulkralmuseum.de/EN/research/library-collections/insights-into-our-collection/ivo-saliger-death-and-girl (accessed 14 December 2023). I am grateful to Christine Slobogin for bringing this work to my attention.
21 Ivo Saliger to Mrs Killpack, 6 December 1973, in the archives of the Dittrick Medical History Center, Case Western Reserve University. For an English translation of the letter, see https://artsci.case.edu/dittrick/collections/images/prints/ (accessed 19 September 2023).
22 Barbara McCloskey, 'Marking time: Women and Nazi propaganda art during World War II', *Contemporaneity: Historical Presence in Visual Culture* 2:1 (2012), 4–5.
23 For starting points, see the work of Paul Weindling, in particular, *Health, Race, and German Politics Between National Unification and Nazism, 1870–1945* (Cambridge University Press, 1989). See also the entry 'Deadly Medicine: Creating the Master Race' in the United States Holocaust Museum's online Holocaust Encyclopedia: https://encyclopedia.ushmm.org/content/en/article/deadly-medicine-creating-the-master-race (accessed 21 September 2023).
24 Christadler, 'From Allegory to Anatomy'.
25 Thomas W. Laqueur, *The Work of the Dead: A Cultural History of Mortal Remains* (Princeton University Press, 2015), pp. 56–7.
26 Charles Baudelaire, 'On the Essence of Laughter' (1855), cited in Christiane Hertel, 'Dis/continuities in Dresden's Dances of Death', *Art Bulletin* 82:1 (March 2000), 101. See Charles Baudelaire, 'On the Essence of Laughter' (1855) in Jonathan Mayne (ed. and trans.),

The Mirror of Art: Critical Studies by Baudelaire (Doubleday Anchor, 1956), pp. 131–53.

27 Hertel, 'Dis/continuities', 102.

28 Baudelaire, 'On the Essence of Laughter' (1855), cited in Hertel, 'Dis/continuities', 101.

29 The commission, from La Société des Cents Bibliophiles, was for a collector's edition of *The Flowers of Evil*. It was cancelled soon after the death of the president of the society a few months later. See Bente Torjusen, 'The Mirror', in *Edvard Munch: Symbols and Images* (National Gallery of Art, 1978), pp. 201–4. Torjusen argues that Munch's notes suggest he may have chosen these two poems himself.

30 Torjusen, 'The Mirror', 202.

31 Charles Baudelaire, *Flowers of Evil*, trans. Jackson Mathews (New Directions, 1955).

32 See: Allison Morehead, 'Hands, Dissection and Embodied Seeing: Strindberg and Munch', in Jonathan Schroeder, Anna Westerståhl Stenport and Eszter Szalczer (eds), *August Strindberg and Visual Culture: The Emergence of Optical Modernity in Image, Text, and Theatre* (Bloomsbury Academic, 2018), pp. 30–1.

33 Baudelaire, *The Flowers of Evil*, 1954.

34 Baudelaire, *The Flowers of Evil*, 1954.

35 Baudelaire, 'On the Essence of Laughter', pp. 140, 143, 144, 152, 153.

36 Hertel identifies a similar oscillation in Alfred Rethel's print series *Another Dance of Death (Auch ein Totentanz)* (1849). Hertel, 'Dis/continuities', 102.

37 Michèle Hanoosh, *Baudelaire and Caricature: From the Comic to an Art of Modernity* (The Pennsylvania State University Press, 1992), p. 41, cited in Hertel, 'Dis/continuities', 102.

38 This likely process is described in Woll, *Edvard Munch: The Complete Graphic Works*, p. 334.

39 The reference to Pop Art is not as out of place as it might seem, given Andy Warhol's series of works appropriating key motifs of Munch's, as well as Warhol's concern for popularised images of death, including his *Skulls* series from 1976. On Warhol's borrowings of Munch, see Patricia G. Berman and Pari Stave, *Munch/Warhol and the Multiple Image* (The American Scandinavian Foundation, 2013). On Warhol's themes of death as engaging with the mass subject seen through the lens of traumatic realism, see Hal Foster, 'Death in America', *October* 75 (Winter 1996), 37–59. Arguably, the joke of 'ladies' underwear' is today available to a large group of people since Munch's work is well documented in catalogues raisonnés and highly accessible online.

40 On the incongruity theory of humour, see John Moreall, 'Philosophy of Humor', in Edward N. Zalta and Uri Nodelman (eds), *The Stanford Encyclopedia of Philosophy* (Summer 2023 edition), https://plato.stanford.edu/archives/sum2023/entries/humor/ (accessed 27 September 2023).

41 See Patricia G. Berman, 'The Many Lives of Edvard Munch', in Woll, *Edvard Munch: Complete Paintings*, vol. 4, pp. 1277–94.

42 The idea of jokes as a transgression of form derives from Sigmund Freud, *Jokes and Their Relation to the Unconscious* (1903), vol. 8 of *The Standard Edition of the Complete Psychological Works of Sigmund Freud*, translated and edited by James Strachey (Hogarth Press, 1960), cited, along with Henri Bergson, *Laughter: An Essay on the Meaning of the Comic*, trans. Cloudesley Brereton and Fred Rothwell (Macmillan, 1911), in Lauren Berlant and Sianne Ngai, 'Comedy Has Issues', *Critical Inquiry* 43:2 (2017), 234. Berlant and Ngai also cite Alenka Zupancic, *The Odd One In: On Comedy* (MIT Press, 2008), as questioning the boundaries between the living and the mechanical.

References

Bale Amundsen, Heidi, and Allison Morehead (eds). *Lifeblood – Edvard Munch*. MUNCH, 2025.

Baudelaire, Charles. 'On the Essence of Laughter' (1855). In Jonathan Mayne (ed. and trans.), *The Mirror of Art: Critical Studies by Baudelaire*, pp. 131–53. Doubleday Anchor, 1956.

Baudelaire, Charles. *The Flowers of Evil* (1857). Translated by William Aggeler. Academy Library Guild, 1954.

Baudelaire, Charles. *Flowers of Evil* (1857). Translated by Jackson Mathews. New Directions, 1955.

Benezit Dictionnaire des peintres, sculpteurs, dessinateurs et graveurs. Vol. 7. Librairie Grund, 1966.

Bergson, Henri. *Laughter: An Essay on the Meaning of the Comic*. Translated by Cloudesley Brereton and Fred Rothwell. Macmillan, 1911.

Berlant, Lauren, and Sianne Ngai. 'Comedy has issues'. *Critical Inquiry* 43 (2017), 233–49.

Berman, Patricia G. 'The Many Lives of Edvard Munch'. In Gerd Woll, *Edvard Munch: Complete Paintings*. Vol. 4, pp. 1277–94. Thames & Hudson, 2009.

Berman, Patricia G., and Pari Stave. *Munch/Warhol and the Multiple Image*. The American Scandinavian Foundation, 2013.

Bond, Anthony, and Joanna Woodall. *Self-Portrait: Renaissance to Contemporary*. National Portrait Gallery, 2006.

Bronfen, Elisabeth. *Over Her Dead Body: Death, Femininity and the Aesthetic*. Manchester University Press, 1992.

Chang, Alison. 'The Art and Science of Observation: *The Women and the Skeleton*'. In Heidi Bale Amundsen and Allison Morehead (eds), *Lifeblood – Edvard Munch*, pp. 131–5. MUNCH, 2025.

Christadler, Maike. 'From Allegory to Anatomy: Femininity and the Danse Macabre'. In Sophie Oosterwijk and Stefanie Knöll (eds), *Mixed Metaphors: The Danse Macabre in Early Modern Europe*, pp. 101–29. Cambridge Scholars Publishing, 2011.

'Deadly Medicine: Creating the Master Race'. In the United States Holocaust Museum's online Holocaust Encyclopedia. https://encyclopedia.ushmm.org/content/en/article/deadly-medicine-creating-the-master-race (accessed 21 September 2023).

Eichberger, Dagmar. 'Close Encounters with Death: Changing Representations of Women in Renaissance Art and Literature'. In Bernard J. Muir, *Reading Texts and Images: Essays on Medieval and Renaissance Art and Patronage in Honour of Margaret M. Manion*, pp. 273–96. University of Exeter Press, 2002.

Forssmann, Eric. 'Tanz und Tod im Werk Edvard Munchs'. In Franz Link (ed.), *Tanz und Tod in Kunst und Literatur*, pp. 299–315. Duncker & Humblot, 1993.

Foster, Hal. 'Death in America'. *October* 75 (Winter 1996), 37–59.

Freud, Sigmund. *Jokes and Their Relation to the Unconscious* (1903), vol. 8 of *The Standard Edition of the Complete Psychological Works of Sigmund Freud*. Translated and edited by James Strachey. Hogarth Press, 1960.

Gertsman, Elina. *The Dance of Death in the Middle Ages: Image, Text, Performance*. Brepols, 2010.

Goodwin, Sarah Webster, and Elisabeth Bronfen (eds). *Death and Representation*. The Johns Hopkins University Press, 1993.

Guthke, Karl S. *The Gender of Death: A Cultural History in Art and Literature*. Cambridge University Press, 1999.

Hanoosh, Michèle. *Baudelaire and Caricature: From the Comic to an Art of Modernity*. The Pennsylvania State University Press, 1992.

Hertel, Christiane. 'Dis/continuities in Dresden's Dances of Death'. *Art Bulletin* 82 (March 2000), 83–116.

Hirsh, Sharon Latchaw. 'Arnold Böcklin: Death talks to the painter'. *Arts Magazine* 55:6 (February 1981), 84–9.

Kerley, Lela. 'Merriment, Medical humor, and masculinity at the Bal de l'Internat, 1897–1911'. *Nineteenth-Century Art Worldwide* 13 (Autumn

2014). www.19thc-artworldwide.org/autumn14/kerley-on-merriment-medical-humor-and-masculinity-at-the-bal-de-l-internat (accessed 27 September 2023).

Kinch, Ashby. 'The *danse macabre* and the medieval community of death'. *Mediaevalia* 23 (2002): 159–202.

Knöll, Stefanie. 'Death and the Maiden'. In Helen Fronius and Anna Linton (eds), *Women in Death: Representations of Female Victims and Perpetrators in German Culture 1500–2000*, pp. 9–27. Camden House, 2008.

Laqueur, Thomas W. *The Work of the Dead: A Cultural History of Mortal Remains*. Princeton University Press, 2015.

Link, Franz (ed.). *Tanz und Tod in Kunst und Literatur*. Duncker & Humblot, 1993

McCloskey, Barbara. 'Marking time: Women and Nazi propaganda art during World War II'. *Contemporaneity: Historical Presence in Visual Culture* 2 (2012), 1–17.

Moreall, John. 'Philosophy of Humor'. In Edward N. Zalta and Uri Nodelman (eds) *The Stanford Encyclopedia of Philosophy* (Summer 2023 edition). https://plato.stanford.edu/archives/sum2023/entries/humor/ (accessed 27 September 2023).

Morehead, Allison. 'Hands, Dissection and Embodied Seeing: Strindberg and Munch'. In Jonathan Schroeder, Anna Westerståhl Stenport and Eszter Szalczer (eds), *August Strindberg and Visual Culture: The Emergence of Optical Modernity in Image, Text, and Theatre*, pp. 19–34. Bloomsbury Academic, 2018.

Neumann, Wolfgang (ed.). *Tanz der Toten – Todestanz: Der monumentale Totentanz im deutschsprachigen Raum*. J.H. Röll, 1998.

Oosterwijk, Sophie. 'Of corpses, constables and kings: the Danse Macabre in late-medieval and Renaissance culture'. *The Journal of the British Archaeological Association* 157 (2004): 61–90.

Oosterwijk, Sophie. 'Dance, Dialogue and Duality: Fatal Encounters in the Medieval *Danse Macabre*'. In Sophie Oosterwijk and Stefanie Knöll (eds), *Mixed Metaphors: The Danse Macabre in Early Modern Europe*, pp. 9–42. Cambridge Scholars Publishing, 2011.

Oosterwijk, Sophie, and Stefanie Knöll (eds). *Mixed Metaphors: The Danse Macabre in Early Modern Europe*. Cambridge Scholars Publishing, 2011.

Rittershuis, Luisa, and Kathrin Eschenberg. 'Black Death, plagues, and the Danse Macabre: Depictions of epidemics in art'. *Historical Social Research* 22 (2021), 330–41.

Torjusen, Bente. 'The Mirror'. In *Edvard Munch: Symbols and Images*, pp. 185–212. National Gallery of Art, 1978.

Warner, John Harley. 'Witnessing Dissection: Photography, Medicine, and American Culture'. In John Harley Warner and James M. Edmonson,

Dissection: Photographs of a Rite of Passage in American Medicine: 1880–1930, pp. 7–29. Blast Books, 2009.

Weindling, Paul. *Health, Race, and German Politics Between National Unification and Nazism, 1870–1945*. Cambridge University Press, 1989.

Wirth, Jean. *La Jeune fille et la mort: Recherches sur les thèmes macabres dans l'art germanique de la Renaissance*. Droz, 1979.

Wolff, Janet. 'Death and the Maiden: Does Semiotics Justify Murder?' In *Resident Alien: Feminist Cultural Criticism*, pp. 59–67. Yale University Press, 1995.

Woll, Gerd. *Edvard Munch: The Complete Graphic Works*. 2nd edition. Philip Wilson, 2012.

Zupancic, Alenka. *The Odd One In: On Comedy*. MIT Press, 2008.

5

Tube pedicles and positionality: The visual humour of a plastic surgery technique

Christine Slobogin

The tube pedicle, or tubed pedicle, is a plastic surgery technique that was invented in the early twentieth century. Its function was to transfer tissue to reconstruct body parts – such as noses, chins or ears – that had been injured or burned.[1] In the tube pedicle procedure, no longer widely practised, the flap of flesh and skin to be transferred was carved from another, healthy part of the patient's body, such as the inner thigh, wrist or forearm, and rolled into a tube to prevent infection. Both ends of the tube were attached to the body by flaps of skin to ensure blood flow, with only the centre of the tube disconnected from the body. Once blood flow was confirmed, one end of the pedicle was removed and reattached to the body closer to the injury. In many cases, this was repeated over periods of days or weeks until one end of the tube pedicle met the wound, thereby slowly moving the desired flesh from one place to another. This procedure, particularly useful to treat wartime facial injuries, was invented almost simultaneously in 1917 by several surgeons, including the British plastic surgeon from New Zealand Harold Gillies (1882–1960), the most prominent practitioner in this field at the time. Tube pedicles were used throughout much of the twentieth century.[2]

When the flesh was slowly transferred from the donor site to the area of reconstruction, in multiple steps and in a rhythm likened to a macabre, protracted waltz, the tube pedicle was sometimes called a 'waltzing' or 'walking stick' pedicle. Patients had to endure extended periods of time with this unnatural-looking appendage on their face or other part of their body, often holding uncomfortable positions and bending their neck or arm to make sure that the pedicle remained where it was needed, all while wounds healed in the places from which the pedicle had been carved. Emphasising the drawn-out nature of this procedure, there were even patients recorded in the surgical literature – probably apocryphally – who were forgotten by surgeons or who put off returning to the hospital, living for years with pedicles dangling from their foreheads or noses. One apparently joined the circus, with the pedicle attached to his nose allowing him to label himself an 'elephant man'.[3] These stories and the use of the term 'waltzing', even – or especially – in official and accepted surgical references to the technique, suggest a commonplace, comical animation of this inert but living piece of almost disembodied flesh.

In part because of its conspicuous strangeness, often positioned in the centre of the face, the tube pedicle was the most visible element of facial reconstruction surgery in twentieth-century Britain – the focus of this chapter. This chapter also homes in on one particular moment of the tube pedicle's popularity: during and shortly after the Second World War, when military personnel and civilians alike suffered from burns and injuries on their faces and bodies that required this nimble grafting technique. Because of its universality in plastic surgery procedures, its peculiar shape and appearance and its visibility, the tube pedicle was a common topic for surgical writers, cartoonists and others commenting on or drawing the medical context of Second World War plastic surgery.

There is intrinsic irony in this procedure: while the tube pedicle was a surgical tool used to make patients' appearances more normative, the tube pedicle was also a temporary disfigurement of the patient's visage that made their facial difference and their injured appearance much more extreme. Rooted partly in this irony, there were seemingly endless ways to play verbally and visually with this striking, fleshy and arguably phallic bodily apparatus; because of this discursive flexibility, it became an object and a procedure that could be understood through humour. And because the humour of the tube pedicle was based so deeply in the strangeness of the appearance of the thing, visual humour was a particularly ripe avenue for making jokes about the surgical technique.

In tube pedicle humour, as with all humour relating to the medicalised body, the positionality of the creator of the visual joke is paramount. This chapter looks at humorous treatments of the tube pedicle from the perspective of the surgeon, the surgical artist and the patient across different reconstructive wards in Second World War England. Through these analyses, this chapter reveals how varied stakeholders used humour in surgical contexts and how they thought about patients' bodies. Showcasing positionalities from three similar but separate contexts highlights the ubiquity of these types of jokes within this medical milieu while also exposing the power relations and hierarchies operating in these surgical spaces. The surgeon's humour – that of the man with the most power in the ward – is the most flippant and tied to the patient's body; the surgical artist's cartoons are still somewhat irreverent, but characterised in a way that removes the 'funny' object from the site of injury and disfigurement; and the patient's humour around the tube pedicle is the most distanced of all, and markedly non-visual.

The surgeon and the irreverent tube pedicle

Harold Gillies's sense of humour was a significant force in twentieth-century plastic surgery, of which he has often been characterised as the 'father'. Examining his written and visual jokes about tube pedicles helps to reconstruct the positionality of the plastic surgeon in relation to patients' bodies in this period. The humour of this surgeon, and that of the many surgeons he influenced or directly trained, was paternalistic; it was likely well-meaning, but it was often irreverent and removed in ways that turned bodies and pedicles into objects.[4]

The 1957 book *The Principles and Art of Plastic Surgery* – styled in Gillies's voice but largely written by his co-author D. Ralph Millard, Jr – communicates, frequently humorously and with eye-catching visuals, the surgeon's anecdotes and techniques. Patients' horrific traumas – not only injuries and long surgical recoveries, but also incidents including a woman's murder by her husband after he saw her surgically altered face – share space with humorous asides, flippant comments, comical cartoons and edited photographs.

One reviewer called it 'a combination of autobiography, an unorthodox text, an informal reference book, filled with the most astounding array of illustrations … as well as a complete drama in the development of plastic surgery'.[5] The foreword of the book classifies Gillies as a 'Puck', and 'an imp in his humor and practical jokes'.[6] As discovered by Andrew Bamji, an editor at Collins declined to publish the book in part because of its distinct brand of off-beat humour. Gillies's humorous side, which was tone-setting and acceptable in the plastics ward, was less appreciated in other professional settings. The editor at Collins stated:

> In our view the fairly long insertions about his personal life and particularly those which deal with his jokes … etc., interrupt the course of the narrative and should be drastically cut. Further, we feel that the book is written in a style which is so elaborate and facetious that it gets between the reader and what the author is saying. Sir Harold does not appear to recognise the difference between a story which is told by him to an appreciative audience of friends and a story written and addressed to a series of unknown people.[7]

The author's facetiousness and jokes, advantageous for facilitating a jovial atmosphere in the hospital and operating room, fell flat for some readers, although an editor did eventually agree to publish the two volumes with these humorous inclusions. The book's tone can in part be explained because it was perceived as 'an autobiography of the outstanding plastic surgeon of the century [Gillies]', thereby inviting the exhibition of his Puckish personality in each chapter.[8]

The infusion of Gillies's personality in *Principles and Art* is aided by the book's artistic additions, the large number of which also posed an issue for potential publishers.[9] In a mixture of edited photographs and small cartoons, characters dance along the paragraphs and line breaks, funny photographs fill the margins and humorous images even supplement the main body of text. For example, on a page in the section on nose surgeries, there is a photograph of a father and son in which the noses of each have been cut and pasted from one face onto the other.[10] Often there are jokes or humorous anecdotes about serious conditions alongside photographs of the actual patients who had them.

The tube pedicle, on its own or as part of other surgical procedures, serves as both a vehicle and a target of humour in this publication. In the 'Tube Pedicles' section of the book, it is stated that 'these flaps are for the patient's good and not our amusement'.[11] However, the way that Gillies wrote about and chose to illustrate these fleshy tubes proves that they were indeed the subject of amusement for Gillies and his perceived audience. At times, they are even referred to as 'sausages'.[12]

A cartoon illustration of a tube pedicle helps to set the tone for the publication. Preceded only by the foreword, acknowledgments and preface, it shows a reproduction of a 'nonsense' drawing by Edward Lear (1812–88), who happened to be a great-great uncle of Gillies's.[13] In the image, a cartoonish man with thin legs and a pot belly walks as if on a tightrope, with his arms outstretched. Before him, his nose extends far longer than the height of his body. Birds of various shapes, some black and some white, are perched atop it. The accompanying limerick goes,

> Edward Lear sketched this man with a nose
> So the birds of the air could repose.
> Dare we be medical,
> Steal his tube pedicle
> For methods we're soon to disclose.[14]

The funniness of the tube pedicle, and the strangeness of seeing such a protrusion on a body, is established from the very beginning of *Principles and Art*. By referring to a figure as prominent as Lear, Gillies firmly placed this ubiquitous surgical technique within the history of British visual humour.

Here and in the rest of his publication, Gillies expounded upon the importance of this technique in plastic surgery. Even though Vladimir Filatov (1875–1956), an ophthalmologist and surgeon from Odessa, Ukraine, has been determined as the true progenitor of the technique, Gillies was 'the evangelist of the tubed flap', and this is clear in the number of times that he mentioned and visualised the tube pedicle across his publications.[15] The tube pedicle became a omnipresent tool for facial reconstruction after it was popularised by Gillies during the First World War at his department in Sidcup, where, in his words in *Principles and Art*, 'the wards soon resembled the jungles of Burma, teeming with dangling pedicles'. Gillies commented on the tube pedicle again later in the book:

> If all the tube pedicles that I have made and those my assistants have made were laid end to end, by calculations at two and a half pedicles per week, they would string like sausages from Buckingham Palace down the Mall, straight on through the Admiralty Arch to Trafalgar Square and half-way up Nelson's monument. It is my ambition that before my last pedicle is made we will reach the top of this famous pinnacle with at least one pedicle left to go into the Admiral's [Nelson's] palate.[16]

Gillies's colleague Archibald McIndoe (1900–60), who treated the patients of The Guinea Pig Club (to be discussed shortly), also spoke in a similarly physical and exaggerated, but detached from patients' bodies, manner about the great number of tube pedicles that he and his team created during the Second World War: '[The Guinea Pig Club] have lost and regained enough skin to paper these walls and could have donated enough pedicles to make a rope sufficient to hang Hitler.'[17]

Gillies's descriptions and illustrations jar with the fact that the tube pedicle is an invasive, uncomfortable object that remains part of the patient's body. Gillies was clearly comfortable with using the grotesque mode of humour to discuss his surgical career as well as the bodies of his patients. In *Principles and Art*, Gillies even mentioned how one procedure resulted in something that looked 'like an anteater's snout and all my colleagues roared with laughter'.[18] This sentence frames the group of surgeons as laughing at the new nose, not the patient, but the joke is still very much attached to the body of a vulnerable individual.

Gillies's visual humour included the patient's body, but in a way that objectified it in a similar fashion to his and McIndoe's descriptions of tube pedicles. The most extreme example of transgressive humour in Gillies's book appears in the section on direct skin flaps, next to an explanation of one called 'The "Marsupial" Flap'. It appears in a chapter called 'Direct Flaps', within the flippantly titled 'Flap Happy' section of the book. This page demonstrates a type of flap that 'may be boldly cut and rolled over like the horizontal tube pedicle'.[19] On a page showing several applications of this flap, the central photograph of an abdominal 'marsupial' flap stands out. In this patient photograph with the patient's face and identity conspicuously missing, an image of a surgeon (it does not appear to be Gillies; perhaps it is J.B. Cuthbert, a surgeon who worked with Gillies and who coined the 'marsupial' name for this technique) has been inserted into the kangaroo-like 'pouch' that the flap has made around the abdomen (Figure 5.1). The absurdity of this image is what makes it funny, the tiny body of the surgeon incongruously inserted into the comparatively massive body of the patient.[20] The insertion of the physician into the patient's body not only adds (questionable) levity to the page, but also, through visual exaggeration, demonstrates the capaciousness of the pouch and therefore its similarity to the pouches of kangaroos and their relatives, from whom it gets its name. There is no explanation of this insertion, although it fits with the tone of the rest of the publication. This is the last page of the section on direct flaps, before the 'Tube Pedicles' chapter.

These are only some of the examples of tube pedicle humour in *Principles and Art*; overall this subset of jokes fits into the wider phenomenon of surgeons' humour. The surgeon can, emotionally and by dint of his power in the hospital, make visual jokes that are shockingly physical. The chipper camaraderie of Gillies and his colleagues (such as McIndoe) had been noted by patients as a positive aspect of their wards, but by some this 'compulsive cheerfulness' was seen as oppressive or inappropriate.[21] Gillies used humour that breached the boundaries of his patients' bodies – something that he did daily with his surgical tools. By doing this, the surgeon illustrated his power not only as the person who crafted the pedicles, but as a person with a normative body fully intact. As sociologist Heather Laine Talley has pointed out, those deemed disfigured by society are often treated and described in this detached, inhuman manner: 'Be it the carnival barker who points to the sideshow performer with facial variance (the "bearded lady" or "elephant man") or the reconstructive surgeon who describes the techniques used on a face ("grafts replace scar tissue"), disfigurement is *talked about* in ways that position people with faces defined as disfigured as objects'.[22] In surgeons' joking descriptions of tube pedicles and in their humorous illustrations of them, there is no attention to, let alone reverence for, the patient's bodily experience.

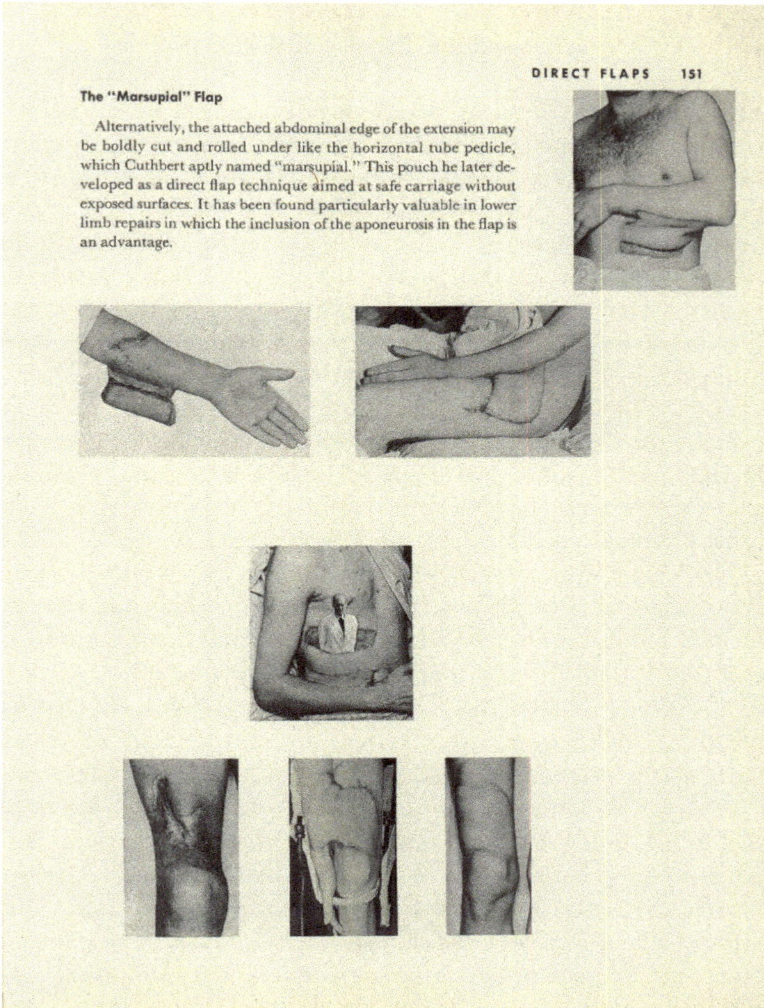

DIRECT FLAPS 151

The "Marsupial" Flap

Alternatively, the attached abdominal edge of the extension may be boldly cut and rolled under like the horizontal tube pedicle, which Cuthbert aptly named "marsupial." This pouch he later developed as a direct flap technique aimed at safe carriage without exposed surfaces. It has been found particularly valuable in lower limb repairs in which the inclusion of the aponeurosis in the flap is an advantage.

Figure 5.1 Harold Gillies and D. Ralph Millard, Jr, *The Principles and Art of Plastic Surgery*, vol. 1, Butterworth & Co., 1957, p. 151.

The artist and the disembodied tube pedicle

The surgical artist was someone involved in patient care in a peripheral manner, spending substantial time with patients: on the wards drawing their portraits and in the theatre drawing the steps of their procedures. Therefore, the positionality of a surgical artist's humour is more nuanced than that of a surgeon orchestrating the operations and calling the shots on the ward. Surgical artists had a more removed sensorial relationship with patients' bodies; they were not cutting into them, but rather were depicting them from a short distance. With examples taken from the *oeuvre* of Diana 'Dickie' Orpen (1914–2008), this section shows how, as an artist, she did not exercise her caregiver power within the hospital through objectifying tube pedicle jokes, as we saw with Gillies's humour. While the surgeon's humour positioned the body and its offcuts as objects, the artist's humour positioned the surgical object as a person.

Working before the 1949 foundation of the Medical Artists' Association of Great Britain (MAA), Orpen and her contemporaries had more freedom to mix the scientific and the humorous in their work than the systematically trained biomedical illustrators of later decades. Often the silly and the serious elements of Orpen's life at Hill End Hospital in St Albans overlapped in her drawings, particularly through the vehicle of the tube pedicle. As Gillies had a tendency to name tube pedicles and hold 'funerals' for those that failed, in her drawings Orpen also performed rituals on these pieces of flesh, anthropomorphising them and individualising them beyond the actual human body from which they originated.[23] But unlike Gillies, Orpen's visual humour did not include the patient's body – that personal side of the surgical treatment and of the joke remained absent from the pedicle's anthropomorphisation.

For example, Orpen created a convergence of religion and humour in a drawing of the stages of the creation of a tube pedicle (Figure 5.2). This page appears as a typical depiction of surgical steps, labelled from step three onward. As the pedicle, with the two flap ends of it still attached to the abdomen, is being lifted from the body and rolled, an additional, smaller tube of flesh – a 'baby' pedicle – is created to the top right of the main structure. At step five,

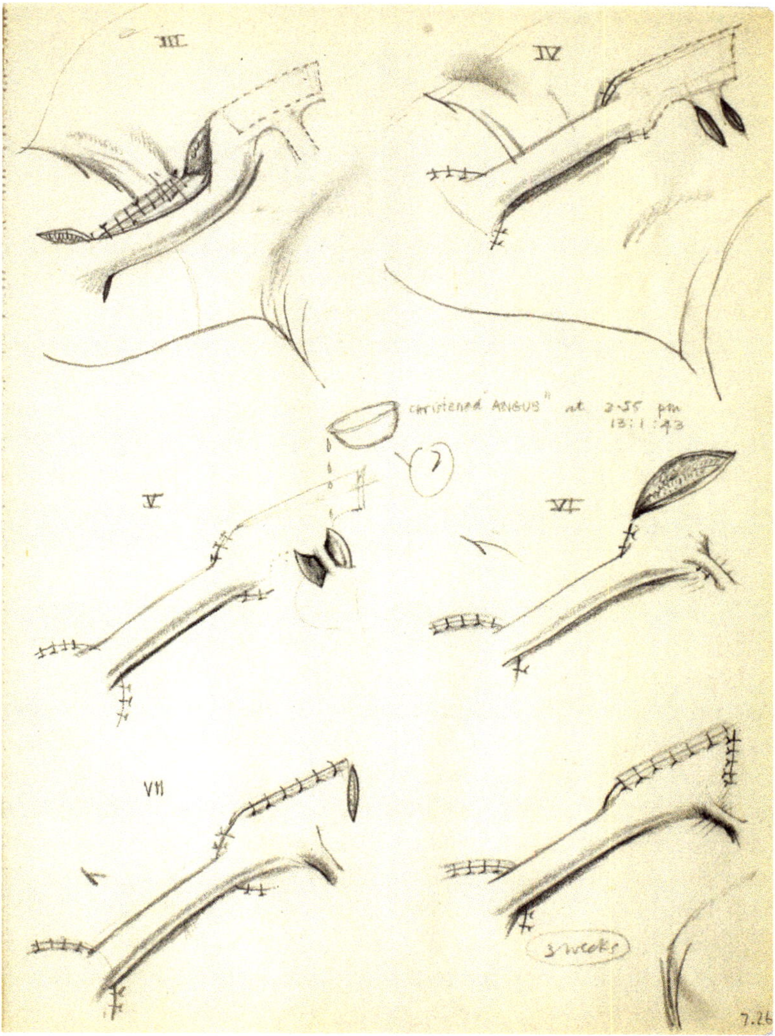

Figure 5.2 Dickie Orpen, BAPRAS/DSB 7.26, 1943, pencil on paper.

Orpen depicted a simple basin pouring four drops of water onto this smaller piece. This represents holy water; she labelled this interaction, 'christened "ANGUS" at 2:55 pm 13:1:43'. Through Orpen's drawing, this tube pedicle became its own Christian entity, separate from the patient from which it was made, gaining the name 'Angus' on 13 January 1943 at 2:55 pm. The annotation circled at the bottom of the page suggested that the patient would need to sit with these surgical sculptures on their body like this for the next three weeks.

As she did with her facetious baptism, Orpen noted the exact time and date of another imagined procedure on a tube pedicle, this time a medical rather than a religious one. In this drawing, titled 'The Plight of the Pregnant Pedicle', Orpen depicted the 'abortion' (excision) of an extra ('baby') tube pedicle from a 'pregnant' one (Figure 5.3). This was performed by the surgeon John Barron (JNB) at 6:20 pm on 16 July 1945. Like the previous illustration, this shows a large tube pedicle with a smaller protrusion branching off at one of its ends. In this case, however, this small piece is to be removed – aborted – rather than baptised.

Both drawings characterise the pedicle as a living being, capable of being 'born', of getting 'pregnant' or of having an 'abortion'. These are, in a way, cartoon 'characters' independent from the reality of the patient whose flesh created them. The baptised pedicle is given the name Angus, and the pedicle pregnancy is framed as being a potential (but eventually unsuccessful) 'brother for Edie', presumably another tube pedicle in this fleshy imagined family. Baptising or aborting a roll of detached but living sculpted flesh – thereby conceptualising the smaller pedicle as an infant – is particularly interesting when used as a visual joke by Orpen, who was a devout Catholic. The fact that this artist blasphemed in this manner in order to get a joke across points to there being something particularly charismatic about this surgical procedure, which Orpen drew hundreds of times during her three years working at Hill End Hospital. This subset of a visual joke cropping up several times in Orpen's *oeuvre* also points to this type of humour being widespread and well accepted in her workplace.

Death and birth, the holy and the profane, and the spiritual and the bodily are collapsed into single images in Orpen's depictions of tube pedicles. For instance, when the religious rite of baptism (held in high regard by the devout Orpen), or when the serious procedure

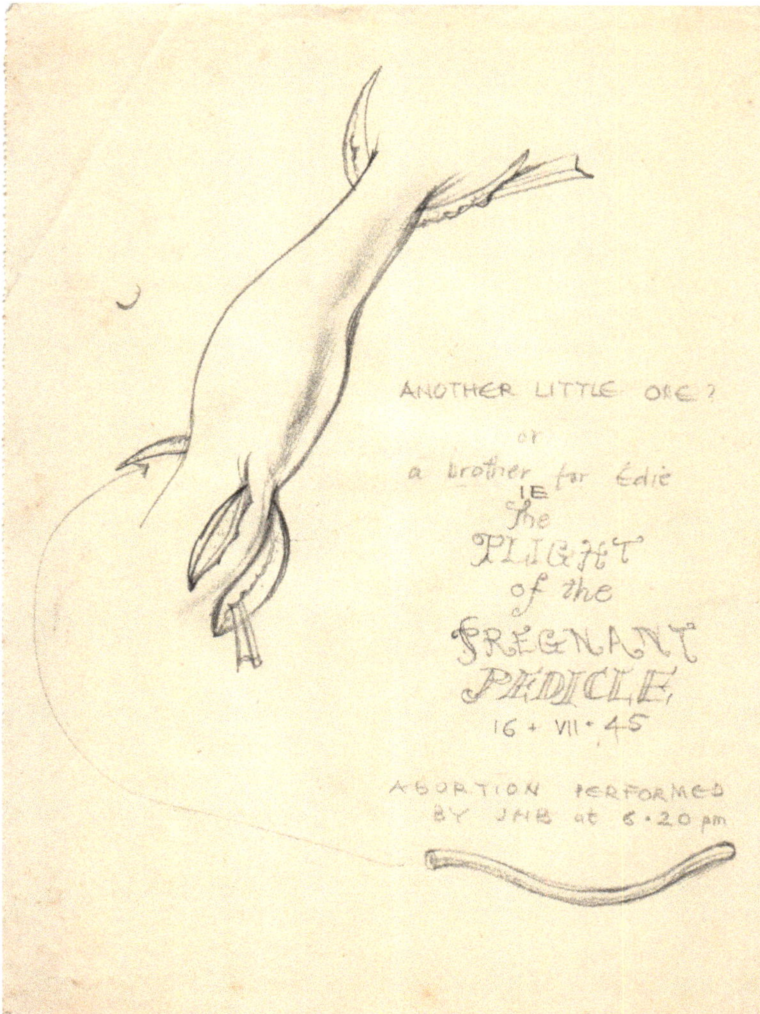
ANOTHER LITTLE ORC ?
or
a brother for Edie
IE
The
PLIGHT
of the
PREGNANT
PEDICLE
16 · VII · 45
ABORTION PERFORMED
BY JHB at 6 · 20 pm

Figure 5.3 Dickie Orpen, *The Plight of the Pregnant Pedicle*, 1945, pencil on paper. From Dickie Orpen's personal papers.

of abortion (presumably looked down upon by the Catholic artist) was performed visually on a soulless piece of flesh, the artist heightened the difference between the clean and holy (baptismal water or a new infant) and the broken and visceral (a surgically created bodily appendage). This contrast results in something that is simultaneously funny and unsettling. Orpen's drawings depict what Mikhail Bakhtin called the 'double-faced fullness of life', resulting in a carnivalesque, grotesque mode of humour and transgression.[24] In these images – which provided relief via humorous release for Orpen and her colleagues – religion, medicine, jokes and the war-broken body meet, and these contradictions accurately portray the complex environment of Second World War surgery and reconstruction.[25]

Another example of Orpen degrading something 'high' (reconstructive surgery and her drawings' supposed purpose of creating medical knowledge) to the 'low' culture of cartoons, jokes and rhymes, can be found in Orpen's writing in her sketchbooks. Alongside pencil drawings of a foot arthroplasty (joint reconstruction), Orpen wrote 'B stands for BONE and BUTCHER and BLOOD'; on the next page she wrote 'C stands for CARTILEDGE [*sic*] and CADAVER and CORPSE.'[26] Here, with an incredibly dark tone, Orpen infantilised the serious matters of surgical reconstruction, injury and death by formatting its morbid vocabulary into the basic structure of an alphabet-themed children's book. As the next section of this chapter shows, this simultaneous morbidity and infantilisation aligned with the way that the patients themselves framed their written tube pedicle humour.

This contrast between the high and the low brings Orpen's drawings into the realm of the medical grotesque. Marie Allitt has framed the 'medical grotesque' within caregiver narratives of the First World War; Orpen herself was a type of caregiver working alongside these patients every day. The medical grotesque is 'characterised by the tensions between bodily protrusions and intrusions' – which the tube pedicle can certainly be considered – and 'it is a vehicle for self-reflection on the conflicting dimensions of caregiving, from the anxieties of repulsion and disgust to dilemmas of medical violence and ethics of intrusion'. Orpen's drawings of tube pedicles can be recognised as one of the medical grotesque 'representational strategies these medics adopt in order to convey the complexities and tensions of medical care'.[27] This mode – the humorous medical grotesque – allowed Orpen to express at the same time detachment and potentially disgust, as well as the empathy and care required in wartime medical spaces. While Gillies's humour could also be framed within the medical grotesque, his positionality as the surgeon with overall power in the ward, and his more irreverent use of the patient's body within his visual humour, removes the potential for reading these jokes and images as self-reflection. While Orpen's representations of tube pedicles create a respectful distance between the joke and the patient's body by placing the agency on the tube pedicle itself, Gillies's tube pedicle humour does not seem to consider, as part of their medical grotesque, the 'ethics of intrusion' inherent in both his opening of the patient's body and his joking about its surgical disfigurement.

Orpen's visualisations of the tube pedicle – that particularly potent vehicle for plastic surgery humour in this period – were removed from the patient's body. In fact, Orpen furnished these tube pedicles with their own functioning 'bodies'. In her visual medical grotesque humour, Orpen created tube pedicle characters that could act within their own physiques separate from the real ones that were being reconstructed in front of her. Anthropomorphising the tubes of flesh that enabled the reconstruction of a person's burned or injured face or body was still potentially irreverent or dark, but Orpen's humour was instead the deferentially detached joking of a medical caregiver dealing with the onslaught of bodies that she saw and drew daily.

The patient and the invisible tube pedicle

Of course, the people with the most 'right' to joke about this subject were the patients who experienced the procedure and who lived for weeks or months with a waltzing tube pedicle attached to some part of their body (Figure 5.4). Talking and exchanging banter with comrades about the singular experience of facial injury and plastic reconstruction was an important part of the physical and psychological recovery process for patients during and after the Second World War in Britain. This was encouraged by Gillies and

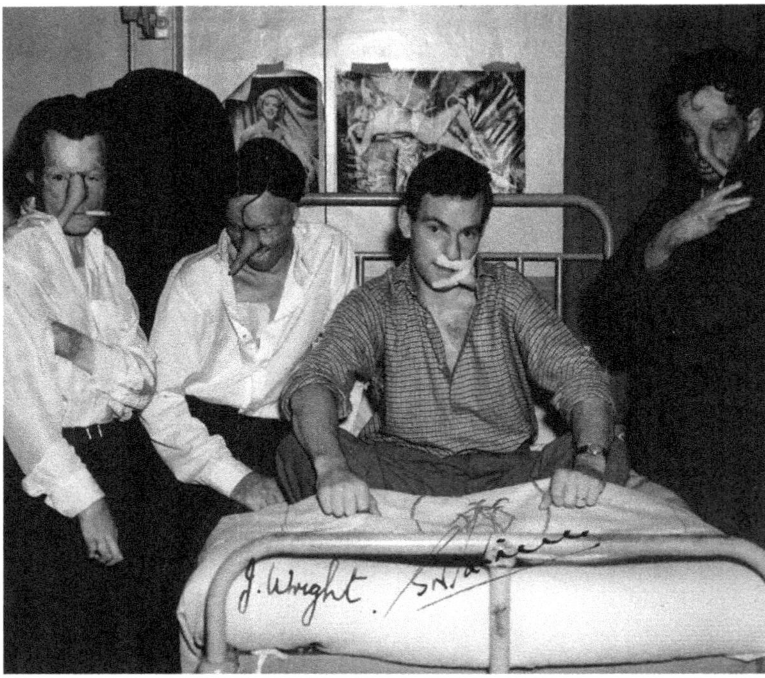

Figure 5.4 Unknown photographer, *Signed Photograph of Guinea Pigs with Tube Pedicles*, 1945, black and white photograph.

the plastic surgeons he trained.[28] At several of the hospitals in which these treatments were offered, patients founded social groups that were connected through shared experiences and, often, drinking and joking at the expense of their own strange conditions and appearances.[29] The Queen Victoria Hospital group was called the Guinea Pig Club, after the patients' pervading but generally good-natured feeling (encouraged by the surgeons in charge) that they were being used as human surgical test subjects. A similar but much less well-known club existed in Scotland during the Second World War; they framed the tube pedicle as their sort of unofficial mascot when they called themselves The Dangle 'Ums Club.[30] To diffuse fear and stigma around the tube pedicles that so many of these men had to wear for weeks as part of their reconstruction, these patients gave the unsightly and uncomfortable apparatus a humorous nickname: 'dangle 'um'. This language trivialised and infantilised the surgical technique, lessening its ability to scare, a tactic that members of the Guinea Pig Club also employed.

The members of the Guinea Pig Club used material culture, cartoons and written humour to stay connected to one another and to cope with their injuries and recoveries in a collective manner. They primarily did this through their club magazine, called *The Guinea Pig*. One story from *The Guinea Pig*'s December 1947 issue made light of the tube pedicle, combining humour with an acknowledgment of the protuberance's frightening effect on the visage. Called 'Ghost Story for Guinea Pigs: As True as I'm Standing Here ...', this two-page story tells of a Guinea Pig with a tube pedicle attached to his nose who visited a friend's house, which happened to be haunted. Inevitably, he encountered the ghosts at night. As soon as the ghosts saw him, 'The sight of that pedicle shook 'em horrible ... The Screaming Nun gave a whimper of fright and vanished through the wall; the Headless Page turned and bolted clean through the wardrobe. Sir Ralph the Ghoul gave a convulsive shudder, snatched up his rusty, trailing chains in his skeletal hands, and dashed headlong from that room.' Dramatically, this Guinea Pig managed to clear the house of ghosts and their noisy disruptions. He 'slept peacefully' after the interaction. He was 'told that not a single ghost has been seen or heard there from that day to this'.[31] This account highlights how visually off-putting a tube pedicle on the face was, but it also likens the tube pedicle to something supernatural with extraordinary powers. By placing the pedicle into a humorous story and giving it the ability to banish ghosts, the author highlighted the strangeness of a Guinea Pig's face while weakening any negative influence that the tube pedicle might have held over a patient to make him feel ashamed or afraid. And yet the tube pedicle is not visualised here; the only illustration that appears is of a chained ghost, presumably Sir Ralph.

Likewise, elsewhere in *The Guinea Pig*, the humorous cartoons showing facial reconstruction avoid visually alluding directly to this surgical object, or to any pathologised facial difference. The bodily elements of reconstructive surgery, when turned into a joke and illustrated in *The Guinea Pig* – by Guinea Pigs themselves and by guest cartoonists – are schematised, distanced and glossed over through the vehicle of the cartoon. When the injuries of the Guinea Pigs, or of other military or civilian patients, are referenced in these cartoons, they are shown only through the occasional cast or X-shaped bandage. The severe facial wounds or bodily burns that placed these patients on their ward, and the very conspicuous techniques used to repair those injuries, are not shown.

Instead of depicting facial wounds or tube pedicles, these *Guinea Pig* cartoons show scenes such a soldier with a very pretty face (with bow-like dark lips, dimples, wide eyes and long lashes) with the caption of one surgeon saying to another, 'Don't you think that's a little *too* good?'[32] Tube pedicles are absent in these cartoons, and yet in written humour, this protuberance facilitated frequent jokes. Perhaps the visual would have been too much of a reminder – too on the nose, if you will – for these patients who had to physically endure the pedicle and other invasive surgical techniques. But in written form, this vehicle for humour was sanctioned and could elicit a chuckle from patients who had experienced the traumatic procedure. The words used to describe, and to joke about, the tube pedicle trivialised it or made it ridiculous. But in the Guinea Pig Club's visual humour, the reality of the tube pedicle was obscured by eliding any representation of it at all.

Photography offers a different perspective. A black-and-white photograph held at the East Grinstead Museum (Figure 5.4) shows four Guinea Pigs with tube pedicles connecting their chests to their faces – three with tubes on their noses and one with a tube attached at the chin. The men are posing for the camera, two looking directly into the lens (one of them with a cigarette in his mouth), one looking down and smiling widely and one looking down in a more reserved manner. These four Guinea Pigs are all in the midst of surgical reconstruction at Queen Victoria Hospital in East Grinstead. They are situated in front of two pin-up posters, and at least two of them have signed the photograph. This is the type of photograph that now illustrates the East Grinstead Museum's website, and that made the rounds, approved of by their surgeon McIndoe, to newspapers and magazines as prominent and international as *Time*.[33] McIndoe was an 'extrovert publicity seeker'; although many have argued that this publicity was for the benefit of his patients, clearly

McIndoe's career saw positive outcomes from the visual and written coverage.[34] Some have called him a 'bully' who 'could and did crush his own staff, his patients, and their families' – and therefore a level of coercion can certainly be read into some of these jokes and publicity photographs.[35] This surgeon-approved photograph not only clearly shows the tube pedicle in use, and attached to the bodies of patients, but the surgical process is framed in a sociable manner – with smiles, signatures and pin-up posters. While the world saw the Guinea Pig Club through these photographs approved of by their surgeon and their hospital administration – and perhaps even by some of the patients, as evidenced by the signatures – the club members themselves expressed their experiences of tube pedicles less visually in their patient magazine cartoons.

The pin-ups in this photograph lead to a final question regarding patients' relationships to tube pedicle humour: did the discomfort in visually representing the tube pedicle in patient-produced visuals have something to do with its phallic shape? In addition to the fact that the tube pedicle made the patients' facial differences even more apparent and dramatic, the particular contours of this surgical technique may have influenced their hesitancy to depict it. As stated by Bakhtin in his major text on Rabelais and the grotesque, historically 'the nose had usually this link with the phallus'.[36] Sander Gilman has shown that this association continued into the nineteenth and twentieth centuries.[37] Perhaps the images of the exaggeratedly phallic temporary tube pedicle nose made this connection too obvious and this grotesque humour too visceral and personal. Part of the potential embarrassment around this surgical object was that the pedicle made the flaccid ridiculousness of the phallus readily apparent (also apparent in the name of The Dangle 'Ums Club), placed prominently on the faces of these men who are then thereby made less sexually desirable while wearing the pedicle. Additionally, in this period in which the Guinea Pig Club was being established and *The Guinea Pig* was being published, plastic surgeons – particularly Gillies – were pioneering the phalloplasty (plastic surgery of the penis) for both injury repair and for gender confirmation surgery.[38] While these men may not have known it, in the 1940s and 1950s similar techniques that were used to reconstruct their faces were also being used to create or reconstruct penises.

The Guinea Pig Club was an intensely masculine space, with the humour of laddish schoolboys pervading the wards, and jokes about sexual virility or at the expense of women working in the hospital were not out of the norm. McIndoe required his nurses 'to be attractive, have a sense of humour, be flirtatious, and never show distaste at men's appearance'.[39] Sexual coercion and assault were commonplace within this ward of men operating both under the literal protection of 'the Boss' McIndoe and under the semantic protection of the pranks and jokes in which this harassment was often cloaked.[40]

Perhaps the emasculating effect of the tube pedicle is why the four men photographed in Figure 5.4 posed in front of pin-up posters: if their masculinity was to be in part questioned by their tube pedicles, then their heterosexuality and virility could be asserted visually in another way.[41] This mirrors, in a more innocuous manner, how actively or previously tube-pedicled men engaged in sexually predatory acts tinged with humour 'to prove that they were still masculine, virile and dominant'. Jasmine Wood has argued that this was done in part 'to cope with the embarrassment of being dependent on female caregivers', but I suggest that it was also in response to the emasculating ridiculousness of having phallic 'sausages' immovable upon their faces for weeks at a time.[42]

This article has thus far positioned patients at the bottom of the hospital power hierarchy by dint of their medical vulnerability, immobility and perceived visual difference, and the ridiculousness caused by the tube pedicle. But these facial injury patients' assertion of masculinity through sexual jokes and assault of the women working on their wards show that the power relations in this medicalised context are complex and dynamic and that humour had the potential to invert typical or expected hierarchies.

Conclusion

As a piece of flesh that is simultaneously of, and removed from, a patient's body, the tube pedicle inhabits an uncomfortable position within the identity and subjective experience of plastic surgery patients in mid-century Britain. The discomfort surrounding this traumatic bodily sculpture protruding incongruously from the injured patient's body could be and was turned into a joke. But, as with all jokes, the positionality of the teller is a vital part of analysing the power and purpose of the humour. When it came to tube pedicles, Gillies could irreverently joke about the tube of flesh in a way that also included the patient's body. Orpen made similar jokes, but without incorporating the vulnerable body of the patient in her humour. Instead, the tube pedicle was metaphorically severed in her drawings, becoming more like a cartoon character in its own right. The patients who wore these pedicles for days, weeks or months excised the procedure from their visual humour, rendering it invisible. Rather than dwelling on the visual grotesquery of surgically manufactured flesh that had adorned their bodies, they instead focused on the written hilarity that the tube pedicle could provoke.

Considerations of power in humour are ever more fraught when the imbalances of authority in the joke are navigated at the sensitive point of a patient's body. When patients banter about their surgeries and disfigurements, they can, at least outwardly, distance themselves from the physical traumas and alien surgical technologies being used on their bodies. The very present and in many ways legendary senses of humour of plastic surgeons like Gillies and McIndoe may be read as a type of genial coercion to encourage wartime stoicism in their patients. The jokes they made at the expense of tube pedicles, and by extension their patients' bodies, could be interpreted as encouraging their patients to do the same: to not bother themselves about the uncomfortable, phallic, bizarre bit of their own flesh attached to their face, but to joke about it instead. While many patients did appreciate the light-hearted atmosphere of the surgical wards, for others it felt oppressive or forced. And while many of the patients seem to have successfully processed their traumas, physical or otherwise, through visual and written humour, it may be that surgeons saw and visualised humour where patients did not: in the tube pedicle.

Humour plays upon and results in emotion, which is influenced by the status and power of the joker, the listener and the butt of the joke. Surgeons had access to patients' bodies through surgery, through photography and through publication. Artists still held a certain power – such as the ability to see and observe procedures – over the patients. But Orpen's position as someone without instrumental power means that her jokes were more democratic than those coming from the surgeons. And finally, patients – even at their most vulnerable – could exercise agency by choosing how to convey humour about their surgical processes, and by choosing which parts of their medicalised bodies or experiences to highlight. But their often-sexual humour could subvert or upend the established hierarchy of the surgical ward in which caregivers – including nurses and surgical artists – had some physical and instructional power over patients. The examples in the final section of this chapter have shown how joking can, at least for a moment, create a new power structure. This chapter's three humorous case studies relating to this popular surgical procedure exhibit not only the role of art and humour in the everyday experiences of the hospital, but they also hint at the levels of comfort, power and agency felt by plastic surgery's different stakeholders.

Notes

1 Although many surgeons and historians now use the phrase 'tubed' pedicle, I use 'tube' pedicle, as this is what appears in my sources.

2 Tube pedicles are still used in some parts of the world. But overall, their popularity dwindled in the 1970s and 1980s. Klaas W. Marck et al., 'The tubed pedicle flap centennial: its concept, origin, rise and fall', *European Journal of Plastic Surgery* 40 (2017), 477. Harold Gillies, 'The tubed pedicle in plastic surgery', *The Lancet* (7 August 1920), 320. Jerome P. Webster, 'The early history of the tubed pedicle flap', *Surgical Clinics of North America* 39:2 (April 1959), 261–75.

3 Harold Gillies and Ralph Millard, Jr, *The Principles and Art of Plastic Surgery*, vol. 1 (Butterworth & Co., 1957), p. 225.

4 Marjorie Gehrhardt has written on the paternalistic aspects of Gillies's patient care in the First World War. Marjorie Gehrhardt, *The Men with Broken Faces: Gueules Cassées of the First World War* (Peter Lang, 2015), pp. 67–71.

5 Albert D. Davis, 'The principles and art of plastic surgery', *California Medicine* 87:1 (July 1957), 67.

6 Jerome Pierce Webster, Foreword to Harold Gillies and D. Ralph Millard, Jr, *The Principles and Art of Plastic Surgery*, vol. 1 (Butterworth & Co., 1957), p. xi.

7 See letter from Mark Bonham Carter to George Greenfield, Gilles's literary agent, 9 July 1957, Gillies's correspondence (Courtesy of Susie Winter). Referenced in: Andrew Bamji, *Faces from the Front: Harold Gillies, The Queen's Hospital, Sidcup, and the Origins of Modern Plastic Surgery* (Helion and Company, 2017), p. 131.
8 Webster, Foreword to *The Principles and Art of Plastic Surgery*, vol. 1, p. xii.
9 D. Ralph Millard, Jr, Preface to Harold Gillies and D. Ralph Millard, Jr, *The Principles and Art of Plastic Surgery*, vol. 1 (Butterworth & Co., 1957), p. xxiii.
10 Gillies and Millard, *The Principles and Art of Plastic Surgery*, vol. 1, p. 200.
11 Gillies and Millard, *The Principles and Art of Plastic Surgery*, vol. 1, p. 165.
12 Gillies and Millard, *The Principles and Art of Plastic Surgery*, vol. 1, pp. 35, 153. For another reference to tube pedicles as 'sausages': Hal G. Bingham and Charles E. Moore, 'Farewell to Queen's Hospital, Sidcup', *British Journal of Plastic Surgery* 29:4 (October 1976), 297–301.
13 Royal College of Surgeons of England, 'Gillies, Sir Harold Delf (1882–1960)', Plarr's Lives of the Fellows, https://livesonline.rcseng.ac.uk/client/en_GB/lives/search/results?qu=gillies&te=ASSET. Gillies wrote, 'One cannot leave the artists without a very honorable mention of the senior author's great-great-uncle–the immortal Edward Lear, one of whose drawings lends a "nosey" pointer to our work', Gillies, acknowledgments in *The Principles and Art of Plastic Surgery*, vol. 1: p. xix.
14 Gillies and Millard, *The Principles and Art of Plastic Surgery*, vol. 1, p. 1. The original Lear poem reads 'There was an Old Man on whose nose, most birds of the air could repose;/ But they all flew away at the closing of day,/ Which relieved that Old Man and his nose.' Victoria & Albert Museum, 'There was an Old Man on whose nose ...', V&A Images, https://www.vandaimages.com/preview.asp?image=2011FD9387&itemw=4&itemf=0001&itemstep=1&itemx=4 (accessed 9 May 2024).
15 Marck et al., 'The tubed pedicle flap centennial', 476.
16 Gillies and Millard, *The Principles and Art of Plastic Surgery*, vol. 1, pp. 37, 153.
17 Archibald McIndoe, 'The Maestro's Message: Speech given by President of the Guinea Pig Club, Sir Archibald H. McIndoe, C.B.E., M.S., M.Sc., F.R.C.S., F.A.C.S., at the Club's Seventh Annual Dinner, East Grinstead, 4th September, 1948', *The Guinea Pig* (Christmas 1948), 4.

18 Gillies and Millard, *The Principles and Art of Plastic Surgery*, vol. 1, p. 40.
19 Gillies and Millard, *The Principles and Art of Plastic Surgery*, vol. 1, p. 151.
20 For more on the incongruity theory, see this volume's Introduction.
21 Ana Carden-Coyne noted this in relation to Gillies's First World War ward. Ana Carden-Coyne, *The Politics of Wounds: Military Patients and Medical Power* (Oxford University Press, 2014), pp. 276–86.
22 Heather Laine Talley, *Saving Face: Disfigurement and the Politics of Appearance* (New York University Press, 2014), p. 10.
23 Andrew Bamji, 'Sir Harold Gillies: surgical pioneer', *Trauma* 8:3 (2006), 152.
24 Mikhail Bakhtin, *Rabelais and His World* (Indiana University Press, 1984), p. 62.
25 I argue elsewhere for the use of Orpen's drawings as convivial humorous relief in the traumatic surgical space in which she worked. Christine Slobogin, '"'E's a Funny Doctor": Dickie Orpen and the Visual Humour of the Second World War Reconstructive Surgery Ward', in Juliette Pattinson and Linsey Robb (eds), *British Humour and the Second World War: 'Keep Smiling Through'* (Bloomsbury, 2023), pp. 111–35.
26 Dickie Orpen, Sketchbook #7, 1943, BAPRAS/DSB 7.46-7.47, Archive of the British Association of Plastic, Reconstructive and Aesthetic Surgeons, London, UK.
27 Marie Allitt, *Medical Caregiving Narratives of the First World War: Geographies of Care* (Edinburgh University Press, 2023), p. 27.
28 Alexander Baldwin, 'Archibald McIndoe's stance against the clinical hospital archetype and the importance of this for the recovery of burnt airmen in the Second World War', *Hektoen International* 8:4 (Spring 2017), https://hekint.org/2017/01/22/archibald-mcindoes-stance-against-the-clinical-hospital-archetype-and-the-importance-of-this-for-the-recovery-of-burnt-airmen-in-the-second-world-war/. John N. Barron, 'McIndoe the Gentle Giant', *Annals of the Royal College of Surgeons of England*, 67:3 (1985), 205. Simon Robert Millar, 'Rooksdown House and the Rooksdown Club: A Study into the Rehabilitation of Facially Disfigured Servicemen and Civilians Following the Second World War' (PhD thesis, Institute of Historical Research, University of London, 2015), pp. 275–82.
29 Emily Mayhew published the primary history of The Guinea Pig Club in 2004, and released an updated version in 2018. Emily Mayhew, *The Reconstruction of Warriors: Archibald McIndoe, the Royal Air Force and the Guinea Pig Club* (Greenhill Books, 2004). Simon Millar has

written a PhD thesis on Rooksdown Club, a similar club based at Park Prewett Hospital. Millar, 'Rooksdown House and the Rooksdown Club' (PhD thesis, Institute of Historical Research, University of London, 2015).

30 Brenda McBryde, *A Nurse's War* (Hogarth Press, 1979), p. 60.

31 'Ghost Story for Guinea Pigs: As True as I'm Standing Here ...', *The Guinea Pig* (December 1947), 6–7. LBY E.81/320.1, Imperial War Museum Archive, London, UK.

32 *The Guinea Pig* (August 1948), 6. LBY E.81/320.1, Imperial War Museum Archive, London, UK.

33 An example of an international magazine article about McIndoe: 'Medicine: The Man Who Makes Faces', *Time*, 27 September 1948, https://time.com/archive/6776460/medicine-the-man-who-makes-faces/.

34 Murray C. Meikle, *Reconstructing Faces: The Art and Wartime Surgery of Gillies, Pickerill, McIndoe, and Mowlem* (Otago University Press, 2013), p. 142.

35 Mayhew, *The Reconstruction of Warriors*, p. 75.

36 Bakhtin, *Rabelais and His World*, p. 87.

37 Sander Gilman, *Creating Beauty to Cure the Soul: Race and Psychology in the Shaping of Aesthetic Surgery* (Duke University Press, 1998), p. 63.

38 Gillies and Millard, *The Principles and Art of Plastic Surgery*, vol. 2, pp. 376–84.

39 Jasmine Wood, '"Lashings of Grog and Girls": Masculinity and sexuality in the rehabilitation of facially disfigured servicemen in the Second World War', *War & Society* 40:4 (2021), 12.

40 Liz Byrski, 'Emotional labour as war work: Women up close and personal with McIndoe's Guinea Pigs', *Women's History Review* 21:3 (2012), 241–61. For more on McIndoe's nickname 'The Boss': Edward Bishop, *The Guinea Pig Club* (Macmillan, 1963); Mayhew, *The Reconstruction of Warriors*, p. 75.

41 For more on masculinity and facial injury in the First World War, see: Joanna Bourke, *Dismembering the Male: Men's Bodies, Britain and the Great War* (Reaktion Books, 1996). Eilis H.L. Boyle, '"An Uglier Duckling than before": Reclaiming agency and visibility amongst facially-wounded ex-servicemen in Britain after the First World War', *ALTER, European Journal of Disability Research* 13:4 (2019), 308–22. Anthea Callen, 'Masculinity and Monstrosity: The Body in Pieces', in *Looking at Men: Anatomy, Masculinity and the Modern Male Body* (Yale University Press, 2018).

42 Wood, '"Lashings of Grog and Girls"', 15.

References

Allitt, Marie. *Medical Caregiving Narratives of the First World War: Geographies of Care*. Edinburgh University Press, 2023.

Bakhtin, Mikhail. *Rabelais and His World*. Indiana University Press, 1984.

Baldwin, Alexander. 'Archibald McIndoe's stance against the clinical hospital archetype and the importance of this for the recovery of burnt airmen in the Second World War'. *Hektoen International* 8:4 (Spring 2017). https://hekint.org/2017/01/22/archibald-mcindoes-stance-against-the-clinical-hospital-archetype-and-the-importance-of-this-for-the-recovery-of-burnt-airmen-in-the-second-world-war/.

Bamji, Andrew. *Faces from the Front: Harold Gillies, The Queen's Hospital, Sidcup, and the Origins of Modern Plastic Surgery*. Helion and Company, 2017.

Bamji, Andrew. 'Sir Harold Gillies: surgical pioneer'. *Trauma* 8:3 (2006), 143–56.

Barron, John N. 'McIndoe the Gentle Giant'. *Annals of the Royal College of Surgeons of England* 67:3 (1985), 203–6.

Bingham, Hal G., and Charles E. Moore. 'Farewell to Queen's Hospital, Sidcup'. *British Journal of Plastic Surgery* 29:4 (October 1976), 297–301.

Bishop, Edward. *The Guinea Pig Club*. Macmillan, 1963.

Bourke, Joanna. *Dismembering the Male: Men's Bodies, Britain and the Great War*. Reaktion Books, 1996.

Boyle, Eilis H.L. '"An Uglier Duckling than before": Reclaiming agency and visibility amongst facially wounded ex-servicemen in Britain after the First World War'. *ALTER, European Journal of Disability Research* 13 (2019), 308–22.

Byrski, Liz. 'Emotional labour as war work: Women up close and personal with McIndoe's guinea pigs'. *Women's History Review* 21:3 (2012), 241–61.

Callen, Anthea. 'Masculinity and Monstrosity: The Body in Pieces'. In *Looking at Men: Anatomy, Masculinity and the Modern Male Body*. Yale University Press, 2018.

Carden-Coyne, Ana. *The Politics of Wounds: Military Patients and Medical Power*. Oxford University Press, 2014.

Davis, Albert D. 'The principles and art of plastic surgery'. *California Medicine* 87:1 (n.d.), 67.

'Ghost Story for Guinea Pigs: As True as I'm Standing Here ...'. *The Guinea Pig*. December 1947. LBY E.81/320.1, Imperial War Museum Archive, London, UK.

Gehrhardt, Marjorie. *The Men with Broken Faces: Gueules Cassées of the First World War*. Peter Lang, 2015.

Gillies, Harold. 'The tubed pedicle in plastic surgery'. *The Lancet*, 7 August 1920, 320.

Gillies, Harold, and D. Ralph Millard, Jr. *The Principles and Art of Plastic Surgery*. Vols 1 and 2. Butterworth & Co., 1957.

Gilman, Sander. *Creating Beauty to Cure the Soul: Race and Psychology in the Shaping of Aesthetic Surgery*. Duke University Press, 1998.

The Guinea Pig. August 1948. LBY E.81/320.1, Imperial War Museum Archive, London, UK.

Marck, Klaas W., Roman Palyvoda, Andrew Bamji and Jan J. van Wingerden. 'The tubed pedicle flap centennial: Its concept, origin, rise and fall'. *European Journal of Plastic Surgery* 40 (2017), 473–8.

Mayhew, Emily. *The Reconstruction of Warriors: Archibald McIndoe, the Royal Air Force and the Guinea Pig Club*. Greenhill Books, 2004.

McBryde, Brenda. *A Nurse's War*. Hogarth Press, 1979.

McIndoe, Archibald. 'The Maestro's Message: Speech given by President of the Guinea Pig Club, Sir Archibald H. McIndoe, C.B.E., M.S., M.Sc., F.R.C.S., F.A.C.S., at the Club's Seventh Annual Dinner, East Grinstead, 4th September 1948'. *The Guinea Pig*, Christmas 1948.

'Medicine: The Man Who Makes Faces'. *Time*. 27 September 1948. https://time.com/archive/6776460/medicine-the-man-who-makes-faces/.

Meikle, Murray C. *Reconstructing Faces: The Art and Wartime Surgery of Gillies, Pickerill, McIndoe, and Mowlem*. Otago University Press, 2013.

Millar, Simon Robert. 'Rooksdown House and the Rooksdown Club: A Study into the Rehabilitation of Facially Disfigured Servicemen and Civilians Following the Second World War'. PhD thesis, Institute of Historical Research, University of London, 2015.

Millard Jr, D. Ralph. 'Preface'. In Harold Gillies and D. Ralph Millard, Jr, *The Principles and Art of Plastic Surgery*, p. xxiii. Butterworth & Co., 1957.

Orpen, Dickie. Sketchbook #7, 1943. BAPRAS/DSB 7.46-7.47, Archive of the British Association of Plastic, Reconstructive and Aesthetic Surgeons, London, UK.

Royal College of Surgeons of England. 'Gillies, Sir Harold Delf (1882–1960)'. *Plarr's Lives of the Fellows* (blog), n.d. https://livesonline.rcseng.ac.uk/client/en_GB/lives/search/results?qu=gillies&te=ASSET.

Slobogin, Christine. '"'E's a Funny Doctor": Dickie Orpen and the Visual Humour of the Second World War Reconstructive Surgery Ward'. In Juliette Pattinson and Linsey Robb (eds), *British Humour and the Second World War: 'Keep Smiling Through'*, 111–35. Bloomsbury, 2023.

Talley, Heather Laine. *Saving Face: Disfigurement and the Politics of Appearance*. New York University Press, 2014.

Victoria & Albert Museum. 'There Was an Old Man on Whose Nose …'. https://www.vandaimages.com/preview.asp?image=2011FD9387&ite

mw=4&itemf=0001&itemstep=1&itemx=4. *V&A Images* (blog), n.d. (accessed 9 May 2024).

Webster, Jerome P. 'The early history of the tubed pedicle flap'. *Surgical Clinics of North America* 39:2 (April 1959), 261–75.

Webster, Jerome P. 'Foreword'. In Harold Gillies and D. Ralph Millard, Jr, *The Principles and Art of Plastic Surgery*, pp. ix–xii. Butterworth & Co., 1957.

Wood, Jasmine. '"Lashings of Grog and Girls": Masculinity and sexuality in the rehabilitation of facially disfigured servicemen in the Second World War'. *War & Society* (October 2021), 1–19.

6

The bittersweet look(s) of AIDS: Consuming the ironic waste of HIV/AIDS imagery (and other butts of the joke) in *Diseased Pariah News*

Jo Michael Rezes

Photographs of suffering offer an intimacy unrivaled by other images.[1]
– Kimberly Juanita Brown

'The rectum is a mixing bowl!'
for a rich medley of disease –
chosen-family favorites,
made for multiple guests with ease.[2]
– Michael Scarce

What a waste!

Tom 'Tommy' Shearer, one of the co-founders and editors of the zine *Diseased Pariah News* (*DPN*), died in his hospital room at the Kaiser Permanente hospital in San Francisco on 8 April 1991. In Issue #3 of *DPN* (Shearer died in the middle of editing the second), his co-founder Beowulf '[Our] Cranky Editor' Thorne, wrote a stylised obituary, published under the glib title 'Darn! One of Our Editors is Dead!' Thorne humorously chronicles the day – from the 'bonding experience of cleaning yogurt from [Shearer's] oxygen hose' the evening before, to the near faux pas of insulting his deceased friend that late, spring morning: 'your colors look terrible! How did you get so jaundiced overnight?'[3] At the age of 33, having dedicated his HIV+ years to writing, editing and curating stories, poems, art and jokes about living with the virus, Tommy lost his battle with AIDS.

True to *DPN*'s style, photographer Marc Geller documents a very different battle, a physical fight between friends, just two weeks prior on 26 March 1991.[4] This one is staged. In a series of portraits, Thorne poses next to Shearer in a hospital bed where the two gay men smile, and gazes directed down the barrel of the lens. Without the medical context, I would assume these are headshots for an editorial feature. As I flick through the negatives at the GLBT Historical Society Archives in San Francisco in their filmic order,[5] the authorial figures begin to play-wrestle (Figure 6.1). Thorne 'strangles' Shearer with his own nasal cannula. In another scene, Shearer poses like a centrefold model (Figure 6.2). This proverbial boudoir series is all enacted near sympathy plants and a bottle of Gatorade. The tone is clear. Even as his body shows signs of disease in front of the camera, Shearer is still performing for his loving audience. For *DPN*'s readers (and critics), most of whom are HIV+ or living with AIDS, this end-of-life visual sees Shearer self-represent not as a 'wasting away' martyr, victim or butt of the joke, but as a sexy, so-alive comedian (who has, admittedly, lost a bit of weight).

Geller photographed the editors of *Diseased Pariah News* for an interview in *The Advocate*, published less than a month after

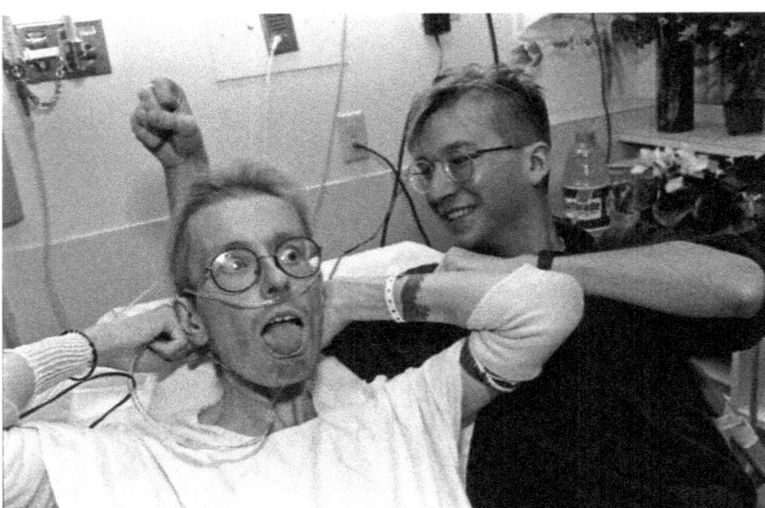

Figure 6.1 Marc Geller, *Untitled*, scan from artist's print.

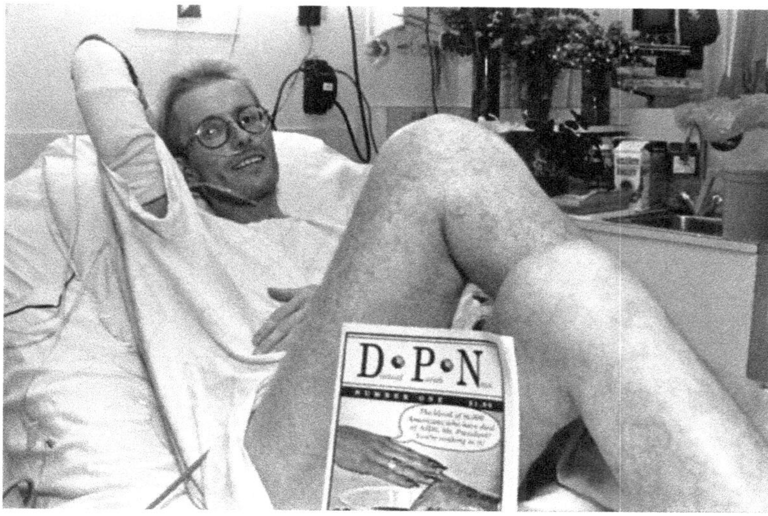

Figure 6.2 Marc Geller, *Tom Shearer*, 1991, scan from photo negative.

Shearer's death (in the infamous X-rated Madonna issue) on 7 May 1991.[6] Though many of the images never appeared in print within the eleven-issue run of *DPN* (1990–99), a strip of negatives were reproduced alongside Shearer's obituary written by Thorne: close-ups of his drawn face, hands clasped gently by his cheeks – as if posing for a glamour shot. His soft smile is framed by wickedly cool arm tattoos and Kaposi's sarcoma lesions which might be considered (by those not in on the jokes which fill *DPN*) to be tasteless. Despite the familiar black-and-white style of Geller's hospital bed portraits, these images defy the sub-genre of visual documentation of HIV/AIDS made famous by the likes of Gideon Mendel, Nicholas Nixon and Nan Goldin due to their ironic tone.[7] No visual foil to Geller's work is clearer than that of Therese Frare's 'David Kirby on his deathbed, Ohio, 1990'. This photograph features the 32-year-old activist in a similar setting to Shearer: laid out on a hospice bed, his body thinned by disease, comforted by loved ones. Kirby's eyes, however, are famously locked upward on something in the middle distance – beyond the present, beyond comprehension. His expression haunts the generations of families who have cared for loved ones with AIDS. Here, the effects of wasting syndrome are seen (and felt) somewhere between anguish and enlightenment. Geller's photographs, and the performances of the editors, similarly blur the lines of affect, though for Tom Shearer, grief and humour traverse the emotional spectrum. The most stirring images of AIDS arouse visual and emotional ambiguity within extant public discourses around the virus. However, as Susan Sontag notes, 'what determines the possibility of being affected morally by photographs is the existence of a relevant political consciousness'.[8] These photographs exist within complex emotional and political contexts, either affirming or challenging a viewer's beliefs on AIDS and its effects on the body, the family and the public.

I do not reproduce the image of Kirby on his deathbed, the 'photo that changed the face of AIDS', at the behest of Frare.[9] The artist lives up to her promise of never using the image for profit and has stated to me, in an act of understatement, that 'the photo has been seen many times'.[10] Kirby's family, however, did not fret about the image's continued circulation. They saw its power not only in commemorating his life, but in challenging the stigma of AIDS at a time when few were willing to look directly at its consequences. When the global fashion retailer Benetton repurposed the image for a 1992 advertisement (logo included), controversy erupted over its supposed exploitation of grief. Kirby's father Bill understood things differently; 'Benetton is not using us, we're using Benetton', he stated, amid his fight to raise awareness around HIV and honour his late son.[11] Thinking with Sontag's claim that a photograph's moral force does not reside solely in its content but in the political consciousness of those who witness it, the image of Kirby invites feeling – but more importantly, it demands context. Its continued circulation is contingent upon the ethical terms of its reception. Frare's refusal to commodify the image mirrors this sensibility: it is not the image alone, but the conditions of its viewing that shape its affective charge.

Benetton's then creative director Oliviero Toscani understood the image of Kirby to signify 'Jesus Christ … dying of AIDS'. But, for Toscani, this black-and-white photograph was not 'realistic' until it was colourised.[12] Toscani's desire to augment the image's emotional realism – by reintroducing the colour drained from

Frare's original photograph – reinforces Sontag's warning about the aestheticisation of suffering: 'To suffer is one thing; another thing is living with the photographed images of suffering.'[13] Photographs that evoke pathos can, in their repetition and stylisation, dull their moral urgency – in Sontag's words, 'images anesthetize'.[14] Has the image of Kirby retained its charge? Has its emotional impact been numbed through oversaturation (pun intended)? Visual power stems not from beauty or even grief alone, but from its anchoring in an activated political consciousness – one shaped by queer caregiving, AIDS activism and the family's own insistence on visibility. The reality of wider publics circulating and consuming images of those dying from AIDS, like Frare's iconic photograph, grounds my chapter, offering much-needed political context for the work of *Diseased Pariah News*.

I begin with Marc Geller's photographs of Tom Shearer and Beowulf Thorne before delving into the visual lifespan of *DPN* to ask: was their hospital room photoshoot a direct act of satire? The 'AIDS' joke they set up is one where David Kirby is not the butt of the joke, no. Rather, the public is. This is an inside joke for those living with HIV and/or AIDS. In staging a fight in portraiture, they too attempt to capture a more 'realistic' look of AIDS: a bittersweet suite of photographs, 're-colorised' with laughter, smiles and gags, like strangling a sick man to death with his own oxygen tube. The peaceful, emotionally ambiguous quality of Frare's photograph is rescripted as the editors humorously critique the visual representation of AIDS across public and medical discourses alike. As the two men play together in their grief, I wonder if they thought of David Kirby staring up at the ceiling, lost and alone in his pain. Did they find irony in that he was surrounded by family, suffering more loudly around him? What a waste! What a different final image of David Kirby we would have if he was invited to their deathbed party! What if wasting bodies were not merely 'images of horror' proliferated! What if those with AIDS died how they wanted to – their bodies depicted on their own terms and not for public consumption?

In this chapter, I turn to case studies found in the Oakland, California-based zine *Diseased Pariah News*, to better understand how HIV/AIDS is illustrated into bodies and photographed for consumption. This publication, 'by, for, and about' people with AIDS, archives the ways in which (predominantly white) gay men navigate depictions of their bodies while living with the virus.[15] Through Thorne's creative direction and his collaborations with political illustrator Kira Od (and others), I explore how 'wasting syndrome' and other 'looks' of AIDS affect sexuality and desire in the bodies of gay people. Following my modes of inquiry into physical archives around this project, I wind case studies through the bowels of AIDS photographic history. I first establish a micro-history of the 'AIDS body' in the cultural imaginary and academic discourses. Specifically, I analyse how the artists and editors of *Diseased Pariah News* exist within (and buck) global visual narratives of symptomatic and suffering (re: wasting) bodies through their staging of jokes. Next, I pull out for a closer look at the anus – that is, I establish how DPN's artists feature butts in their ironic bodily representations of AIDS: as sites of both pleasure and pain, good taste and waste, liberation and potential contamination. I then end this chapter returning to Marc Geller's photography of Tom Shearer in his hospital bed.

After Shearer's passing, Thorne continued to lead the zine until his own untimely death, before the release of the eleventh and final issue. Threat of contagion follows the many appearances of 'AIDS bodies', even his own. The creators of *DPN* address this nuance through comic strips, illustrations and a popular cooking column, 'GET FAT, don't die!' The featured column, with bylines by Biffy Mae (a drag character created and sustained by Thorne), attends to readership questions regarding weight loss in People with AIDS (PWAs), offering comedic self-help style advice for combating nausea, avoiding acid reflux and gaining weight through high-calorie diets. Building on theories of humour in HIV/AIDS circulated media, *DPN*'s strength of community building for audiences is in camp: '[their] prime mode is in fact humor … [not] simple "levity", but instead … a biting, even a bitter, edge'.[16] The visual gags – about survival, food and sex (anal and oral) – are sprinkled throughout the issues, featuring 'wasting' bodies due to AIDS. The humour at the core of *DPN* is based in acts of collective care, intimacies of shared aesthetics and experience, but who is at the *butt* of the joke?

'What does a person with AIDS look like?'

Visual changes, or perceived aesthetic shifts, in those living with AIDS trigger phobias and panic among broader publics. Kaposi's sarcoma (cancerous, purple lesions), 'wasting syndrome' (bodies succumbing to malnutrition), 'AZT Butt' (weight loss due to the prevailing antiviral side-effects) and more appear in and on the performing bodies of those living with HIV/AIDS. Images are circulated worldwide in photojournalism and safer sex pamphlets which warn the public about the threat of AIDS on their families and lives. Owing to the repeated association of image and action, the 'AIDS body' becomes synonymous with the 'gay body' within American culture: 'the most pervasive image of AIDS remains the bedridden, emaciated "homosexual body"; weight loss means something very different in American culture when its subject is a gay man'.[17]

Historically, 'wasting' has marked a body in decline across multiple diseases – tuberculosis, syphilis and even cancer – where visible emaciation signified loss: of life, of agency, of the moral self. In the late nineteenth and early twentieth centuries, tuberculosis was so common among poor and racialised populations that physicians dubbed its manifestations in Black communities 'Black tuberculosis', a racialised variant of the 'White Plague' that reinforced hierarchies of purity.[18] These earlier associations between thinness, contagion and deviance primed the public imagination for later readings of HIV/AIDS, where visible wasting again indexed both illness and perceived moral decline. What happens when the visual signification of AIDS is attributed to weight loss in communities of white gay men in coastal cities in the United States? Where is attention to care turned? How do HIV and AIDS become (de)racialised and sexualised through imagery?

The image of the 'AIDS body' within the United States is constructed in parallel to the circulation of images featuring sick and malnourished images of African people (especially children) during the 1960s and 1970s with Biafran War photography.[19] The colonial gaze re-emerged with further imagery of wasting bodies triggered by 'slim disease' in Africa during the onset of the HIV/AIDS epidemic – geographically grounding images of 'AIDS' symptoms within (and from) 'Africa'. Cindy Patton, in *Globalizing AIDS* (2002), argues that mapped webs of logic around geography, bodies and AIDS result in power dynamics across the social order, rendering bodies (regardless of HIV status) racialised and sexualised due to layered associations of virus. Patton navigates the specific othering of African bodies, as wrapped up in 'epidemiological thinking' of stereotypes of place (i.e. if AIDS originated in Africa, Black bodies must be prone to carry AIDS). Patton argues that these stereotypes of 'African AIDS' are easily perpetuated through logics of racism and space, when the ideology is lodged in '*I don't live/go there*' or '*I'm not one of those*' thought frameworks.[20] Through her work, Patton distinctively marks the globalisation of the HIV/AIDS crisis as one that must also contend with the virus's inherent racialisation. These discourses do not merely reflect public health messaging; they are sustained by the repetition of specific images – emaciated, wasting bodies that mark the 'AIDS body' as a racialised figure. As such, visual manifestations of wasting syndrome – losing weight, attempts to gain weight, etc. – cannot be viewed outside of the racialised history of disease and foreign aid.

As Sontag reminds us, in *On Photography*, needing 'to have reality confirmed and experience enhanced by photographs is an aesthetic consumerism to which everyone is now addicted'.[21] The photographic image is more than documentation; it becomes a substitute for direct experience, a visual surrogate for empathy. The desire to *see* suffering becomes entangled with its consumption. Likewise, Kimberly Juanita Brown, in her essay 'Regarding the Pain of the Other', builds on Sontag's arguments, interrogating how visual representations of Black suffering in famine and war photography induce a type of affective transfer. She argues that there is a racialised violence of *looking* – where the Black body is too often read as a suffering object, its visibility tied to its disposability. 'Images of famine', for Brown, do not merely show symptoms of violence on bodies, but 'reiterate the rhetoric of human "wasting" – people discarded by other people like waste, and bodies wasting away from malnourishment'.[22] Following Brown, I argue that representations of bodily wasting associated with AIDS-related complications continues this rhetoric of disposability. As more images of 'wasting syndrome' are consumed, the more physical and symbolic violence is done towards those showing signs of disease.

This concept is illustrated by Lukas Engelmann in his chapter 'Seeing Bodies with AIDS'. Engelmann argues that the optics of the AIDS epidemic began (around 1981) as a crisis of representation where doctors, gay men and wider publics were seeking visual clarity around the virus: 'grasping, defining and seeing the "person with AIDS" was the single most important way to perceive the epidemic in its first decade'.[23] Medical publications like *A Colour Atlas of AIDS* (1986) used clinical photography to portray symptoms, notably Kaposi's sarcoma, as diagnostic tools rather than as portraits of individuals. Engelmann notes that these photographs 'were not included to strengthen a public empathy with persons who had developed AIDS, nor was their purpose to raise public awareness of the disastrous effects of the disease'.[24] Thorne himself was a fan of the *Colour Atlas of AIDS*, using the shocking images as inspiration for his own drawings, especially later in the eleven-issue run of *DPN*. Gay activists in organisations like Survive AIDS (formerly the AIDS Coalition to Unleash Power (ACT UP) Golden Gate) operated in the San Francisco Bay Area like the writers of *Diseased Pariah News*. Many of their visual public health warnings, found in a series of posters all beginning with the phrase 'THIS COULD BE YOU[R] ...' feature patients with wasting syndrome, perivulval and perianal herpes simplex, papilliferous tumours on a penis and a severe case of shingles.[25] Graphic medical images of 'wasted' or otherwise symptomatic bodies were eventually deployed in these 'scare tactic' interpolations.

The 'look of AIDS' is transposed from such instances of photographic capture, echoed in public health illustrations and marketing through the early 1990s. One such instance, a graphic with many copycats found across HIV/AIDS public health archives, centres a core philosophical (and physiological) question: 'What Does a Person with AIDS Look Like?'[26] In this circulated poster, starving Black bodies are staged in children's school-book-style boxes with descriptors like 'AIDS or Malnutrition?' and 'AIDS or Cancer?' to highlight the conflation that many diseases (especially viruses) have in their effects on the body. These drawings are designed to stir viewers, to warn them of the potential harm caused by AIDS.

Depictions out of African countries, in this instance Uganda, prompt viewers to draw a conclusion that AIDS does not 'look' one way, rather 'AIDS can look like many diseases'. Semiotically, this implies that AIDS and other diseases do in fact 'look' similar, and that the *look* is based on the bodily features of emaciated Black figures. These materials were circulated and consumed by Western audiences concurrently to famine photography, thus a circumscribed 'look' to AIDS pervades the (white) cultural imaginary.

Conversely, the Center for Disease Control and Prevention (CDC) ran a multiracial campaign where 'healthy-looking' adults (not visually symptomatic) stand in front of a portrait background, smiling with their eyes directed towards the viewer with a tagline: 'They show all the signs of having HIV.' In this campaign, AIDS 'looks' like a type of 'idealized "self" – healthy, empowered and possessing options'; these figures are full of hope, gently cautioning viewers.[27] Engelmann argues that this visual shift is due to the 'growing availability of anti-retroviral treatment [and] photography of people with HIV infections[, which] became invested in picturing healthy, normal, and capable persons, with bodies that have "HIV under control"'.[28] In this way, an American and/or European body with AIDS is presumed to be 'healthy-looking', and when bodies deviate from that look – white or otherwise – therein lies a crisis of representation.

Through the 1990s, AIDS photography moved from focusing on visible symptoms in Western gay men to visualising risk in global health contexts – notably poverty, sex work and maternal transmission: 'AIDS photography accordingly diversified to become a practice as complex and manifold as the epidemic.'[29] These frames are crucial to understanding how photographs like Frare's widely circulated image of Kirby – a white, gay man dying of AIDS, surrounded by family – unsettled white American visual norms. The photo was lauded as 'the photo that changed the face of AIDS', precisely because it redirected the public gaze away from imagined racialised others toward the domestic, white, middle-class interior. As Kimberly Juanita Brown notes, proximity (visual, emotional, racial) reshapes how suffering is received: certain bodies become more grievable, more worthy of public mourning.[30] HIV transmission, the threat of AIDS to white, straight, middle-class families, becomes synonymous with Black African bodies. I frame bodily figurations within *DPN* as manifestations of the global impact of HIV/AIDS on weight loss, connecting their readers with the ongoing realities of living with HIV/AIDS in the 1990s (and their own internalised phobias). Predominantly white audiences (and mostly white creators) of the zine grapple with food insecurities and the effects of HIV/AIDS in the Greater San Francisco Bay Area. Through humour, they negotiate external constructions of the 'AIDS body', disrupting and disintegrating public perception away from a monolith, but there are limits to *DPN's* brand of camp.

For the editors of *DPN*, sympathetic portraits – like Frare's (and even Geller's) – were not sufficient in relaying the truth of living with AIDS to an avid gay readership. Nor were the medicalised photographs or 'scare tactic' illustrations viable for their publication. Thorne is credited with illustrating most of the comics in *DPN*, finding joy in politically incorrect (though bitingly political) humour. Taking an art form conventionally reserved for the most conservative and restrained American families over Sunday breakfast, the editors, illustrators and contributors make an inflammatory, dark humour zine, peppered with flippant and casual references to, and representations of people's relationships with, death. 'The cremains of your Dusty Deaditor (Tom Shearer)… have been ground up and mixed into the ink of this issue', Thorne declares in Issue #5,[31] with accusatory illustrations of conservative men dying from disease ('the thought is positively un-Christian!')[32] and hundreds of deliberately vulgar features littered elsewhere in the eleven issues.

The artwork laughs in the face of disease and despair, with articles like 'Top Ten Ways to Avoid Bruises from Sitting with a Bony Ass' and 'Pariah Chase: Hunting Serocloseted Republicans' (Figure 6.3), helping to shift the 'look of AIDS' away from outsider gazes or social diagnoses. Figure 6.3 appears in Issue #7 (1992), with the comic illustrations drawn by Thorne. I place Thorne's illustrations in the same category as the 'underground comix' styles of the 1960s and 1970s, which pushed forward social commentary through adult themes and conflated youthful drawings with serious political content. Not unlike the 'look of AIDS' being illustrated in cartoon imagery of emaciated Black Ugandan bodies in posters,

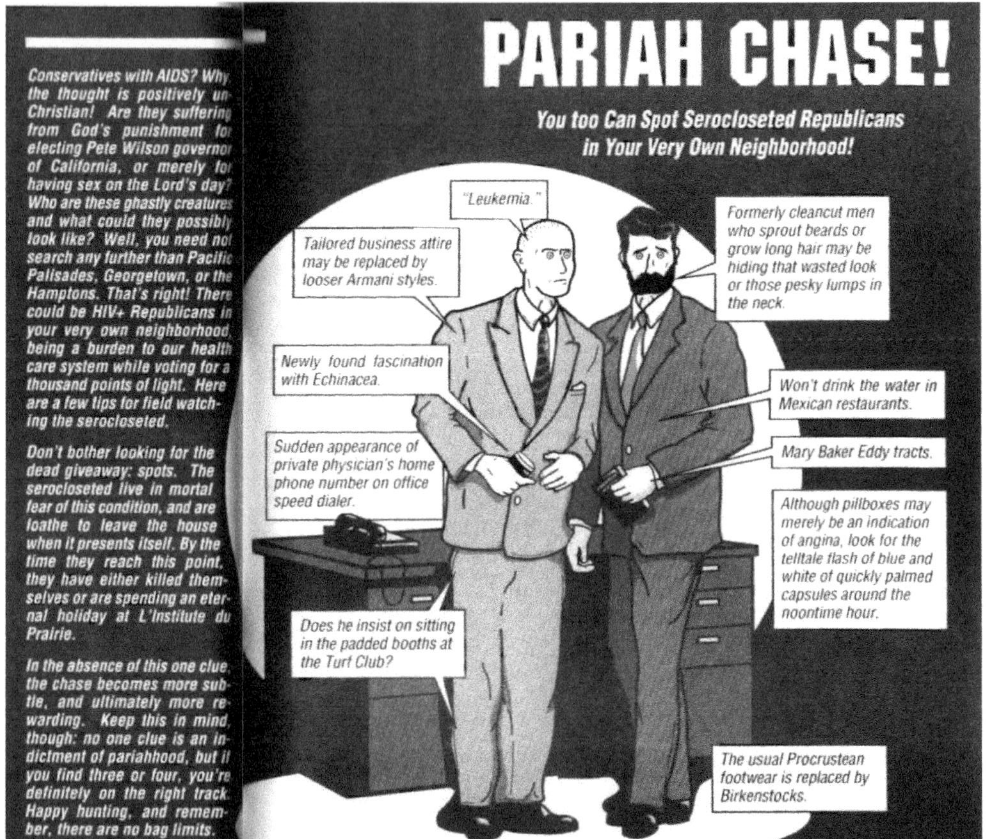
PARIAH CHASE!
You too Can Spot Serocloseted Republicans in Your Very Own Neighborhood!
Conservatives with AIDS? Why, the thought is positively un-Christian! Are they suffering from God's punishment for electing Pete Wilson governor of California, or merely for having sex on the Lord's day? Who are these ghastly creatures and what could they possibly look like? Well, you need not search any further than Pacific Palisades, Georgetown, or the Hamptons. That's right! There could be HIV+ Republicans in your very own neighborhood, being a burden to our health care system while voting for a thousand points of light. Here are a few tips for field watching the serocloseted.
Don't bother looking for the dead giveaway: spots. The serocloseted live in mortal fear of this condition, and are loathe to leave the house when it presents itself. By the time they reach this point, they have either killed themselves or are spending an eternal holiday at L'Institute du Prairie.
In the absence of this one clue, the chase becomes more subtle, and ultimately more rewarding. Keep this in mind, though: no one clue is an indictment of pariahhood, but if you find three or four, you're definitely on the right track. Happy hunting, and remember, there are no bag limits.
"Leukemia."
Tailored business attire may be replaced by looser Armani styles.
Newly found fascination with Echinacea.
Sudden appearance of private physician's home phone number on office speed dialer.
Does he insist on sitting in the padded booths at the Turf Club?
Formerly cleancut men who sprout beards or grow long hair may be hiding that wasted look or those pesky lumps in the neck.
Won't drink the water in Mexican restaurants.
Mary Baker Eddy tracts.
Although pillboxes may merely be an indication of angina, look for the telltale flash of blue and white of quickly palmed capsules around the noontime hour.
The usual Procrustean footwear is replaced by Birkenstocks.

Figure 6.3 Beowulf Thorne, 'Pariah Chase!', 1992, *Diseased Pariah News*, issue #2, scan from personal copy.

Thorne's 'serocloseted figures' are also 'wasted' in their look. Here, the objectified 'look of AIDS' is turned on white conservative 'heterosexual' men hiding not just their serostatus, but also their sexuality. Just like the 'self-help' style of the CDC's public health campaigns, Thorne creates an ad to protect families and neighbourhoods by signalling a new 'look of AIDS' of which to be wary: oversized business suits, hair loss and 'beards or … long hair … hiding that wasted look or those pesky lumps in the neck' (inflamed lymph nodes). This comic, designed and written by self-proclaimed 'pariahs', recycles bodily associations with HIV/AIDS, flipping the script on the presumed 'look of AIDS'. Symptoms like wasting, taste aversion, nausea and early death are converted into the tongue-in-cheek, readily consumed (but not easily stomached) humour zine.

Thorne and Shearer capture a level of campiness which connects communities of those living with HIV and AIDS to all the bodily functions of survival, especially sight, smell and taste. Humour in this zine performs through illustration and photography. Contributing artists, writers and editors achieve ironic connection through a touching feast of visual potpourri. Shared lived experience as PWAs (and those living with or with the threat of HIV) is performed through a niche brand of comedy that is inflected in the visual: zine illustrations and collage. Shared experiences of bodily function, however, are captured through an affectual relationship to zine materials: trying new recipes, masturbating into the centrefold or crying onto the pages. I position these artists in a practice of world-building in a shared humour. Their bitter humour refuses to let outsider audiences be 'touched' by their pariah status. After the death of Shearer, Michael Botkin, Tom Ace and Thorne, fellow editors and contributors follow the logic of 'it's my party and I'll die if I want to'. A riff like that is exactly the sort of comedy which plagues *DPN*. Editors recycle pop culture from the past, literally layering trash and filth ephemera on top of high-art and mainstream media through collage. They abjectly embrace bitter irony and disgust which cut through the stinging sweetness of mainstream media. *DPN* does not attempt to play the victim card but rather opts to recycle it for a more interesting dance card: tracking the many 'feelings of AIDS' in their community with the publication, rather than the totalising 'look of AIDS' within mainstream discourses and circulations. I cannot help but think of David Román's comments on the circulation of humour in his chapter also named '... and I'll Die if I Want To'. He states that artists (and those living with HIV/AIDS) frequently invoke the humour aesthetic of camp as a survival strategy to communicate and thrive in theatrics which invert the horrors of daily life.[33]

I ground my camp reading of *DPN* in José Esteban Muñoz's disidentification model which claims that camp 'scrambles and reconstructs the encoded message of a cultural text in a fashion that both exposes the encoded message's universalizing and exclusionary machinations and recircuits its workings to account for, include, and empower minority identities and identifications'.[34] I see the embrace of 'AIDS feelings' by HIV-positive performers, activists, artists and writers within *DPN* as performances of disidentification which can re-fashion taste within queer communities and, specifically, people living with HIV or AIDS. The editors welcome sexualisation, disgust and pariah status into their visual vocabulary and use of bodily representation. *DPN* uses visual humour to undo social constructions of how the 'AIDS body' is represented to the public. Simon Watney, with his concept of the *spectacle of AIDS*, theorises about bodily associations made through media moralism, wherein homosexuality – as an action, an embodied lifestyle – becomes synonymous with HIV/AIDS: a threat to the family, a threat to life. The 'AIDS victim' as an aesthetic gesture in media is also critiqued in Watney's work, highlighting how the 'homosexual' figure in media becomes a metaphor for the impossibility of homosexuality within culture:

> [H]omosexuality, understood by AIDS commentary as the 'cause' of AIDS, is always available as a coercive and menacing category to entrench the institutions of family life and to prop up the profoundly unstable identities those institutions generate. [...] In this manner the axiomatic identification of AIDS as a sign and symptom of homosexual behavior reconfirms the passionately held view of 'the family' as a uniquely vulnerable institution.[35]

This is the spectacle of AIDS, an 'embodied ... drama, relayed between the image of the miraculous authority of clinical medicine and the faces and bodies of individuals who clearly disclose the stigmata of their guilt. The principal target of this sadistically punitive gaze is the body of "the homosexual"', the Other, the pariah.[36] David Román highlights acts of refusal of queer bodies entrenched in the *spectacle of AIDS*, highlighting the political interventions made by gay men through protest performance and community-based AIDS education. I bring this cultural frame to my reading of *DPN*. While gay sex, and those who practise it, have become associated with HIV/AIDS since the 1980s, Román argues that 'all gay male ... acts of intervention ... contribute, immeasurably and in ways impossible to register effectively, to the continual negotiations of AIDS, sexuality and citizenship in the local, regional and national spheres'.[37] From this vantage point, performance and humour offer a space to liberate those living with HIV/AIDS from metaphors of bodily contagion, stigma and other violent associations wrapped up into Watney's *spectacle of AIDS* theory. I understand *DPN*, and the community of artists it created, as directly combating the *spectacle of AIDS*. A reclamation of bodily autonomy and embrace of pariah status through comics and community health via nutrition adds to an alternative genealogy to AIDS history, in which 'gay male performers representing, or conjuring, AIDS allowed other gay men vulnerable to AIDS to locate themselves on a new ... identificatory continuum'.[38] Performing bodies offer alternative histories (and futures) to dominant discourses on HIV/AIDS as a virus, as an epidemic, and as a queer metric through humour. But jokes – *sick jokes*, specifically – do not always land.

'A recipe for rectal tarts', and other anal art

People living with HIV/AIDS, as they are depicted through the eleven issues of *DPN*, feel a sense of community in their shared sensations and symptoms of nausea, taste aversion and *hunger*. Faced with malnutrition (and unwanted celibacy), this zine satiates readers' desire for food and sexual stimulation. Biffy Mae (Beowulf Thorne) serves her brand of comedy to the sour-stomached in the recurring recipe feature 'GET FAT, don't die!' hoping they keep it all down. But her cuisine, rich as it is, often goes right through them. Thorne similarly stirred the pot of butt jokes during Geller's photoshoot of Shearer in his hospital bed. These boudoir images (Figure 6.2), in my interpretation, were intended for Shearer's feature as a centrefold model in the next issue (which he did not live to read). By placing the first issue of the zine over his 'AZT Butt' and genitals, Tom Shearer laughs in the face of the objectifying camera lens. He renders himself not the butt of an 'AIDS joke', nor a victim living in only a 'wasting' body, but rather an object of desire. I situate this humour within the context of centrefold images found throughout *DPN* which are buttressed by anal art in an attempt to subvert the visual associations of AIDS on the body.

However, re-interpretations of the 'AIDS body' often fall behind, failing to address race and globalisation in the history of gay culture, anal sex and HIV/AIDS in *DPN*. Editors care for their readers through a shared humour aesthetic but unintentionally exclude people of colour through a reliance on 'white trash' and American and European tastes. A strong sense of 'counterpublicity' forms within *DPN*'s readership, 'though the erotic mode of corporeality was often constituted in part through strategic rhetorics of whiteness … that render White racial identity invisible or under-interrogated'.[39] The nude models – with their white, centrefold rumps – are seropositive fans of *DPN* but are rarely people of colour. And, when they are, they are rendered inscrutable:

> [W]hen men of color did appear, qualities of their appearances sometimes marked racial difference while protecting whiteness from interrogation. Byl Hulse's appearance in a two-page *DPN* centerfold spread differed considerably from all other *DPN* centerfolds … the image of Hulse's naked body was digitally distorted almost beyond recognition into a circular blur; the only way that a reader could have seen his body clearly was by viewing the image at about a 458 angle in a reflective cylindrical surface.[40]

Gay seropositive men of colour in *DPN* are often wrapped in depictions which 'dehumanize, exoticize, or fetishize' them.[41] This affective transfer is not unlike the aforementioned consumption of famine photography about which Brown writes: 'visual interest manifested in a collective desire to see black bodies in varying states of corporeal chaos and decay'.[42] I argue that Hulse's body in its contortion, and other bodies of colour that are circulated and consumed throughout *DPN*, are relegated to visual flux. Meanwhile, the *sexy* 'AIDS body' is sequestered into frames of 'healthy-looking', white models. Their butts – white, round, plump and centred – are digitally laid out in the zine by Thorne and other editors with the explicit purpose of seducing the readership; there is no 'AZT Butt' in sight! While some jokes (especially ones about butt sex) are placed next to the centrefold models' bottoms, the tone is predominantly that of sensuality.

The creators of *DPN* refer to butts quite often throughout the eleven-issue run of the zine – even beyond the centrefolds' rumps. Whether a special column on lubricant or first-hand accounts of incontinence, poop jokes abound in the publication. While the jokes are often self-defecating – sorry, self-deprecating – the diseased pariahs are never 'butts of the joke'. Their campiness elevates their position, and their bodies, beyond derision. Sex is baked into the *DPN* brand of comedy. What powers led them (writers living with HIV/AIDS) to drop the kids (faeces jokes) off at the pool (*Diseased Pariah News*)?

While it may not be a medical diagnosis, assuming that a queer body is diseased is not new to the medical community or to histories of medicine surrounding sexually transmitted diseases. Identity indicates action, according to protocols of diagnosis. Michael Scarce, public health activist and writer, covers this in his book *Smearing the Queer: Medical Bias in the Health Care of Gay Men* (1999).[43] His work – deconstructing an array, a cocktail, of sexually transmitted diseases and syndromes associated with anal sex acts among gay men as 'gay bowel syndrome' – confirms that medical professionals have historically used an associative style of diagnostics in the early treatment and identification of disease. The performing bodies of gay men face scrutiny due to their history of sexual experiences. What is more, anal sex is a totalising force on this style of diagnostic. Once a person has anal sex with someone of the same gender, namely cisgender men with cisgender men, 'Gay' as a label is immediately placed on this patient. These early associations with gay men and unknown diseases due to gay sex continues through the HIV/AIDS crisis.

An illustration from Issue #10 of *DPN* features a naked figure, rear-end up to the sky (Figure 6.4). At first glance it looks as if the

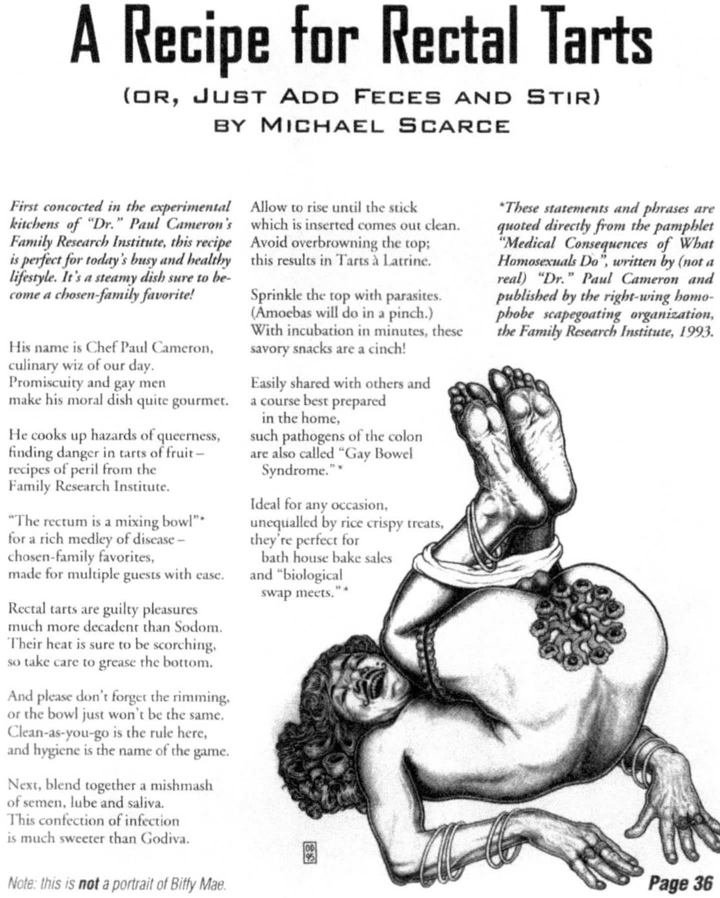

A Recipe for Rectal Tarts

(OR, JUST ADD FECES AND STIR)
BY MICHAEL SCARCE

First concocted in the experimental kitchens of "Dr." Paul Cameron's Family Research Institute, this recipe is perfect for today's busy and healthy lifestyle. It's a steamy dish sure to become a chosen-family favorite!

His name is Chef Paul Cameron,
culinary wiz of our day.
Promiscuity and gay men
make his moral dish quite gourmet.

He cooks up hazards of queerness,
finding danger in tarts of fruit –
recipes of peril from the
Family Research Institute.

"The rectum is a mixing bowl"*
for a rich medley of disease –
chosen-family favorites,
made for multiple guests with ease.

Rectal tarts are guilty pleasures
much more decadent than Sodom.
Their heat is sure to be scorching,
so take care to grease the bottom.

And please don't forget the rimming,
or the bowl just won't be the same.
Clean-as-you-go is the rule here,
and hygiene is the name of the game.

Next, blend together a mishmash
of semen, lube and saliva.
This confection of infection
is much sweeter than Godiva.

Allow to rise until the stick
which is inserted comes out clean.
Avoid overbrowning the top;
this results in Tarts à Latrine.

Sprinkle the top with parasites.
(Amoebas will do in a pinch.)
With incubation in minutes, these
savory snacks are a cinch!

Easily shared with others and
a course best prepared
in the home,
such pathogens of the colon
are also called "Gay Bowel
Syndrome."*

Ideal for any occasion,
unequalled by rice crispy treats,
they're perfect for
bath house bake sales
and "biological
swap meets."*

**These statements and phrases are quoted directly from the pamphlet "Medical Consequences of What Homosexuals Do", written by (not a real) "Dr." Paul Cameron and published by the right-wing homophobe scapegoating organization, the Family Research Institute, 1993.*

*Note: this is **not** a portrait of Biffy Mae.*

Page 36

Figure 6.4 Michael Scarce, illustration by Kira Od, 'A Recipe for Rectal Tarts', 1995, *Diseased Pariah News*, issue #10, scan from personal copy.

anus is prolapsed, or is full of pustules, or worse. But these protrusions are fruits, arranged delicately as decorations on a dessert. Michael Scarce submits, to this contributor section of poetry and illustrations, 'A Recipe for Rectal Tarts: Just Add Feces and Stir', a humour poem based on a pamphlet 'The Medical Consequences of What Homosexuals Do' from 1993: 'First concocted in the experimental kitchens of "Dr." Paul Cameron's Family Research

Institute, this recipe is perfect for today's busy and healthy lifestyle. It's a steamy dish sure to become a chosen-family favorite.'[44] The poem itself is almost too rich in food references, exposing Cameron's possibly subconscious deployment of food metaphors around gay sex acts. Scarce captures this, pinpointing a quote from the pamphlet ('The rectum is a mixing bowl'), and taking the reader on a journey through the creation of gourmet *rectal tarts*. These 'guilty pleasures' are cooked hot in a well-greased anus, hygienically made through a process of anal rimming. Ingredients include semen, lube and saliva, which – when mixed – are 'sweeter than Godiva'. Chefs are warned of overbrowning, but if instructions are followed carefully, 'Tars à Latrine' can be topped with parasites, '(Amoebas will do in a pinch.)', and shared with others, though 'best prepared at home'. Scarce ends the poem with another quote from Cameron, abjectly embracing the homophobic institute's language around gay sex as 'biological swap meets', by adding that rectal tarts are perfect for 'bath house bake sales'.[45]

This single page exemplifies the camp of *DPN*. The poem exists as a standalone entry illustrated by Kira Od, who worked as a designer and 'defender of traditional media' for *DPN*.[46] The figure accompanying the parodistic recipe has a dandy style – flowing hair, mole-marked lips and a moustache waxed to a curl. His eyes are closed, locked in an expression of delight, relishing his own position. Bracelets adorn his feet and ankles, a garter hugs the lower right thigh, and pineapple slices, berries and cream surround the anus: 'Wulf had a photo of a guy in that position, and we brainstormed camping it up … our focus was on horsing around with the "tart" double entendre.'[47] The style of the illustration, Od tells me, was inspired by Soviet and Nazi graphic design ('though NOT in their philosophies', she affirms). In fact, all things 1950s-retro seem to have inspired the visual vocabulary of Thorne's layout and imagery: from the recipe illustrations to layered photo-editing.

By visualising the rectum as a mixing bowl, Paul Cameron claims that homosexuals threaten public health at large: 'With the rise of new contagious diseases, homosexuality not only raises our medical costs, it increases the hazards of giving and getting medical care, receiving blood, *and eating out*' (emphasis mine). Cameron perpetuates the moral panic around AIDS by a process of identitarian transference, claiming that the true victims of AIDS are heterosexual family units; their way of life, everyday acts like eating at a restaurant, are threatened by homosexuality. The 'AIDS victim' as an aesthetic gesture in media is also critiqued in Watney's work, highlighting how the 'homosexual' figure in media becomes a metaphor for the impossibility of homosexuality within culture. Homosexuality is not only the cause of AIDS, but also 'the axiomatic identification of AIDS as a sign and symptom of homosexual behavior reconfirms the passionately held view of "the family" as a uniquely vulnerable institution'.[48] Scarce writes, Od designs and Thorne, Ace and Botkin edit a spread which reconstructs the anxiety and paranoia of contracting 'gay bowel syndrome' within the camp aesthetic of *Diseased Pariah News*. 'Rectal tarts' may be a form taken by shame, concoctions which are not 'distinct "toxic parts", of a group or individual identity that can be excised; they are instead integral to and residual in the processes by which identity itself is formed'.[49] In this way, readers of *DPN* may identify with the figure who is acting as the rectal tart mixing bowl/serving platter, or find themselves as potential (and willing) consumers. Thinking with Eve Sedgwick, I read Scarce's poem alongside Kira Od's illustration as artistic re-manifestations of *shame:* that of both 'Dr.' Paul Cameron and the people with AIDS reading the zine. Sedgwick notes that shame, 'living as it does, on and in the muscles and capillaries of the face – seems to be uniquely contagious from one person to another'.[50] What sense, then, can be made of Od's dandy, supine figure whose face is contorted, not in shame, but rather in a visage overcome by shameless pleasure? Does shame manifest before or after audiences feast (their eyes) on the 'rectal tarts?'

This collaborative (and militantly stylised) parody of the Family Research Institute's scientific findings – a humorous portrayal of gay sex acts as a delicious dessert – ruptures the shame/performativity dialectic set forth by Sedgwick. They move their visual satire away from identity politics and into the body. However, the parodies embedded within *DPN* are so tied to feelings of desire and hunger – despite the potential threat of contagion – that shame is not part of their aesthetic palate. Rather, shared taste motivates *DPN*'s camp. Pleasure and disgust coexist, mirroring the lived experience of people with AIDS. Shame may arrive after the 'rectal tarts' are eaten, or after a disease is contracted, but the performance still entices with a confused mixture of good and bad flavours.

Od's illustration similarly blends opposite aesthetic qualities which span the invisible divide between beautiful and grotesque. In fact, read together, I understand how one may see 'rectal tarts' as a concept in bad taste – politically incorrect for its eroticisation of 'unsafe' sex. This camp performance is erotic in description and design, but is that possible within parody? Leo Bersani writes (in his aptly titled *Is the Rectum a Grave?*) that 'parody is an erotic turn-off, and all gay men know that. Much campy talk is parodistic, and while it may be fun at a dinner party, if you're out to make someone you turn off the camp'.[51] Bersani makes this comment, citing a scenario in which someone licks a man's leather boots as a joint turn on, remarking that parody, subversion of macho masculinity, cannot exist in this dynamic. However, the humour and style of *DPN* allows for performances in which 'sexual pleasure generates politics'.[52] Camp, then, has the capacity for erotics, especially as a mechanism for nourishing people living with HIV/AIDS. 'Butts' of jokes are corporeally able to arouse audiences of *DPN* through affecting tastes. And what about licking boots?

For one final example of a 'butt joke' in *DPN*, I return to Issue #10, but this time to the cover (Figure 6.5). Going in for a lick, one might miss Od's signature, encased in a rectangle near the heel of a cowboy boot – almost completely overshadowed in the umbrage of a wrinkled, veiny depiction of Senator Jesse Helms's bare bottom. Taking the homophobic shame tied to anal sex and the political rhetoric of Helms on how gay men contract AIDS ('deliberate, disgusting, revolting conduct'), the artists begin visually representing the senator for *DPN*'s readers. Flipping through the Thorne papers at the GLBT Archives, I notice a note written in purple pen, and recognise Thorne's handwriting about a digitally edited piece of erotica or pornography still (Thorne was known to do both): 'My initial reliance on vericose [*sic*] veins and stretchmarks was due to the limited amount of wrinkles I could add.' Od's reply is a pen-over-pencil draft featuring Helm's face looking over the nude cowboy's shoulder. An entire pack of cigarettes are jammed up his anus, and the 'butts' are just beginning to smoke. Drawn as an

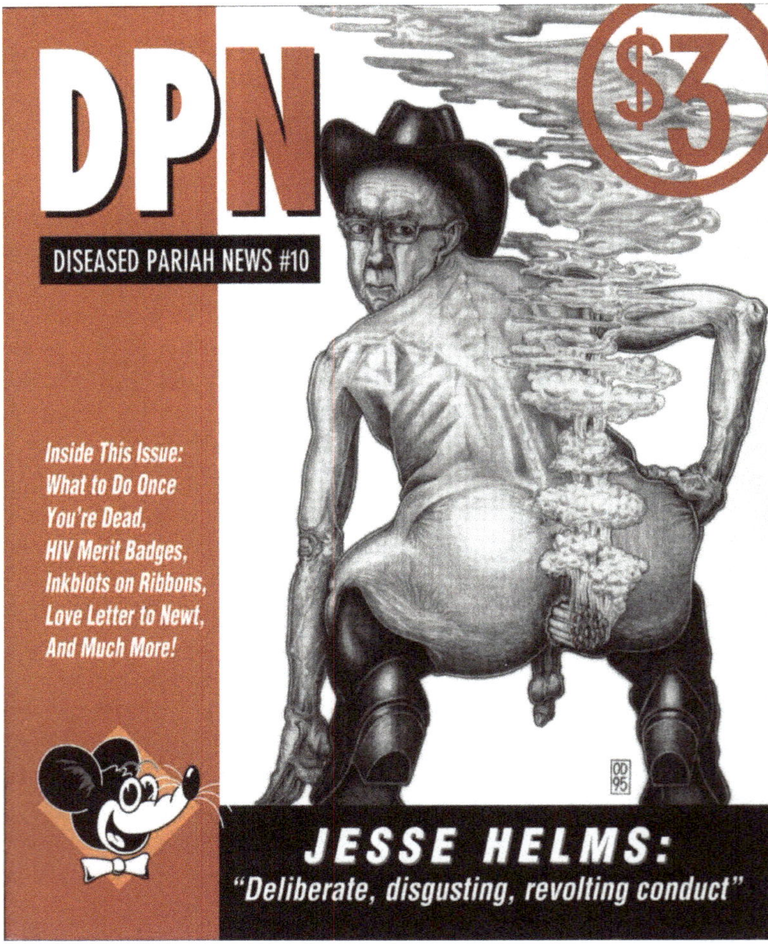

Figure 6.5 Kira Od based on digital image edits by Beowulf Thorne, Cover of *Diseased Pariah News*, issue #10, 1995, scan from personal copy.

image pairing for an article titled 'Jesse Helms Makes Me Sick', Od and Thorne are able to campily recycle the conservative rhetoric of a senator, gay sex acts and an absurdity to comment on the politics of the day: Helms is the literal 'butt' of their 'AIDS joke'. The artists physically transport shame from gay sex acts into the body of a homophobe. Herein lies the visual parody of *DPN* at its sharpest wit and use of ironic waste. Coincidentally, this visual magnum opus was printed in Thorne's final issue.

A sweet 'look' at AIDS from the bitter (rear) end

Beowulf Thorne was not in the hospital room when his friend Tom Shearer died. But he was there, on Shearer's bed, for a photoshoot just two weeks before. Most of these images, including the two of them smiling and playing together, were never published.

Towards the end of Thorne's life, and while working on the final issue of *DPN* that he never got to see in print, his eyesight began to fail due to AIDS, as reported in his piece 'How I Fought CMV Retinitis and Lost'.[53] While I combed the GLBT Archives one last time, I made special note of Thorne's scribbles, doodles and notes which contributed to his final full *DPN* article. Swirling images of plants and eyeballs – his attempts at drawing their cell structure at a macro and microscopic level jump out at me in blurry, frenetic pen sketches. I think I've seen that plant before: an oxalis gifted to Tommy Shearer by Tom E. ('his erstwhile boyfriend'). Thorne writes in Shearer's obituary that it was a 'special ornamental variety with red and purple leaves, and during a really bad night Tommy hallucinated it into some menacing creature made of slabs of liver'.[54] From the look of these sketches, I think Thorne was attempting to make sense of a similar visual hallucination, or of that very plant in his personal collection of his friend's life. Even with a cursory glance, I see the exact sympathy plant behind the dynamic duo, resting on a shelf near Shearer's hospital bed.

I open another folder and locate the photo negatives of Geller's portraits of Shearer – oxygen cannula in place, a faint smile playing on his lips (Figure 6.6). I imagine Thorne turning these pieces of plastic over in his fingers, debating their publication. Brown reminds us of the precious quality that 'film negative gifts us with' – a 'translucence of texture that mimics the fragility of skin. You can peer into it or cut it to pieces. It belongs to the viewer, never the subject.'[55] Is that how Thorne felt, eyesight getting fuller with retinal 'crumbs' looking at these images of his friend? That to touch

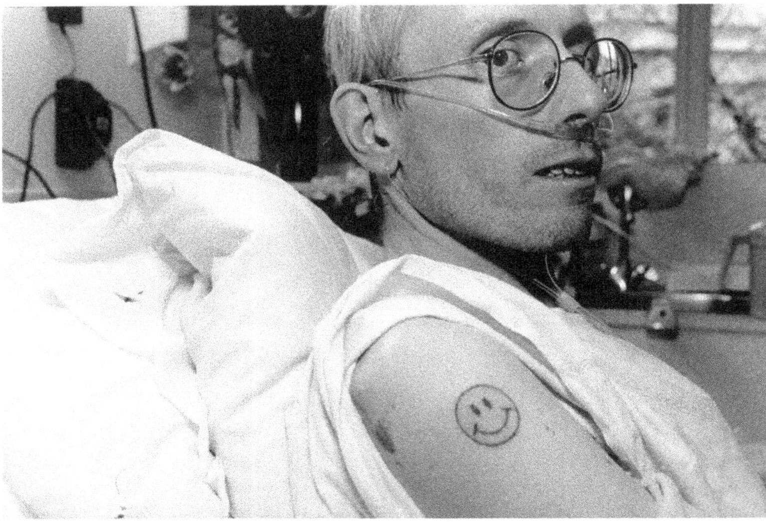

Figure 6.6 Marc Geller, *Tom Shearer*, 1991, scan from artist's print.

these negatives, to look at them up close, meant he had ownership over his image, memory or body? I doubt it; what a waste of precious time!

Power resides in Shearer's direct, unwavering gaze into the camera. He does not look away, not into a middle-distance of metaphysical abstraction, but at us, the viewers. This is not a look of resignation; it is knowing and charged with irony. Shearer's eyes, framed by both a smiley-face tattoo and Kaposi's lesions, challenge the genre of AIDS deathbed photography by refusing to take up its usual emotional cues. Shearer is not serenely departing nor tragically wasted – he is posing. In this gesture, he flips the script on the viewer: if Frare's David Kirby became an icon of loss and the moral cost of looking, Shearer insists we laugh and grieve with his image on different terms. This is an image for those who can read the joke and feel the intimacy in it. Shearer is both performer and patient, camp icon and dying friend, holding eye contact with a public that too often looked away or looked only to feel righteous sadness. Shearer's stare refuses the anaesthetising effect of repetition; it does not sentimentalise suffering but satirises the frameworks through which it is made visible. His look is the punchline, an invitation into a world of queer resistance and humour aesthetic that *DPN* built. Even at death's door, his body speaks back – eyes daring you to make him the 'butt' of any joke.

Notes

1 Kimberly Juanita Brown, 'Regarding the Pain of the Other: Photography, Famine, and the Transference of Affect', in Elspeth H. Brown and Thy Phu (eds), *Feeling Photography* (Duke University Press, 2014), p. 193.

2 Michael Scarce, *Smearing the Queer: Medical Bias in the Health Care of Gay Men* (Haworth Press, 1999), p. 113.

3 Beowulf Thorne, Tom Ace and Tom Shearer (eds), *Diseased Pariah News*, no. 3 (FOG Press, 1991), p. 3.

4 This date was offered to me via personal email correspondence with photographer Marc Geller on 10 January 2025.

5 Special thanks to (now Acting Director of Archives and Special Collections) Isaac Fellman at the GLBT Historical Society for his help locating materials for this chapter. And to Lee Mandelo and Candace Hansen for their companionship while co-researching in the archives.

6 Glen Helfand, 'Not a Laughing Matter: Fanzine Editor Tom Shearer [of DPN – Diseased Pariah News] Prescribes AIDS Humor as Medicine', *The Advocate*, 7 May 1991, 70.

7 For more on queer portraiture of subjects living with HIV/AIDS in this period, see Fiona Johnstone, *AIDS & Representation: Queering Portraiture during the AIDS Crisis in America* (Bloomsbury, 2023).

8 Susan Sontag, *On Photography* (Farrar, Straus and Giroux, 1977), p. 19.

9 Ben Cosgrove coins Therese Frare's image of David Kirby as the 'photo that changed the face of AIDS' in his *LIFE* article. Ben Cosgrove, 'The Photo That Changed the Face of AIDS,' *LIFE*, 25 November 2014, https://www.life.com/history/behind-the-picture-the-photo-that-changed-the-face-of-aids/.

10 This quote was sourced from personal LinkedIn correspondence with Therese Frare on 16 September 2024.

11 Alexandra Genova, 'The Story Behind the Colorization of a Controversial Benetton AIDS Ad', *TIME*, 14 December 2016, n.p.

12 Genova, 'The Story Behind the Colorization of a Controversial Benetton AIDS Ad'.

13 Sontag, *On Photography*, p. 20.
14 Sontag, *On Photography*, p. 20.
15 Greg Lugliani, 'Last Laughs', *POZ*, 1 October 1997, https://www.poz.com/article/Last-Laughs-1754-5803.
16 Steven Kruger, '"GET FAT: don't die!": Eating and AIDS in Gay Men's Culture', in Ron Scapp and Brian Seitz (eds), *Eating Culture* (SUNY Press, 1998), p. 49.
17 Kruger, '"GET FAT: don't die!"' p. 37.
18 See Samuel Kelton Roberts Jr, *Infectious Fear: Politics, Disease, and the Health Effects of Segregation* (University of North Carolina Press, 2009) for a discussion of the limits of racialised medicine; and Randall M. Packard, *White Plague, Black Labor: Tuberculosis and the Political Economy of Health and Disease in South Africa* (University of California Press, 1989) for an account of how political economies construct race within the demographics of public health and, by extension, diagnostics.
19 For more on the formation of postcolonial humanitarianism see Lasee Heerten, *The Biafran War and Postcolonial Humanitarianism: Spectacles of Suffering* (Cambridge University Press, 2017).
20 Cindy Patton, *Globalizing AIDS* (University of Minnesota Press, 2002), p. 120.
21 Sontag, *On Photography*, p. 24.
22 Brown, 'Regarding the Pain of the Other', pp. 188–9.
23 Lukas Engelmann, 'Seeing Bodies with AIDS', in *Mapping AIDS: Visual Histories of an Enduring Epidemic* (Cambridge University Press, 2018), p. 37.
24 Engelmann, 'Seeing Bodies with AIDS', p. 50.
25 San Francisco Public Library, San Francisco History Center, 'Survive AIDS—ACT UP Golden Gate Records' (oversize folder 10) .
26 University of California, Los Angeles, UCLA Library Digital Collections, AIDS Posters Collection, no. 306, item UG00, poster by AIDS Control Programme (Uganda), Uganda Ministry of Education, and UNICEF, https://digital.library.ucla.edu/catalog/ark:/21198/zz0002kzpn.
27 Rodney H. Jones, 'Marketing the damaged self: The construction of identity in advertisements directed towards people with HIV/AIDS', *Journal of Sociolinguistics* 1:3 (1997), 399.
28 Engelmann, 'Seeing Bodies with AIDS', pp. 95–6.
29 Engelmann, 'Seeing Bodies with AIDS', p. 96.
30 Brown, 'Regarding the Pain of the Other'.
31 Thorne, *Diseased Pariah News*, no. 5 (FOG Press, 1992), p. 2.
32 Thorne, *Diseased Pariah News*, no. 7 (FOG Press, 1992), p. 8.

33 For further reading on gay men's interventions in 'AIDS Performance' and the circulation of camp humour see: David Román, '"It's My Party and I'll Die if I Want To!" – AIDS Performance and the Circulation of Camp in the Late 1980s and Early 1990s', in *Acts of Intervention: Performance, Gay Culture, and AIDS* (Indiana University Press, 1999), pp. 88–115.
34 José Esteban Muñoz, *Disidentifications: Queers of Color and the Performance of Politics* (University of Minnesota Press, 1999), p. 31.
35 Simon Watney, 'The Spectacle of AIDS', *October* 43 (1987), 77.
36 Watney, 'The Spectacle of AIDS', 78.
37 Román, *Acts of Intervention*, p. 10.
38 Román, *Acts of Intervention*, p. 48.
39 Daniel C. Brouwer, 'Counterpublicity and corporeality in HIV/AIDS zines', *Critical Studies in Media Communication* 22:5 (2005), 360.
40 Brouwer, 'Counterpublicity and Corporeality in HIV/AIDS Zines', 360.
41 Brouwer, 'Counterpublicity and Corporeality in HIV/AIDS Zines', 360.
42 Brown, 'Regarding the Pain of the Other', p. 190.
43 Scarce, *Smearing the Queer*.
44 This comment was sent by Kira Od to me in personal email correspondence on 14 August 2023.
45 Paul Cameron, chairman of the Family Research Institute published 'Medical Consequences of What Homosexuals Do' online as early as 2009 according to the Internet Archive. It was removed from the website (in English) in 2023 in the same month I first presented on this research at the Visual Histories of Humor and Health: A Virtual Symposium on 6 September 2023 at the Johns Hopkins Center for Medical Humanities & Social Medicine.
46 GLBT Historical Society Archives, San Francisco, CA. Beowulf Thorne Papers, uncategorised folder, uncategorised pages, n.d.
47 This comment was sent by Kira Od to me in personal email correspondence on 14 August 2023.
48 Watney, 'The Spectacle of AIDS', 77.
49 Eve Kosofsky Sedgwick, *Touching Feeling: Affect, Pedagogy, Performativity* (Duke University Press, 2003), p. 63.
50 Sedgwick, *Touching Feeling*, p. 64.
51 Leo Bersani, 'Is the Rectum a Grave?', in *Is the Rectum a Grave? and Other Essays* (University of Chicago Press, 2009), p. 14.
52 Bersani, 'Is the Rectum a Grave?', p. 14.
53 Beowulf Thorne, 'How I Fought CMV Retinitis and Lost', *Diseased Pariah News*, no. 11 (FOG Press, 1999), p. 11.

54 Beowulf Thorne, 'Obituary for Tom Shearer', *Diseased Pariah News*, no. 3 (FOG Press, 1991), p. 4.
55 Brown, 'Regarding the Pain of the Other', p. 193.

References

Allen, Mark. 'That's Not Funny, Or Is It?' *Vice*, 31 December 2010, https://www.vice.com/en/article/that-s-not-funny-663-v18n1/

Bersani, Leo. "Is the Rectum a Grave?" In *Is the Rectum a Grave? and Other Essays*. University of Chicago Press, 2009.

Brouwer, Daniel C. 'Counterpublicity and corporeality in HIV/AIDS zines'. *Critical Studies in Media Communication* 22:5 (2005), 351–71.

Brown, Kimberly Juanita, 'Regarding the Pain of the Other: Photography, Famine, and the Transference of Affect'. In Elspeth H. Brown and Thy Phu (eds), *Feeling Photography*. Duke University Press, 2014.

Cooter, Roger, and Claudia Stein. 'Visual Imagery and Epidemics in the Twentieth Century'. In David Serlin (ed.), *Imagining Illness: Public Health and Visual Culture*. University of Minnesota Press, 2010.

Cosgrove, Ben. 'The Photo That Changed the Face of AIDS'. *LIFE*, 25 November 2014. https://www.life.com/history/behind-the-picture-the-photo-that-changed-the-face-of-aids/

Engelmann, Lukas. 'Seeing Bodies with AIDS'. In *Mapping AIDS: Visual Histories of an Enduring Epidemic*. Global Health Histories, Cambridge University Press, 2018.

Genova, Alexandra. 'The Story Behind the Colorization of a Controversial Benetton AIDS Ad'. *TIME*, 14 December 2016, https://time.com/4592061/colorization-benetton-aids-ad/

Helfand, Glen. 'Not a Laughing Matter: Fanzine Editor Tom Shearer [of DPN – Diseased Pariah News] Prescribes AIDS Humor as Medicine'. *The Advocate*, 7 May 1991, 70–1.

Heerten, Lasse. *The Biafran War and Postcolonial Humanitarianism: Spectacles of Suffering*. Cambridge University Press, 2017.

Johnstone, Fiona. *AIDS & Representation: Queering Portraiture during the AIDS Crisis in America*. Bloomsbury, 2023.

Jones, Rodney H. 'Marketing the damaged self: The construction of identity in advertisements directed towards people with HIV/AIDS'. *Journal of Sociolinguistics* 1:3 (October 1997), 315–472.

Kauffman, Jonathan. 'Get Fat, Don't Die'. *Hazlitt*, 28 April 2020. https://hazlitt.net/longreads/get-fat-dont-die

Kruger, Steven. '"GET FAT: Don't Die!": Eating and AIDS in Gay Men's Culture'. In Ron Scapp and Brian Seitz (eds), *Eating Culture*, 36–59. SUNY Press, 1998.

Lugliani, Greg. 'Last Laughs', *POZ*, 1 October 1997. https://www.poz.com/article/Last-Laughs-1754-5803

Muñoz, José Esteban. *Disidentifications: Queers of Color and the Performance of Politics*. University of Minnesota Press, 1999.

Packard, Randall M. *White Plague, Black Labor: Tuberculosis and the Political Economy of Health and Disease in South Africa*. University of California Press, 1989.

Patton, Cindy. *Globalizing AIDS*. University of Minnesota Press, 2002.

Roberts, Samuel Kelton. *Infectious Fear: Politics, Disease, and the Health Effects of Segregation*. University of North Carolina Press, 2009.

Román, David. *Acts of Intervention: Performance, Gay Culture, and AIDS*. Indiana University Press, 1998.

Scarce, Michael. *Smearing the Queer: Medical Bias in the Health Care of Gay Men*. Haworth Press, 1999.

Sedgwick, Eve Kosofsky. *Touching Feeling: Affect, Pedagogy, Performativity*. Duke University Press, 2003.

Sontag, Susan. *On Photography*. Farrar, Straus and Giroux, 1977.

Thorne, Beowulf, Tom Ace and Tom Shearer (eds). *Diseased Pariah News*, no. 3. FOG Press, 1991.

Thorne, Beowulf, Tom Ace and Tom Shearer (eds). *Diseased Pariah News*, no. 5, FOG Press, 1992.

Thorne, Beowulf, Tom Ace and Tom Shearer (eds). *Diseased Pariah News*, no. 10, FOG Press, 1997.

Watney, Simon. 'The Spectacle of AIDS'. *October* 43 (1987), 71–86.

7

Irony, assisted dying and the Disabled Avant-Garde

Laura Cowley

See note[1]

In 2007, the artists Katherine Araniello (1965–2019) and Aaron Williamson (b. 1960) set out to use irony as a tool to critically engage with what they perceived as a cavernous gap between their own experiences of disability and wider society's understanding of disabled lives.[2] Operating under their collaborative name, 'the Disabled Avant-Garde', Araniello and Williamson performed and documented *Assisted Passage*, a satirical piece of performance art that combined Araniello's long-term artistic and activist engagement with the politics of assisted dying and Williamson's expertise in mischievous yet confronting site-specific interventions.

Documentation of this performance piece shows a mock protest, with Araniello and Williamson inviting passers-by to sign a petition on a table decorated with comedically illustrated posters (Figure 7.1). Their ostensible aim was to gather signatures in support of Araniello's right to access medically assisted dying in Switzerland, which they claimed had been curtailed by 'budget' airline companies banning her from flying out of the UK, through some vague but sinister process of blacklisting. *Assisted Passage*, which they described as Live Art – a subset of practices exploring performance as research – proceeded with the hypothesis that their audience would be unable to identify their guerrilla art as satirical.[3] It is impossible to judge from the video documentation the motivations of each signatory who chose to approach the table and engage with the petition. However, in Araniello's estimation, the participating audience was sincere and unquestioning in their support.[4] The petition, rain soaked and replete

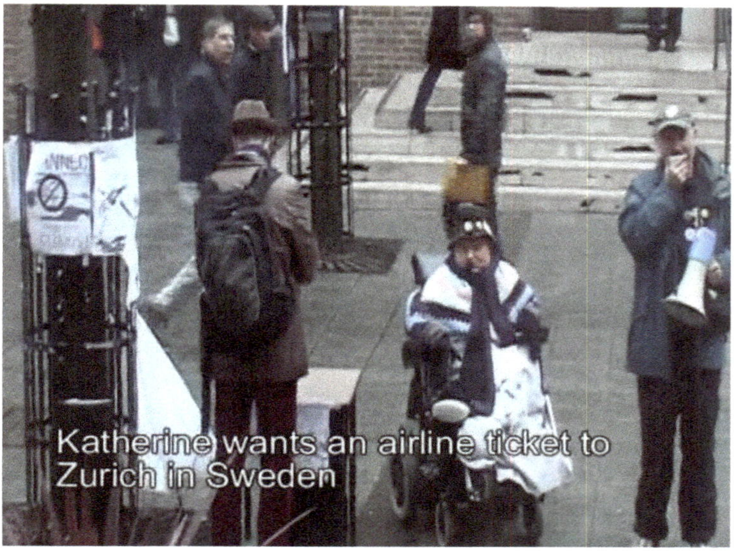

Figure 7.1 The Disabled Avant-Garde, Still from *Assisted Passage*, 2007 in *Bite the Hand that Feeds!* (Live Art Development Agency, 2012) PAL-DVD, (01.08).

with exclamation points, was surprisingly successful and was ultimately signed by thirty-seven people. The text of the petition read as follows:

> We, the undersigned, believe that it is a gross infringement of human rights to blacklist individuals from travelling to any destination assuming they intend to harm no-one but themselves. We the undersigned believe that Katherine Araniello, and others who so wish, have the right to fly to Zurich and other destinations in order to purchase an assisted demise. Airlines have no right to block their passage!!![5]

Araniello and Williamson named their inspiration for *Assisted Passage* as the sustained irony of Jonathan Swift's satire *A Modest Proposal* (1729).[6] In *A Modest Proposal*, Swift's narrator made an account of the hunger and poverty experienced by the people of Ireland and arrived at systematic cannibalistic infanticide as a reasonable response. This was an absurd proposition, but it was disguised within an indirect satire, which emerged gradually and remained ambiguous to some of Swift's audience.[7] This style of satire relies on deploying ironic communication as a device.[8] Araniello and Williamson's ironically stated position was that we should support Araniello's wish to access medically assisted dying overseas. It is possible that this and the above petition statement do not read to you, as they do not read to me, as particularly absurd. This chapter thoroughly considers how, and to a lesser extent why, *Assisted Passage* presents this position as risible.

To that end, I make use of the pretence theory of irony. This theory holds that ironic communicators pretend to be unwise people speaking to uninitiated audiences.[9] In this understanding of irony, there is no 'true' and opposite meaning secreted within an ironic statement which we might uncover as audience or analysts. Instead, the ironic pretence of expressing a particular position has just 'one purpose': 'the illustration of the deficiencies in that point of view'.[10] Araniello and Williamson used irony, not to convince their audience that Araniello wanted to live, but to ridicule the view that she should want to die. If their communication failed, it was because they addressed an audience who was not party to the pretence, being genuinely uninitiated. This is the dynamic that Araniello and Williamson set out to exploit, explore and evidence. A successful satire does, by most definitions, involve a ratification of the satire by some members of an audience.[11] In *Assisted Passage*, however, that moment is deferred to the video documentation. Araniello and Williamson's investment in the live experiment was in observing where their ironic communication failed. Immediately, this reading of *Assisted Passage* raises two final points of importance for defining ironic communication: hostile feeling and the direction of this emotion towards part of an audience.[12] In the following analysis, I examine these two ideas, arguing that Araniello and Williamson convey feelings of contempt for many narratives about disabled lives and for those that uncritically accept these narratives.

Little analytical attention has so far been given to this performance.[13] Bree Hadley located *Assisted Passage* among performances by other disabled artists. Hadley concluded that public performances allow disabled artists to interrupt 'the mechanisms of imag(in)ing disability' by 'asking people to reflect on how they, too, act as an unconscious performer, how they, too, intervene in public perceptions of disability, and how a change in their own perceptions might change the order of things'.[14] This chapter gives new attention to Araniello and Williamson's subversion of that moment of potential intervention. Eleanor Roberts's recent article found that crip humour – meaning anarchic jokes from disabled communities – was used by Araniello and Williamson to critique disability arts institutions. This chapter examines the construction and specifically ironic nature of their critical humour.[15] My close reading of Araniello and Williamson's satire first observes the debates that impacted their position, contextualising their humour in the traditions and communities from which it emerged. I then explore how Araniello and Williamson used visual humour to create ironic distance from their pretended position, potentially signalling to their audience that the performance was satirical. This then leads me to a discussion of the participating audience's broad failure to read these signs and recognise the work as ironic. This discussion will allow for expanded insights into the critical potential of humour to hold contradictions and complex emotionality, while subverting autobiography in communication around charged medical narratives.

Tragic, pitiable and poor: Ersatz discursive positions

Assisted Passage intervened into the well documented public conversation over access to assisted dying in the UK, to which audiences would have likely felt they had ample context. The *Assisted Passage* documentary video, publicly hosted on Araniello and Williamson's shared YouTube channel, is still available at the time of writing (spring 2025). The video identifies the documented performance as a satire, providing context unavailable to the live audience of 2007. The video begins with a slow slideshow of white text on a black background, setting a sombre tone: thirty-seven people had signed their petition 'without question or debate' and what follows will be a grim accounting of public support for Araniello's right to 'fly/die'.[16] For passers-by this ruse only needed to be confusing in the way that communication and legality around assisted dying was – and is – already confusing in the UK. The BBC has a news topic tag for 'Euthanasia and assisted dying', which is regularly updated with personal stories alongside political reporting.[17] This news tag is particularly active as I edit this chapter (in autumn 2025). In the UK, the legality of assisted dying is in flux. In November 2024, Members of Parliament voted in favour of a bill that proposed legalising medically assisted dying for terminally ill adults in England and Wales. Now, the bill is being further scrutinised in Parliament and in the public eye, on its uncertain progression towards becoming law. Questions of dignity, autonomy and institutional distrust are at the core of these conversations, as are proclamations about disabled people's views on assisted dying. But for now, as in 2007, there continue to be no legal routes to physician-assisted dying within the country.[18]

Travel across borders to access medically assisted dying or 'suicide tourism' of the sort that Araniello and Williamson reference in *Assisted Passage* was – and remains – live in the cultural imagination of UK audiences. By travelling to Switzerland, non-residents – including UK citizens – are able to access medical assistance in dying, if they are able to raise the significant private funds necessary to cover their medical and travel expenses.[19] The most recognisable Swiss clinic is called Dignitas, a name which conjures associations of autonomous, reasoned choice and the inalienable human dignity of the patient.[20] Death, or suicide, in this form has long occupied a legally – and morally – ambiguous space in the UK, accessible in limited circumstances to a fraction of the population. Araniello and Williamson intervened into this context with elaborate irony, sowing uncertainty and positioning themselves as individuals caught up in a difficult medical, legal and political arena.

Williamson categorised the personas he and Araniello adopted for this performance as 'medical-model cripples', situating the performance within longstanding, but lesser-known debates about the extent to which disability is a medical 'problem'.[21] The medical model describes a paradigm where disability is discussed as individual impairment, best 'understood and addressed in medical terms'.[22] Disability activists and scholars defined the medical model in opposition to the 'social model', which first emerged in the late 1990s, describing disability as innately political and created by societal attitudes and barriers to access.[23] Affirmative models also emerged at the turn of the twenty-first century, defining disability (encompassing impairment) as neither an entirely medical nor social experience but instead as an alternative, 'non-tragic' way of living in the world.[24] Key to reading the irony in *Assisted Passage* is an understanding that the view of disability as an individual tragedy and a medical problem is widely critiqued, alongside associated ideas of curative medicine, pity and charity. This history gives context to debates among disabled people about assisted dying legislation and its many potential implementations. There is unsurprisingly no consensus on the topic among disabled people or disabled activists: there are disabled people and disability groups advocating both against and for assisted dying legislation, from many different perspectives.[25] Objections often coalesce around a keen awareness of how definitions of disability, illness and terminal illness are changeable, contested and subjective.

During the 2024 legislative push, major advocacy group Disability Rights UK (DRUK) diverged from their previously neutral stance on assisted dying and made a strong statement: 'assistance to die should not be easier to access than assistance to live'.[26] The choice to live, they argue, cannot be certain in the context of ongoing austerity politics.[27] Disabled scholar Tom Shakespeare, who advocates for assisted dying legislation and equitable access for terminally ill disabled people, sees austerity as a separate fight, writing that, 'dying people should not be held hostage to systemic failures'.[28] In these debates we can see why definitions of disability as medicalised sickness are so strongly contested: changing medical rights and medical norms are dependent on such definitions. Araniello made public statements against assisted dying legislation in 2014, which followed similar lines, arguing that 'we are all terminally ill'.[29] In *Assisted Passage*, Araniello and Williamson pretended to agitate for Araniello's disability to be viewed as a medical problem. They described their adopted position as that of 'medical-model cripples' because their personas believed in the inevitability of their own suffering and the need for professionalised, commercialised medical intervention.

Their vocal performances, costuming and petition all contributed to this effect. As documented in the video, Araniello's performance was deeply subdued. Posed between Williamson and a table housing her petition, her demands for 'assisted passage, now!' were quiet and quavering. She softly asked that people 'just queue up please, please take your turn and sign the petition' for this was a 'worthy cause, thank you so much'.[30] Her protest was polite and grateful. The emphasis on 'budget' airlines also indicated the precarity of Araniello's pretended situation. Oriana Fox, an artist, researcher and friend of Araniello said that personas, absurdity, deadpan delivery and playing the victim were some of Araniello's key tools and talents as an artist.[31] These were all components in *Assisted Passage*. Her persona was demurely thankful, but also unhappy, wrapped up against what was clearly dreary weather (while it added to her put-upon persona, she likely wasn't pretending to be cold; it can be unpleasant to sit outdoors for many hours in a wheelchair). Her signature hairstyle, always dyed boldly and brightly, was disguised under a woolly hat, complemented by a crocheted blanket draped around her shoulders. This was an unusually homely and shrinking costuming for Araniello, emphasising that her 'medical-model cripple' persona was unfit for the public square. Her performance and costuming played deadpan to the idea that her disability eliminated all pleasure from her being, and it satisfied the expectation that she perform for others as an object of pity, best returned post haste to the medical sphere.

Any humour we can find in Araniello's meek and 'mewling' performance is bone dry.[32] The humour in Williamson's persona, for all its brash exuberance, is only slightly less subtle. He presented himself as an agitator for Araniello's cause, shouting vigorously into a broken megaphone throughout the performance, feigning obliviousness to the lack of amplification. This referenced both Williamson's deafness, which may or may not have been legible to their passing audience, but also created a broader slapstick performance of public incompetence. This functioned as a pantomime of what disability studies scholar Rosemarie Garland-Thomson called a 'misfitting' in her theorisation of disability as a way of being in an environment.[33] Like Araniello, Williamson's persona failed to fit in this arena of street protest, as the apparent incompatibility of the megaphone and his disability appeared to preclude him from full competence and control in his environment. Williamson's pretended lack of self-awareness made him a potential object of derision or pity, but by performing into the anticipated misreading he had the last laugh.

Both artists' personas indulged in widely recognised stereotypes. They presented themselves as being in the grip of tragedy, desiring pity and in need of medical intervention. In doing so they echoed familiar narratives about disability that could be used to non-ironic ends. The credulity of their audience suggests that these ideas continued to be ubiquitous, and that the performers' knowledge of contemporary debates about disabled people were politically out of step with their audience. Performance art specialist Petra Kuppers addressed the inaccessibility of 'purity' in contemporary performances of disability by disabled artists. On Bill Shannon (b. 1970) and his intensively physical street performances, Kuppers wrote that his 'street actions are not performances of disability, but a performance of the readings, visceral effects, social embodiments, and public nets surrounding the meeting of different bodies'.[34] Araniello and Williamson, who were always conscious of the melodrama in the public existence of their disability, approached this performance of disability similarly and also performed into these 'nets'. By doing so they privately asserted control of these predicted (mis)perceptions of their lives and bodies, and seized the opportunity to make themselves superior through their pretence. They also created a fertile ground for satire, by echoing familiar positions and provoking ongoing discourses. However, as I address in the next section, for a satire to succeed, ironic distance from these discourses needs to be signalled by the satirist to the audience.[35]

Signalling satire: Intertextual strategies

A satirist can signal distance from the pretended position through exaggeration, absurdity and the presentation of unexpected ideas or unfamiliar reasoning.[36] This strategy undermines their pretended position from within, signalling to the audience that the satirist does not mean what is said. This was true of *Assisted Passage*, even if the audience in the square failed to read those signs. The video documents moments where the exaggeration and absurdity become more obvious. Hadley marks as particularly farcical Araniello and Williamson's sung variation of *Ticket to Ride* by the Beatles, which changed the lyrics from 'she's got a ticket to ride' to 'she's got a ticket to die'.[37] This element of the performance took the familiar strategy of singing at protests and distorted it with incongruous flippancy that signalled insincerity. It is this re-mixing of familiar discourse structures that allows audiences to identify ironic statements.[38] In *Assisted Passage*, the audience's failure to read what is, as the following analysis will detail, in many ways a fairly conventional satire, suggests either an unlikely unfamiliarity with the conventions of protest or, more convincingly, an unfamiliarity with the art, activism and broader culture of disabled people in the UK.

As a researcher of images of disability, I am drawn to the posters designed by Araniello and Williamson. The posters were prominently displayed and taped to nearby fencing, their table and Araniello's legs, suggesting that all three could be considered by the audience to be similarly inanimate accessories to the protest. The posters were part of every sighted interaction with the work. Clear photographs of the posters were inserted into the video, indicating their importance to the performance. Posters, handmade or otherwise, are expected components of street protest, and comic practices are similarly established and observed strategies for protesters.[39] In these posters, broad stereotypes and precise comic deviations occurred. There were three posters, two of which made comic, but deliberately confusing, references to airlines, illustrated by images of wheelchair-using stick figures (more officially called International Symbols of Accessibility and familiar from public signage) tumbling from easyJet branded planes. The visual effect is somewhere between a grimly slapstick mass suicide and an assault by uniformed, wheelchair-using paratroopers. The remaining poster illustrated Araniello's 'wish' to access assisted dying with a rough, diagrammatic image of a resurrection (Figure 7.2). In this image a hand-drawn styling of the International Symbol of Accessibility lies in a coffin in a grave, but – fear not – this figure can be liberated from disability by death. This liberation was illustrated by an instructional arrow, showing a neat transformation into a normative standing stick figure (the international symbol of men's public lavatories). This poster was charged with an irreverent

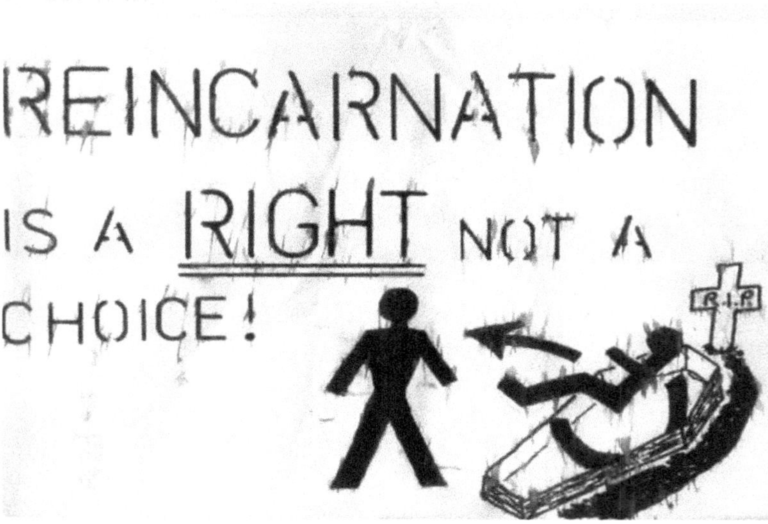

Figure 7.2 The Disabled Avant-Garde, Still from *Assisted Passage*, 2007 in *Bite the Hand that Feeds!* (Live Art Development Agency, 2012) PAL-DVD, (04.23).

comedy and made crudely and expertly visible the framing of disabled people as perpetually and naturally desiring to be other than what they are, pursued to an absurd and illicit limit: the desire to be other as the desire to be dead. This is underlined by the large, capitalised caption: 'Reincarnation is a right not a choice!'

Philosopher of aesthetics Gregory Currie has written that the success of communicative pictorial irony is limited because the images must contain a large amount of representative detail and can therefore be heavy-handed. They may either fail due to a lack of expressive indicators of irony, meaning that the irony is dependent on extra-pictorial aspects of the pretence. Or, if the image does contain the necessary stylistic indicators, Currie writes that it may be impossible to attribute to it the 'straight-faced' pretence best suited to the ironic mode.[40] The 'reincarnation' poster was certainly both heavy handed and already integrated into a broader ironic performance but in this case inelegance was elegantly harnessed by Araniello and Williamson. The poster employs a favourite strategy of Araniello and Williamson, who enjoyed creating a 'low-fi aesthetic' and deliberately demonstrating an affected 'lack of skills and professionalism'.[41] The poster was 'low-fi' and stylistically juvenile, produced via marker pen and careful stencilling, but this was consistent with Araniello and Williamson's self-presentation as clumsy and inept street protesters. The use of these materials signalled a (false) naivety which only heightened the pathos of the image. The exaggeration had a double function, continuing to play down to stereotypes, but also presenting a reasoning of assisted dying that was unexpected, remaking the familiar as ultimately risible. The irony of the poster, as an extension of other aspects of the performance, was an ever present signal of satire.

Williamson and Araniello also played towards ideas of incompetence, adjacent to Araniello's performance of juvenility and meekness. A return to Figure 7.1 shows that Williamson called early and loudly for Araniello to receive a ticket to 'Zurich in Sweden'.[42] Fox and Araniello, jokingly sensitive to Williamson's feeling that audiences would not be able to tell whether they were truly 'pathetically stupid', has since clarified the joke: Williamson and Araniello were aware of the location of Zurich (a city in San Marino, as we all know).[43] The choice to signal 'stupidity' is doubly intriguing in this context. It situates the personas adopted for *Assisted Passage* in the midst of debates around capacitated consent. Is your petition for medical intervention undermined if you make errors of geography, or cannot satisfactorily describe where the procedure will take place? Additionally, signalling satire through the infantile and the 'stupid' stood in for unreliability, and introduced the idea of the untrustworthy disabled person who may be twisted in body and mind, making a killing on benefit fraud, or indeed lying to you about their wish to end their life as part of an elaborate, documented art experiment which they filmed and later posted online. Although Araniello and Williamson did signal satire, as we have seen, they were able to do so in ways that were not wildly differentiated from their straight-faced presentation of themselves as disabled. The live audience's reliance on stereotypical images of disability, and their unfamiliarity with contemporary debates about disability meant that they were unprepared to make these slightly granular differentiations. Their acceptance of these images of disability became part of the performance, successfully proving the Disabled Avant-Garde's 'point'; there was a gap between their and their audience's perception of disability.

Williamson has written that when 'mainstream' audiences encounter the broader scene of disability arts, they may ask 'are [the artists] really as crazy/ infantile/ pathetically stupid as they're trying to make out, or are they trying to get a rise out of us?'[44] *Assisted Passage* exploited this dynamic. Humour has long been an important feature of disabled art-making and disabled protest in the UK. Beginning in the late 1970s, the disability arts movement produced work across many forms and institutions, creating theatre, dance, cabaret, visual arts, poetry and protest songs, which developed an irreverent brand of humour that focused 'on the absurd way our society treats disabled people' and made 'sense of the senseless'.[45] The use of humour is also an observed tactic in disability activism and is listed as one of fifty key topics in *Disability Studies: A Student's Guide*, where humour is described as sometimes angry but also deployed to 'soften critical insights with amused understanding'.[46] For disabled people, displaying a good sense of humour is not necessarily revolutionary. 'To be granted fully human status by normates', wrote Garland-Thomson, 'disabled people must use charm, intimidation, ardor, deference, humor, or entertainment to relieve nondisabled people of their discomfort.'[47] To be entertaining, to joke and to serve as fools is therefore a dynamic that has historical precedence for disabled people. Activists have also historically used humour that offers relief from discomfort, leaving their targets more willing to accept critical commentary on disability. Here, Araniello and Williamson decisively disrupt that context and caution, finding pleasure in playing down to the wide net of stereotypes available to them, with a humour that is alienating and neither entertaining, persuasive nor understanding.

This brand of humour is described as developing from and alongside an awareness of a more expected power dynamic, where disabled people are the victims of denigrating 'sick jokes'.[48] Joking at the expense of disabled people is theorised in disability studies as a tool of superiority and social correction in harmony with racist, sexist and homophobic humour, where an objectified 'other' is made comical in their denigrated difference. Tom Shakespeare and other disabled scholars have questioned whether jokes at the expense of disabled people are truly in any way taboo, querying the extent of their proscription, largely in social situations but also in visual culture, from the dwarfs of Diego Velasquez's *Las Meninas* (1656) to the recurring character who used but did not need a wheelchair in Matt Lucas and David Walliams's *Little Britain* (2003–6).[49] Disabled comedienne and organiser Barbara Lisicki tidily brought these ideas together, suggesting that it is the same anxieties and embarrassments which provoke jokes at her expense – or 'school boy laughter' at '"spastic" nonsense' – that then prevent audiences from laughing at her deliberate, crafted jokes.[50] Araniello and Williamson are keenly aware of their audience's potentially limited understanding of this tension and its history in disability arts.

Their satire explores the resulting dynamic, testing the limits of an audience's polite public refusal to acknowledge the ridiculous in the context of disability, and using their caution against them. This is also noted by Hadley, who begins to consider the mechanics of Araniello's other satirical work on assisted dying in this context, observing that 'some people find it so difficult to believe a woman as severely disabled as Araniello would make fun of her own assigned identity position in this way that they can dismiss this possibility'.[51] This should not be taken as an argument for reductive binaries of disabled and 'abled' subjectivities, which cannot be proven by this experiment; the video makes careful note of a wheelchair user approaching the tableau and signing the petition.[52] However, Araniello and Williamson could here signal satire on their own terms and be reasonably certain that their audience would lack the necessary cultural acumen to make a successful reading. Araniello once said with characteristic wit that their collaborative work as the Disabled Avant-Garde was 'ultimately / taking the piss, but Aaron's very good at / intellectualising anything that we do'.[53] Araniello and Williamson were not surprised to have their satire missed. By taking the piss, you hope to have some fun, but you also seize the power to make someone else look ridiculous.

Victims: The right audience for the wrong audience

Irony can have two victims: first, a person or group who holds the view that is being ridiculed, and second, the audience who fails to identify the pretence.[54] In *Assisted Passage*, the video documentation showcases members of the audience missing the comedically exaggerated pretence, and concludes that this failure occurs because they endorse the idea being ridiculed. They are doubly victimised by the irony. It is this dynamic that Araniello and Williamson wish for secondary, online audiences to view. But *Assisted Passage* does also contain a disconcerting mockery of a disabled person who wishes to die. Araniello and Williamson could have chosen to avoid this discomfort, and delivered a gentler satire by pretending to be kindly activists agitating on behalf of disabled people who wished to access assisted dying. But how available was this position to Araniello and Williamson should they have wanted to take it up? As observably disabled performers, they were not able to pretend themselves into an embodied performance of an imagined 'abled' subjectivity. Unintuitively, they were constrained in their performance of disability. But this willingness to be harsh and direct is also a reflection of their strength of conviction on this issue, and a reminder that hostile feeling for the pretended position is an essential and potentially fraught part of ironic communication.

This hostility is also apparent in the presentation of the live audience to the online audience. Hadley observed that 'secondary spectators' have a much clearer view of performances than the live audiences, who are made 'unwitting co-performers'.[55] With the introduction of video documentary they become unknowing co-stars. In an interview with Hadley, Araniello denied that the piece operated like a candid camera. Hadley agreed and wrote that, 'though prankish in some ways, the point was not to make fun of a passer-by's potentially troubling assumptions about disabled people'.[56] There is undoubtedly an urge to distance the piece – part of a largely under-theorised disability arts – and its high-stakes subject matter from discomforting and low status contexts like 'gotcha' candid camera television. However, this is a context that must come to mind when viewing the covert and unsteady shots compiled for the video. The videographer used a handheld camera, usually at some distance from anyone approaching the petition, and focused in on shoulders that were hunched over the petition table, capturing their faces as they turned away. A photograph of the petition clearly displaying names and signatures is featured in the video. In the context of Williamson's very strong condemnation of the signatories and Araniello's statement that they had 'happily signed [her] life away', this exposure is a little shocking.[57] While the 'point' of the initial performance and the documentation was certainly more nuanced than a 'prank', the nature of satire and ironic communication must mean that 'making fun' of people's assumption about disabled people was an inevitable and powerful product of the performance.

'Making fun', like 'taking the piss', may contain controlled or constrained anger. While humour can offer conditional space for empathy in shared laughter, in the performance of *Assisted Passage* this was not taken up, partly because Araniello and Williamson wielded this potential solidarity harshly. Successful satire does, by most definitions, involve a ratification of the satire by some members of an audience.[58] In *Assisted Passage*, this process appears entirely absent in the live audience, with neither video documentation nor Araniello and Williamson's separate reflections revealing anyone who recognised the joke. Those who missed the irony were not only unable to access the feeling of superiority shared between satirists and those hypothetical audience members who might successfully read the satire, but also left open to Araniello and Williamson's ridicule in the public eye. By joking, Araniello and Williamson did not explain or persuade; instead they took revenge. This conclusion follows the findings of Cynthia Willett and Julie Willett in their chapter on 'fumerism', where they argued that in feminist stand-up, humour can be a type of revenge fuelled by both anger and joy, that 'deals a new hand', allowing the joker to play a game that reframes expected dynamics of authority and control.[59] This allows the angry joke teller and their – in *Assisted Passage* absent – laughing audience to create a new power dynamic where exclusion from the joke remakes the previously assured insider as a newly victimised outsider. The humour of *Assisted Passage* therefore left conciliatory 'amused understanding' to one side and abandoned the comic as an effective vehicle for political seduction, perhaps aiming instead for social correction. Araniello and Williamson's 'crip' humour embraced non-conformity and offence and operated beyond a disability arts that was wary of bad taste, discomfort and anger, instead embracing modes that excluded and jeered.

Significant to this discussion is that these victims, co-stars and the primary targets of Araniello's and Williamson's hostile feeling, were not an ill-defined 'public' but a university population. The performance was staged in a popular location for student activists: in a communal square amidst buildings belonging to various devolved institutions of the University of London. The building framed behind Araniello and Williamson in Figure 7.1 was – and is – part of the School of Oriental and African Studies (SOAS). The text at the beginning of the video names their location as Birkbeck, University of London, the institution I currently attend. The hypothesis of their experiment was that their experience of disability would be dangerously different from wider societies' views of disability, and they anticipated that this would be just as true in this particular place. As part of establishing this university setting, the video highlights that the work was part of a 'diversity week', an event that would usually aim to celebrate the inclusion of marginalised people in a community or workspace, and draw attention or 'awareness' to their voices. This context framed Araniello and Williamson as 'othered' ambassadors from the world of disability so immediately and fully that I initially considered that this might have been an elaborate continuation of the satire.

However, anecdotal recollections from staff at Birkbeck and surrounding academic institutions suggest that this was a real, recurring and now sadly defunct event.[60] A diversity week framed Williamson and Araniello – who were both professional artists with postgraduate qualifications – as temporarily celebrated participants, while implicitly recognising that their knowledge was marginal in a university setting, requiring a separate, specific and contained week in which to showcase them and their work. This marginality is termed more strongly as 'critical avoidance' by literary disability scholar David Bolt, who has suggested that disability – among other 'marked' bodies and identities – is either avoided in the academy or contained within disability studies contexts.[61] This suggests that beyond an unfamiliarity with the conventions of disability arts, *Assisted Passage* exposed a disinclination towards critical thought around disability. The audience was unprepared to do anything but take the words of these 'diverse voices' at face value. Uncritical, charitable support made up the central drama of *Assisted Passage*, which rested on the audience ignoring the clues that signalled satire. It is this lack of criticality that Araniello and Williamson highlight to their secondary audience.

Impersonal narrative

Assisted Passage aimed to demonstrate a gulf between the perception of disabled people and the experience of disability. And yet the performance itself revealed little about Araniello and Williamson's own lives, other than their unsurprising knowledge of disability stereotypes. This is a consequence of irony. If irony operates only to denigrate a particular, pretended point of view, a satirist can then only reliably let us 'know what they deplore, and not what they endorse'.[62] The live performance interjected into normative narratives deplored by Araniello and Williamson, but could not immediately promote another narrative in place for as long as the irony was sustained. The live audience therefore experienced a reinforcement of the very narratives Araniello and Williamson were mocking. This was tolerated by Araniello and Williamson, who wanted to showcase the miscommunication. Their intended intervention into public perceptions of disability – and any more didactic revelations about Araniello and Williamson's experiences – was deferred to unironic post-mortem arguments, like those presented in the YouTube video. For Araniello and Williamson an explanation was necessary for at least two reasons. First, the framing of the performance as research necessitated the discussion of both the hypothesis and the results. The video was only the beginning of a long process, which this chapter now contributes to, of ruining the joke. Second, strongly held political convictions motivated the performance, and continued ambiguity was a potential risk to their activism. However, while it was sustained, irony allowed Araniello and Williamson to ridicule negative perceptions, with no accompanying obligation to argue the opposite by demonstrating their own potential 'model minority' status or denying their own – or their community's – complexities.

This is a significant conclusion for disability studies, which often vests substantial weight on the need to publicly produce the personal narratives (and personal bodies) of disabled people to disrupt critical avoidance and displace societal misconceptions perpetuated with undue authority.[63] Roberts found that the work of the Disabled Avant-Garde moved 'away from the autobiographical subject (which can drift towards essentialist interpretations), and towards the actively inauthentic, ironic, and punk'.[64] Williamson and Araniello have largely mistrusted both the efficacy and dignity of sharing much about their own lives in their art. In a 2023 interview in an academic journal, Williamson outlined elements of his childhood experiences of disability 'in slightly reluctant terms to address "prurient curiosity"', an inescapable impulse that he describes satirising in his work with Araniello as the Disabled Avant-Garde.[65] Many more elements of Araniello's 'life story' are now part of the narrative of disability arts in the UK, featured in archives, in poet Allan Sutherland's oral history of the movement, *Electric Bodies: Travels in Life History* (2011) and now in obituaries and tributes from many friends.[66] The blurring of terminal and chronic diagnosis within Araniello's childhood medical experiences might perhaps give insight into her interest in and public position on physician-assisted dying.[67] And yet I am uncertain as to their usefulness to this chapter, where instead her ironic 'disclosure' of her wish to die might lead us to alternatives to confessional, individual narratives.

Medical humanities scholarship has complicated the usefulness of the personal narrative. Angela Woods has written on the limited value of the linear narrative, which may be inaccessible or inauthentic to many experiences of ill health.[68] Stuart Murray, in his 2023 introduction to *Medical Humanities and Disability Studies* finds potential in more complex narratives, writing that 'life stories in and through critical frames and vice versa' have the potential to disturb even as they clarify, beyond the simplicity of the confession, or the elevation of a suppressed 'voice'.[69] His text culminates in a passage that narrativises Murray's own relationship with debility and death, in explanation or perhaps justification of his project. He places poems and vignettes throughout his text, although none are as combative and resistant to interpretation as the performance of *Assisted Passage*. Araniello and Williamson prematurely answered Murray's call for (writing) practices that 'misdirect', 'complain', 'despair' and move through other uncomfortable spaces of feeling. In their performance, Araniello and Williamson mislead their audience as to the nature of their complaint. Why, after all, should you perform generously or vulnerably to an audience that, as you are demonstrating, is not really engaging with care? Instead Araniello and Williamson use ironic communication in order to exercise anger at a charitable but careless audience, exorcise despair as to how to communicate with them and find some measure of enjoyment as the audience was made vulnerable in turn and exposed to potential judgement. All of these states of feeling are undoubtedly complex, and at times difficult to view, but they are also carefully set out in both the performance and presentation of the performance in video documentation.

Despite this, *Assisted Passage* is unlikely to be persuasive on the overarching question of legal access to assisted dying in the UK. In all my engagement with this piece, it has not convinced me. But it is a compelling demonstration that there is – or very optimistically that there was in 2007 – a gap between Araniello and Williamson's experience of disability and the understanding of Araniello's disability in an academic audience. They extrapolate from there to argue that a gulf between their experience and their audiences' perception means that we cannot trust their wider social context to maintain Araniello's right to live, should she have the right to die. They highlight disconnects which equally apply to naturally fallible gatekeepers and safeguarding agents for publicly and privately funded medical and social aid. In two of their posters Araniello and Williamson called for 'choices and rights'. The phrase 'choices and rights' is a prominent slogan for the disability rights movement in the UK.[70] It also echoes rhetoric used by campaigners for assisted dying and around other matters of medical autonomy (for example abortion procedures and gender confirmation surgeries) delimited variously in the UK.[71] In the video of *Assisted Passage* Araniello and Williamson demonstrate to their audience that our ways of perceiving – or indeed not perceiving – disability and disabled lives prevent these two positions from comfortable compatibility.

For Araniello and Williamson, irony was an effective tool for critical engagement with these ideas. In *Assisted Passage*, satire and the ironic voice did two things in the context of personal narrative. They presented a mode of live research for disabled artists that angrily rejected satisfying the curiosity of the audience and asked for something more than a polite, supportive encounter. Araniello and Williamson were able to perform disability inauthentically, defying their audience's presumptive assurance as to how to read their publicly disabled bodies. The personal, political and the collective body are always in tension in disability arts and while not trying to speak collectively or individually about the endless, absurdly banal experiences in this open space, Araniello and Williamson also chose not to fill this gap with their own personal narratives. The piece punished the audience by cheerfully ridiculing them for their lack of critical engagement and cultural blindspots. This inversion of the surface-level power relationship at play in their tableau of faux vulnerability is uncompromising, but it is also illicitly and unexpectedly fun.

The video ends by revealing that Araniello and Williamson are both 'making fun' and having fun. The final clips chosen for the video are of Araniello and Williamson singing *Somewhere Over the Rainbow*, a song that is incongruously saccharine and sentimental, but with lyrics apt to Araniello's reportedly thwarted wish to fly towards her death.[72] Their singing becomes almost immediately too ridiculous for Williamson and Araniello to stomach, and their unplanned laughter briefly breaks into their performance. Laughter also physically transforms the literal framing of the performance; just before the video ends by cutting to black, the frame begins to shake and muffled breathy laughter can be heard. This laughter comes either from Araniello's microphone or, more likely, from the until now invisible figure of the camera operator, whose feeling is made visible through the shaking frame. This break for laughter also makes the separation between the laughing artists and the pitiable personas briefly visible. Disability studies has considered how disabled people are able to show that they have lives 'full, rich and well worth living' through humour and humorous personal narrative, largely attending to everyday communication or stand-up comedy, as opposed to humorous visual art.[73] In the video, Araniello and Williamson have already implicitly demonstrated that they have full professional and creative lives as artists and satirists. This disruption of their otherwise uncompromisingly severe position feels less like a plea for recognition of their humanity and more like a reminder that their performance did contain the potential for shared laughter.

If visual humour can, for the medical humanities, be about emotion as knowledge transfer, complexity and ambiguity, then I suggest that *Assisted Passage* becomes significant for its contradictions, hostility and its refusal to communicate accessibly. If we want to look at jokes from (and not just about) disability, we have to consider the unspeakability of anger and our inability to facilitate it as a communicative tool in most settings, including the medical. Humour can make anger visible, but this visibility is not necessarily set up for our easy viewing. Disabled humour is here an ironic wit that attempts to make known the murky space between perception and experience, and attempts to unmake dominant discourses into uncertainties, without offering new positions of authority in their place.

Acknowledgements

With thanks to Dr Aaron Williamson for generously granting me permission to use these images.

Notes

1 This work was supported by the Wellcome Trust [223350/Z/21/Z].
2 Aaron Williamson, *Aaron Williamson: Performance/ Video/ Collaboration* (Live Art Development Agency, 2008), p. 92.
3 For more on the history of Live Art in the UK see Deirdre Heddon and Jennie Klein (eds), *Histories and Practices of Live Art* (Bloomsbury Press, 2012); Dominic Johnson, *Critical Live Art* (Routledge, 2013); RoseLee Goldberg, *Performance: Live Art 1909 to the Present* (Harry N. Abrams, 1979). For more on Live Art and disability in the UK

see Lois Keidan and C.J. Mitchell (eds), *Access All Areas: Live Art and Disability* (Live Art Development Agency, 2012). For more on Live Art and comedy see Maria Chatzichristodoulou, *Live Art in the UK: Contemporary Performances of Precarity* (Bloomsbury, 2020).

4 Oriana Fox, *Performance Art Can Change Your Life! Shame Attacking and Parrhesia as Feminist Practices of Freedom* (PhD thesis, Goldsmiths, University of London, 2019), p. 239.

5 The Disabled Avant-Garde (@Disabledavantgarde), 'Assisted Passage', YouTube, 28 November 2007 [1:38], https://www.youtube.com/watch?v=SvgVv-nEEIs (accessed 19 August 2024).

6 Williamson, *Aaron Williamson: Performance/ Video/ Collaboration*, p. 92; Jonathan Swift, *A Modest Proposal for Preventing the Children of Poor People from Being a Burthen to Their Parents or the Country, and for Making Them Beneficial to the Publick* (S. Harding, 1729).

7 Dustin Griffin, *Satire: A Critical Reintroduction* (University Press of Kentucky, 1994), p. 173.

8 Roger Kreuz and R.M. Roberts, 'On satire and parody: The importance of being ironic', *Metaphor and Symbol* 8:2 (1993), 97–109; Cate Watson, *Comedy and Social Science: Towards a Methodology of Funny* (Routledge, 2017), p. 70.

9 Herbert Clark and Richard Gerrig, 'On the pretense theory of irony', *Journal of Experimental Psychology*, 113:1 (1984), 121.

10 Gregory Currie, 'The Irony in Pictures', *British Journal of Aesthetics* 51:2 (2011), 151.

11 Craig Stewart, 'Strategies of verbal irony in visual satire: Reading *The New Yorker*'s "Politics of Fear" cover', *Humour* 26:2 (2013), 203.

12 Clark and Gerrig, 'On the pretense theory of irony', 122.

13 Bree Hadley, *Disability, Public Space Performance and Spectatorship: Unconscious Performers* (Palgrave Macmillan, 2014); Bree Hadley, Jelena Rajak, Andrew Filmer, Rebecca Caines and Alan Read, 'The "Dirty Work" of the lie', *Performance Research* 15:2 (2010), 123–9; Angharad Butler-Rees and Bree Hadley, 'Exploring the Role of the Disabled Body as a Vehicle and Art Form within Anti-Austerity Protest', in *Politics as Public Art* (Routledge, 2022); Fox, *Performance Art Can Change Your Life.*

14 Hadley, *Disability, Public Space Performance and Spectatorship*, p. 183.

15 Eleanor Roberts, 'Disability art is dead, long live disability art!: The sick crip Disabled Avant-Garde', *Contemporary Theatre Review* 34:3 (2024), 262–79.

16 The Disabled Avant-Garde [0:37].
17 Euthanasia and Assisted Dying, *BBC News*, https://www.bbc.co.uk/news/topics/cljev4r3zgxt (accessed 29 June 2024).
18 The Suicide Act, 1961 decriminalised the act of suicide, but detailed the enabling or assisting of suicide as criminal. See, Suicide Act, 1961, sec 1–2 (England and Wales). Although punishable by a prison sentence of up to fourteen years, recent guidelines for prosecutors advise against pursuing conviction where the assistance was motivated 'wholly by compassion' and the determined consent of the suicide can be confirmed. However, cases are still investigated and prosecutions occur. Guidelines for leniency make clear exceptions for individuals with authority: carers and anyone acting in a capacity of care. See Criminal Prosecution Service (2014), 'Suicide: Policy for Prosecutors in Respect of Cases of Encouraging or Assisting Suicide' sec. 43.14, https://www.cps.gov.uk/prosecution-guidance/suicide-policy-prosecutors-respect-cases-encouraging-or-assisting-suicide
19 Lloyd Riley, 'The cost of dying overseas', dignityindying.org.uk, 13 November 2017, https://features.dignityindying.org.uk/true-cost-dignitas/ (accessed 22 August 2024).
20 Dignitas, 'Welcome to Dignitas', 25 August 2024, https://dignitas.ch/en/ (accessed 26 August 2024).
21 Williamson, *Aaron Williamson: Performance/ Video/ Collaboration*, p. 93.
22 Alison Kafer, *Feminist, Queer, Crip* (Indiana University Press, 2013), p. 5.
23 Mike Oliver, 'A Sociology of Disability or a Disablist Sociology?' in Len Barton (ed.), *Disability and Society: Emerging Issues and Insights* (Routledge, 2018 [1996]), 18–42.
24 John Swain and Sally French, 'Towards an affirmation model of disability', *Disability & Society* 15:4 (2000), 569–82.
25 There are disability groups advocating for assisted dying legislation, for example Disabled People for Dignity in Dying (2013–). See Harriet Sherwood, 'Disability Rights Campaigners Urge MPs and Peers to Back Assisted Dying Bill', *Guardian*, 24 October 2024; Araniello protested with the disability-first advocacy organisation Not Dead Yet UK, which campaigned against legalising assisted dying. Not Dead Yet UK argues that assisted suicide dangerously diminishes the need for assisted living as well as palliative care. For these palliative care and disability activist perspectives see Harvey Max Chochinov and Catherine Frazee, 'Finding a balance: Canada's law on medical assistance in dying', *The Lancet* 388:10044 (2016), 543–5.

26 Disability Rights UK, 'Position on Assisted Dying', disabilityrightsuk.org, https://www.disabilityrightsuk.org/news/disability-rights-uk%E2%80%99s-position-assisted-dying (accessed 3 April 2024).
27 For insight into UK austerity and the Disabled Avant-Garde see Roberts, 'Disability art is dead, long live disability art!', 262–79.
28 Tom Shakespeare, 'A quiet majority of disabled people support assisted dying. I'm one of them', *Express*, 21 November 2024, https://www.express.co.uk/news/politics/1979063/assisted-dying-bill-disabled-tom-shakespeare (accessed 3 April 2025).
29 John Pring, 'Assisted dying bill: Disabled activists warn of bill's threat', *Disability News Service*, 25 July 2014, https://www.disabilitynewsservice.com/assisted-dying-bill-disabled-activists-warn-of-bills-threat/ (accessed 3 April 2025).
30 The Disabled Avant-Garde, [3:38], [2:43].
31 Oriana Fox, 'Satire and subversion with Katherine Araniello', *Multiple Os*, podcast, 30 November 2021.
32 Williamson, *Aaron Williamson: Performance/ Video/ Collaboration*, p. 93.
33 Rosemarie Garland-Thomson, 'Misfits: A feminist materialist disability concept', *Hypatia* 26:3 (2011), 591–609.
34 Petra Kuppers, *Disability and Contemporary Performance: Bodies on the Edge* (Routledge, 2003), Chapter 3, subheading 'Involving the public scene', para 3. ebookcentral.
35 Stewart, 'Strategies of verbal irony in visual satire', 203.
36 Paul Simpson, *On the Discourse of Satire* (John Benjamins, 2003), p. 9.
37 Hadley, *Disability, Public Space Performance and Spectatorship*, p. 100.
38 Stewart, 'Strategies of verbal irony in visual satire', 203.
39 Alister Wedderburn, *Humour, Subjectivity and World Politics* (Manchester University Press, 2021), p. 3.
40 Currie, 'The Irony in Pictures', 167.
41 Queen Mary University of London Archives, Live Art collection, Katherine Araniello, Reference KA/13, printed material, loose pages, page beginning 'Taken from website …', n.d., lines 14–15.
42 The Disabled Avant-Garde, [01:09].
43 Fox, 'Satire and subversion with Katherine Araniello'; Williamson, *Aaron Williamson: Performance/ Video/ Collaboration*, p. 14; Araniello appears to have been attuned to the potential risks in being seen as 'stupid' in public presentation and weighed them carefully when making art. Shortly before her death she expressed concern, for example,

that a poetry collection featuring oral history style interviews with her and favouring a fragmented, naturalistic style through transcription would make her 'look stupid'. She weighed this concern carefully against her desire to honour the process of the poet Allan Sutherland. Allan Sutherland, 'Disabled Avant Garde', *A Different Way of Engaging* (D4D: 2020), p. 3, https://d4d.org.uk/wp-content/uploads/2019/05/Katherine-A-Poems-A-Different-Way-of-Engaging.pdf

44 Williamson, *Aaron Williamson: Performance/ Video/ Collaboration*, p. 14.

45 Colin Barnes, *Disabling Imagery and the Media* (Ryburn Publishing; British Council of Disabled People, 1992), p. 29.

46 Colin Cameron, *Disability Studies: A Student's Guide* (Sage, 2014), pp. 69–72.

47 Rosemarie Garland-Thomson, *Extraordinary Bodies: Figuring Physical Disability in American Culture and Literature* (Columbia University Press, 1999), p. 13.

48 Beth Haller and Sue Ralph, 'John Callahan's Pelswick cartoon and a new phase of disability humor', *Disability Studies Quarterly* 23:3 (2003), 4–16.

49 Tom Shakespeare, 'Joking a part', *Body and Society* 5:4 (1999), p. 48; Rebecca Mallett, 'Claiming comedic immunity, or what you get when you cross contemporary comedy with disability', *Review of Disability Studies* 6:3 (2014), 5–14.

50 Elinor Rowlands, 'Bringing the legacy of NDACA into focus: Feminist Arts News June 1989', *disabilityarts.online*, 3 May 2020, https://disabilityarts.online/magazine/opinion/bringing-the-legacy-of-ndaca-into-focus-feminist-arts-news-june-1989/ (accessed 21 August 2024).

51 Hadley, *Disability, Public Space Performance and Spectatorship*, p. 135.

52 The Disabled Avant-Garde, [3:34–4-12].

53 This quotation is from a poem and the forward slashes denote line breaks. Sutherland, 'Disabled Avant Garde', *A Different Way of Engaging*, p. 63 (18–20).

54 Stewart, 'Strategies of verbal irony', 204.

55 Hadley, *Disability, Public Space Performance and Spectatorship*, pp. 26, 102.

56 Hadley, *Disability, Public Space Performance and Spectatorship*, p. 100.

57 Hadley, *Disability, Public Space Performance and Spectatorship*, p. 99.

58 Stewart, 'Strategies of verbal irony', 207.

59 Cynthia Willett and Julie Willett, *Uproarious: How Feminists and Other Subversive Comics Speak Truth* (University of Minnesota Press, 2019), pp. 30, 35.

60 Mark Pimm, Disability Officer at Birkbeck, University of London, asked another staff member who worked for the university at that time, and they recalled Diversity Week anecdotally. Pimm relayed that the work of organising Diversity Week at Birkbeck and SOAS should be credited to Deborah 'Deb' Viney, who worked as Diversity Advisor at SOAS, University of London and passed away in June 2014 (Mark Pimm, 'Research enquiry about a disability arts event in 2007!' email to author, 21 October 2022). Viney did organise art events, but SOAS does not have records of the commissioning process, organisation and funding of the event, and the extent to which the college co-signed the nature of the Disabled Avant-Garde's intervention.

61 David Bolt, 'Social Encounters, Cultural Representation and Critical Avoidance', in Nick Watson, Alan Roulstone and Carol Thomas (eds), *Routledge Handbook of Disability Studies* (Routledge, 2012).

62 Griffin, *Satire*, p. 172.

63 David Bolt, *Metanarratives of Disability* (Routledge, 2021).

64 Roberts, 'Disability art is dead, long live disability art!', 278.

65 Aaron Williamson and Larry Lynch, 'Situating deaf-gain: Performance and writing in the work of and Aaron Williamson', *Journal of Visual Art Practice* 22:2–3 (2023), 291–305.

66 Allan Sutherland, *Electric Bodies: Travels in Life History* (Disability Arts Online, 2011).

67 Sutherland, 'Disabled Avant Garde', pp. 23–4.

68 Angela Woods, 'The limits of narrative: Provocations for the medical humanities', *Medical Humanities* 37:2 (2011), 73–8; Woods, 'Beyond the Wounded Storyteller: Rethinking Narrativity, Illness and Embodied Self-Experience', in Havi Carel and Rachel Cooper (eds), *Health, Illness and Disease: Philosophical Essays* (Taylor & Francis Group, 2014).

69 Stewart Murray, *Medical Humanities and Disability Studies: In/Disciplines* (Bloomsbury, 2023), p. 15.

70 For example, the unofficial anthem of the movement was *Choices and Rights* by punk-poet performer Johnny Crescendo (aka Alan Holdsworth).

71 Disability studies scholar, sometime stand-up comedian and assisted dying campaigner Tom Shakespeare wrote that the public cannot understand why activists against assisted dying within the disability movement support choice, control and assistance in every aspect of life but this. Tom Shakespeare, 'Memorandum by Tom Shakespeare',

parliament.uk (House of Lords, Assisted dying for the terminally ill bill, Volume II: Evidence, 4 April 2005), https://publications.parliament.uk/pa/ld/ldasdy.htm (accessed 23 January 2025), pp. 245–7.

72 The Disabled Avant-Garde, [06:55].

73 Kim Reid and Edy Hammond Stoughton, 'The humorous construction of disability: "Stand-up" comedians in the United States', *Disability & Society* 21:6 (2006), 629–43; see also, Teresa Milbrodt, '"Today I had an Eye Appointment, and I'm Still Blind": Crip Humour, storytelling, and narrative positioning of the disabled self', *Disability Studies Quarterly* 38:2 (2018).

References

Barnes, Colin. *Disabling Imagery and the Media*. Ryburn Publishing; British Council of Disabled People, 1992.

BBC News. 'Euthanasia and Assisted Dying', https://www.bbc.co.uk/news/topics/cljev4r3zgxt (accessed 29 June).

Bolt, D. 'Social Encounters, Cultural Representation and Critical Avoidance'. In Nick Watson, Alan Roulstone and Carol Thomas (eds), *Routledge Handbook of Disability Studies*. Routledge, 2012.

Bolt, David. *Metanarratives of Disability: Culture, Assumed Authority and the Normative Cultural Order*. Routledge, 2021.

Butler-Rees, Angharad, and Bree Hadley. 'Exploring the Role of the Disabled Body as a Vehicle and Art Form within Anti-Austerity Protest'. In *Politics as Public Art*. Routledge, 2022.

Cameron, Colin. *Disability Studies: A Student's Guide*. Sage, 2014.

Chatzichristodoulou, Maria. *Live Art in the UK: Contemporary Performances of Precarity*. Bloomsbury, 2020.

Chochinov, Harvey Max, and Catherine Frazee. 'Finding a balance: Canada's law on medical assistance in dying'. *The Lancet* 388:10044 (2016), 543–5.

Clark, Herbert, and Richard Gerrig, 'On the pretense theory of irony'. *Journal of Experimental Psychology*, 113:1 (1984), 121–6.

Corker, Marian. '"Disability" the unwelcome ghost at the banquet … and the conspiracy of "normality"'. *Body & Society* 5:4 (1999), 75–83.

Currie, Gregory. 'The irony in pictures'. *British Journal of Aesthetics* 51:2 (2011), 149–67.

Dignitas. 'Welcome to Dignitas'. 25 August 2024, https://dignitas.ch/en/

Disability Rights UK. 'Position on Assisted Dying'. disabilityrightsuk.org, https://www.disabilityrightsuk.org/news/disability-rights-uk%E2%80%99s-position-assisted-dying (accessed 3 April 2024).

The Disabled Avant-Garde (@Disabledavantgarde). 'Assisted Passage'. YouTube, 28 November 2007, https://www.youtube.com/watch?v=SvgVv-nEEIs

The Disabled Avant-Garde. 'Assisted Passage'. In Katherine Araniello and Aaron Williamson (dirs.) *Bite the Hand that Feeds!* PAL-DVD. Live Art Development Agency, 2012.

Fox, Oriana. *Performance Art Can Change Your Life! Shame Attacking and Parrhesia as Feminist Practices of Freedom*. PhD thesis, Goldsmiths, University of London, 2019.

Fox, Oriana. 'Satire and subversion with Katherine Araniello'. *Multiple Os Podcast*. Season 1, Episode 16, 30 November 2021.

Garland-Thomson, Rosemarie. *Extraordinary Bodies: Figuring Physical Disability in American Culture and Literature*. Columbia University Press, 1999.

Garland-Thomson, Rosemarie. 'Misfits: A feminist materialist disability concept'. *Hypatia* 26:3 (2011), 591–609.

Ginsburg, Faye, and Rayna Rapp. '"Not Dead Yet": Changing Disability Imaginaries in the Twenty-First Century'. In Veena Das (ed.), *Living and Dying in the Contemporary World: A Compendium*. University of California Press, 2015.

Goldberg, RoseLee. *Performance: Live Art 1909 to the Present*. Thames & Hudson, 1979.

Griffin, Dustin. *Satire: A Critical Reintroduction*. University Press of Kentucky, 1994.

Hadley, Bree, Jelena Rajak, Andrew Filmer, Rebecca Caines and Alan Read. 'The "Dirty Work" of the lie', *Performance Research* 15:2 (2010), 123–9.

Hadley, Bree, Jelena Rajak, Andrew Filmer, Rebecca Caines and Alan Read. *Disability, Public Space, Performance and Spectatorship: Unconscious Performers*. Palgrave Macmillan, 2014.

Haller, Beth, and Sue Ralph. 'John Callahan's Pelswick cartoon and a new phase of disability humor'. *Disability Studies Quarterly* 23:3 (2003), 4–16.

'Health in the age of disinformation'. *The Lancet* 405:10474 (2025), 173.

Heddon, Deirdre, and Jennie Klein (eds). *Histories and Practices of Live Art*. Bloomsbury, 2012.

Johnson, Dominic. *Critical Live Art*. Routledge, 2013.

Kafer, Alison. *Feminist, Queer, Crip*. Indiana University Press, 2013.

Keidan, Lois, and C.J. Mitchell (eds). *Access All Areas: Live Art and Disability*. Live Art Development Agency, 2012.

Kreuz, Roger, and R.M. Roberts, 'On satire and parody: The importance of being ironic'. *Metaphor and Symbol* 8:2 (1993), 97–109.

Kuppers, Petra. *Disability and Contemporary Performance: Bodies on the Edge*. Routledge, 2003.

Mallett, Rebecca. 'Claiming comedic immunity, or what you get when you cross contemporary comedy with disability'. *Review of Disability Studies* 6:3 (2014), 5–14.

Milbrodt, Teresa. '"Today I had an Eye Appointment, and I'm Still Blind": Crip humour, storytelling, and narrative positioning of the disabled self'. *Disability Studies Quarterly* 38:2 (2018). https://doi.org/10.18061/dsq.v38i2.6163

Murray, Stewart. *Medical Humanities and Disability Studies: In/Disciplines*. Bloomsbury, 2023.

Oliver, Mike. 'A Sociology of Disability or a Disablist Sociology?' In Len Barton (ed.), *Disability and Society: Emerging Issues and Insights*. Routledge, 2018.

Pring, John. 'Assisted dying bill: Disabled activists warn of bill's threat'. *Disability News Service*, 25 July 2014. https://www.disabilitynewsservice.com/assisted-dying-bill-disabled-activists-warn-of-bills-threat/ (accessed 3 April 2025).

Reid, Kim, and Edy H. Stoughton. 'The humorous construction of disability: "Stand-up" comedians in the United States'. *Disability & Society* 21:6 (2006), 629–43.

Riley, Lloyd. 'The cost of dying overseas'. dignityindying.org.uk, 13 November 2017, https://features.dignityindying.org.uk/true-cost-dignitas/

Roberts, Eleanor. 'Disability art is dead, long live disability art!: The sick crip Disabled Avant-Garde'. *Contemporary Theatre Review* 34:3 (2024), 262–79.

Rowlands, Elinor. 'Bringing the legacy of NDACA into focus: Feminist Arts News June 1989'. *Disability Arts Online*, 3 May 2020, https://disabilityarts.online/magazine/opinion/bringing-the-legacy-of-ndaca-into-focus-feminist-arts-news-june-1989/

Shakespeare, Tom. 'Joking a part'. *Body and Society*, 5:4 (1999).

Shakespeare, Tom. 'Memorandum by Tom Shakespeare'. parliament.uk (House of Lords, Assisted dying for the terminally ill bill, Volume II: Evidence, 4 April 2005), pp. 245–7. https://publications.parliament.uk/pa/ld200405/ldselect/ldasdy/86/4120223.htm

Sherwood, Harriet. 'Disability Rights Campaigners Urge MPs and Peers to Back Assisted Dying Bill'. *Guardian*, 24 October 2024.

Simpson, Paul. *On the Discourse of Satire* (John Benjamins, 2003).

Stewart, Craig. 'Strategies of verbal irony in visual satire: Reading *The New Yorker*'s "Politics of Fear" cover'. *Humour* 26:2 (2013), 197–217.

Swain, John, and Sally French. 'Towards an affirmation model of disability'. *Disability & Society* 15:4 (2000), 569–82.

Swift, Jonathan. *A Modest Proposal for Preventing the Children of Poor People from Being a Burthen to Their Parents or the Country, and for Making Them Beneficial to the Publick*. S. Harding, 1729.

Sutherland, Allan. 'Disabled Avant Garde'. *A Different Way of Engaging* (D4D, 2020), p. 63 (18–20), https://d4d.org.uk/wp-content/uploads/2019/05/Katherine-A-Poems-A-Different-Way-of-Engaging.pdf

Sutherland, Allan. *Electric Bodies: Travels in Life History*. Disability Arts Online, 2011.

Watson, Cate. *Comedy and Social Science: Towards a Methodology of Funny*. Routledge. 2017.

Willett, Cynthia, and Julie Willett. *Uproarious: How Feminists and Other Subversive Comics Speak Truth*. University of Minnesota Press, 2019.

Wedderburn, Alister. *Humour, Subjectivity and World Politics*. Manchester University Press, 2021.

Williamson, Aaron. *Aaron Williamson: Performance/Video/Collaboration*. Live Art Development Agency, 2008.

Williamson, Aaron, and L. Lynch. 'Situating deaf-gain: Performance and writing in the work of and Aaron Williamson'. *Journal of Visual Art Practice* 22:2–3 (2023), 291–305.

Woods, Angela. 'The limits of narrative: provocations for the medical humanities'. *Medical Humanities* 37:2 (2011), 73–8.

Woods, Angela. 'Beyond the Wounded Storyteller: Rethinking Narrativity, Illness and Embodied Self-Experience'. In Havi Carel and Rachel Cooper (eds), *Health, Illness and Disease: Philosophical Essays*, 113–28. Taylor & Francis Group, 2014.

Part III

Comical health communications

8

'Doctor, Are You Speaking in Tongues?': Humour and the health humanities of Selma and Lois DeBakey

Jeffrey S. Reznick

See note[1]

Press play…

The video begins silently. A snow glitch – an artefact of the pre-digital age – briefly interrupts before a black screen segues to a blue background. A title appears in white capital letters: 'DOCTOR, ARE YOU SPEAKING IN TONGUES?' Details of the presenter follow: 'Lois DeBakey, PhD, Professor of Scientific Communication, Baylor College of Medicine, Houston, Texas'. The video briefly fades to black before Dr DeBakey herself appears, speaking directly to her audience (Figure 8.1): 'I'm pleased to have the opportunity to address the question, "Doctor, are you speaking in tongues?" Even if you have not given your language much thought until now, I hope to show you that verbal dexterity can enhance your effectiveness as a physician or scientist.' With this cordial introduction, Dr DeBakey signals her intention to address the question not as a debatable observation but rather as a hallmark of professional behaviour by her audience with whom she seeks to ingratiate herself by magnifying their efficacy. She is easing into a subtle combination of verbal and visual humour designed to deliver palatable rebukes to change their behaviour while avoiding blunt assessments that might offend them.

The construction and intention of this video reflected a lifelong initiative by Lois DeBakey (1920–2016) and her sister, Selma DeBakey (1915–2013): using humour to call out poor medical communication, primarily by physicians but also by biomedical

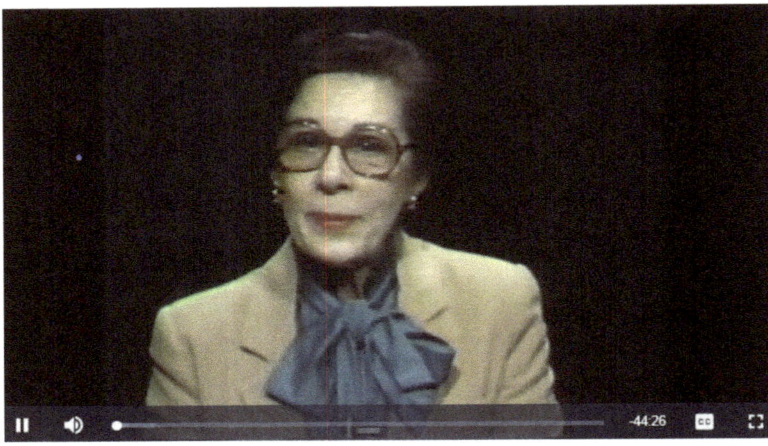

Figure 8.1 Lois DeBakey, in her 1981 video lecture 'Doctor, are You Speaking in Tongues?'

researchers and medical journalists. They sought to help them remedy this poor communication for the benefit of their respective professions and the individuals they served. Together and independently over the course of five decades, the DeBakeys coined their own terminology for the problem they sought to address, delivering their techniques and critiques of medical communication with charm, gentility and wit while carefully establishing themselves as change agents in a field which was not necessarily amenable to reform. Moreover, they published dozens of scholarly articles, designed and taught hundreds of classes across the United States and around the world and they cultivated a unique professional self-image in the eyes of their audience and in the media.[2] Their work overall was of a piece with contemporary conversations about the role of language in modern medicine and its potential to obscure or clarify reality, and, more fundamentally, about achieving lucid medical writing as an ethical and professional imperative.[3] However, their work was as unique as they were, their character, experiences and observations of humour being essential ingredients in their medical education to help medical professionals understand how to achieve the best of their expertise and service.

Across the trajectory of their early lives and later professional achievements, the DeBakey sisters participated in a complex ecosystem of private intimacy and public influence comparable to that through which the prominent Canadian researcher-physician Maude Abbott (1868–1940) shaped her own career. Like the story of Abbott that Annmarie Adams uncovered through 'friendship archeology' – the work of 'digging deeply at specific sites and times to uncover layers of relationships' which 'destabilizes ... earlier biographical accounts' – the story of the DeBakey sisters navigating the male-dominated field of medicine, and using humour to empower themselves and their arguments, involves their private and public relationships with each other and with their famous brother, whose support and fame had an effect on the currency of their arguments.[4] Examining the lives and work of the sisters through this professional and familial prism, and focusing on their visual outputs of films and cartoons, situates their story within the broader themes of this volume. More immediately, this focus foregrounds their story rather than, as elsewhere, subordinating it to their famous brother's narrative.[5] Indeed, it makes clear that Lois and Selma DeBakey deserve their own spotlight and analysis to appreciate their legacy in the context of the health humanities.

Background, family and brother Michael

Lois and Selma, along with sisters Goldie (1912–52) and Selena (1914–98), and brothers Ernest (1910–2006) and Michael (1908–2008), were born and raised in Lake Charles, Louisiana. Their Lebanese immigrant parents, Shaker and Raheeja Dabaghi (later anglicised to DeBakey), actively fostered their children's education and encouraged all of them to attend college.[6] Lois attended Sophie Newcomb College where, in 1940, she earned her undergraduate degree in mathematics. She subsequently attended Tulane University where she earned her master's and doctoral degrees in English and then joined the institution's English department. Selma also attended Sophie Newcomb College where, in 1937, she earned her undergraduate degree in French. She subsequently pursued graduate studies in linguistics and philosophy and went on to work as an editor, director of medical communications at the Alton Ochsner Foundation and founding editor of its *Cardiovascular Center Bulletin*.[7]

In 1960, the leadership of the American Medical Writers' Association named Lois and Selma co-editors of *The Quarterly Bulletin*, the official publication of the association.[8] Four years later, at Tulane, they began the first curriculum-approved communications course ever offered at a medical school.[9] In 1968, the leadership of Baylor College of Medicine recruited them to serve as professors of scientific communications, and soon thereafter, at Methodist Hospital adjacent to Baylor, they began to serve on the editorial board of the *Methodist DeBakey Cardiovascular Journal*. Selma continued to serve as an editor for professional writing organisations as she took on guest editorships of special issues. She was also a guest editor of special issues, as well as a member of advisory committees of the Friends of the Texas Medical Center Library.

Throughout their lives, Lois and Selma embraced values and viewpoints rooted firmly in their upbringing. As they recalled, 'in addition to [their] abundant love, our parents instilled in us their own high Christian values and human principles of honesty, integrity, discipline, compassion, and the commitment to give more than we received from society'.[10] While the sisters' intention to contribute to society would become central to their future work, their strong sibling relationship with their brother Michael – indeed their shared intimacy, familial history and professional support – was a fundamental influence and supportive force in their early lives and later professional path. 'When he saw a need in medical education', Lois and Selma explained, 'he pointed us in its fruitful direction.'[11] As young college graduates, they recalled further:

> we began to help [him] and other medical authors prepare their manuscripts for publication. We soon realized that physicians and bioscientists had had no instruction in this subject and no guidelines to follow. As a result, they simply mimicked the articles they had read in medical journals, often replicating the errors, frozen style, and other flaws. Lacking instruction in critical reasoning as well, they often accepted as gospel all published results instead of critically analyzing and evaluating the conclusions.[12]

Selma recalled this trajectory involving 'our brother notic[ing] that his colleagues, who were some of the brightest and most learned people in the country, had problems speaking and writing simple, clear English', and he therefore 'suggested that with our education and training, [we] could pursue a career in helping physicians communicate better'.[13] Michael himself characterised the intimacy of his relationship with Lois and Selma: 'Deep down, you really depend on your siblings for the kind of support that is very subtle, but, nonetheless, is there. You share your thoughts with them, even though you might not be able to share them with others. You don't feel alone.'[14] Later in life, Lois and Selma reflected on their treasured relationship with Michael by recalling one of their 'most cherished possessions ... a message accompanying [their] Christmas gifts in 2005', shortly before Michael became ill and passed away: 'Dear Selma and Lois, First, Merry Christmas. Second, and equally important, I love you both dearly, and I thank God. He blessed me with two angel sisters. I pray He will continue to shower us with His Blessings. Your loving brother Michael.'[15] Reflecting on these sentiments, the sisters explained that 'those few, highly evocative words define our relationship. The implicit bond in that exquisite Christmas missive was forged early in life by our parents and remained sacrosanct, impervious to even the most unpropitious forces, and it remains intact today, for its home is in the inaccessible recesses of our innermost hearts.'[16] This lifelong sibling bond, as well as that between the sisters themselves, are key to understanding the origins, development and shape of what Lois and Selma achieved.[17]

Michael eventually excelled in his own education and became a globally appreciated surgeon, educator and medical statesman. Privately along the way to his own success, he was his sisters' biggest champion. Publicly along their own trajectory to fame in medical circles, Lois and Selma embraced their individual professional identities and goals even as their common surname associated them with Michael. An article in the *Des Moines Tribune*, '2 Other DeBakeys Do Word Surgery' reflected this duality as it foregrounded the sisters' distinct professional identity and advocacy and their impactful work in addressing 'the pompous, confusing, vague, monotonous and ambiguous medicalese that so often turns up in learned journals of medicine and in the conversations of physicians'.[18]

The deep-rooted and mutually supportive relationship between the sisters and their brother shaped how the pair thought critically together about their ideal approach to using humour to help cure the problem of poor medical communication. As they designed their instruction for their 'target population' of 'physicians and biomedical researchers who had already devoted several decades to formal education', they understood that it was 'somewhat audacious' to suggest that this group needed to improve their writing and speaking. In light of this understanding, the sisters gradually realised that they 'needed an appealing entrée' to their instruction:

> We were timorous at first, but as we continued to read articles in peer-reviewed journals critically, there appeared in our mind's eye graphic representations of the specious arguments; the invalid data; the pretentious, incomprehensible language; the somnifascient expressions; and the inadvertently humorous or otherwise faulty prose.[19]

The sisters' acknowledgement of 'an appealing entrée', and their initial but soon overcome 'timorousness' registered their awareness of the gendered dimension of their foray as change agents in the largely male-dominated field of medicine that was not necessarily open to reform. From this awareness grew their ability to spotlight and make significant meaning of the 'inadvertently humorous or otherwise faulty prose' of physicians, adopting and adapting it strategically to soften their blow of criticism and to communicate multiple messages simultaneously and succinctly. For the DeBakeys, therefore, tactful humour became a key ingredient in 'the appealing entrée' to be consumed by their audience whose communication practices the sisters sought to change. Rather than seeing humour as a distraction to medical education – and no evidence in current research suggests that they thought it could be so – the DeBakeys understood it to be integral to learning, and especially to their own method of teaching medical professionals.

As Lois and Selma worked to achieve this change, they viewed themselves as a team even as they published independently and were frequently cited, quoted and seen publicly apart from each other. Testifying to their mutual respect and support, Lois described Selma as 'my preceptor, professional partner, and alter ego' who had offered 'unstinting support and sororal devotion'.[20] Selma reflected similarly: 'Our parents taught us not to compete with others, but to compete with ourselves. To do better tomorrow than we did today.'[21] A 1977 *Houston Post* photograph of the sisters reflected their close partnership as it depicted them sitting together in their shared office – notably on the same chair – smiling amidst their common books and files which informed their highly collaborative work (Figure 8.2). A description of their lifelong partnership serves as a powerful caption to this image: 'Selma and Lois DeBakey grew up together, went to school and college together, and worked together. They could be seen walking arm in arm to Houston Methodist Hospital, where their offices were adjacent to their iconic brother's. Throughout their lives, their love for their parents, siblings, and profession remained foremost and unabridged.'[22]

Such was the deep intimacy – rooted in their upbringing and their close relationship with each other and with their

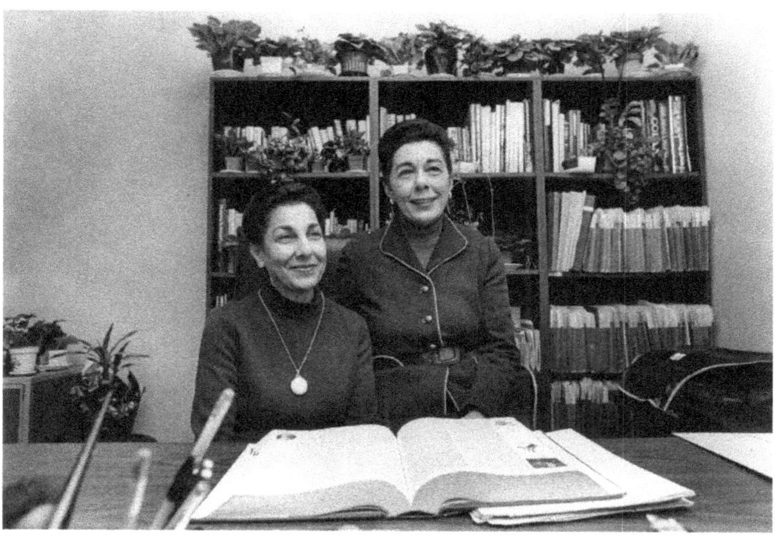

Figure 8.2 *Houston Post* press photo, labelled on reverse 'DeBakey, Lois, Prof. Baylor College of Medicine (left is sister – Selma DeBakey, a speech and writing teacher) © The Houston Post, 26 January, 1977. Photo by Danny Connolly'.

brother – which informed the sisters' private lives and moral values while shaping their public service mission to improve medical communication. The fact that Lois and Selma described their sibling relationship as a 'collegial family triad' and a 'durable triad' testified directly to its foundational role in their personal and professional lives.[23]

'Let's begin …'

Immediately following her polite and carefully calibrated introduction in 'Doctor, Are You Speaking in Tongues?', Lois pivots to her first example of such communication by focusing on 'the definition of paper-writing from a scientific journal'. She reads the definition aloud as it scrolls from the bottom to the top of the screen:

> Given Freud's structural point of view … paper-writing can no longer be conceptualized without considering the intersystemic complications which threaten it from within. The conclusion, then, is inescapable. The paper-writing function of the ego is not always the only ego function instrumental in paper-writing. Under circumstances which still await psychoanalytic elucidation scientific papers are sometimes written in a complementary part–object relationship between the paper-dictating function of the writer's ego and the dictation-taking function of a scribe or secretary.

The scrolling text disappears, the camera returns to Lois, and she flashes a subtle smile. 'You're puzzled', she states, and then refers to herself in the third person – anticipating the thoughts of her viewers – before returning to the first person and explaining her approach: 'Is she going to be speaking in that kind of gibberish? You're wondering. Let me reassure you that I am not. I opened with that passage merely to illustrate an affliction of epidemic proportion among today's presumably educated people.' Paradoxically and very intentionally, her approach will be the opposite: she is indeed planning to speak more in 'that kind of gibberish' to her physician audience as a way to convince them to be better representatives of 'today's presumably educated people' and to 'correct their ways'. Lois continues, choosing a series of uncommon words to demonstrate the ridiculousness of the epidemic she sees as plaguing the field of medicine: 'What may be called in the lingo characterizing it, lalopathy, logorrhea, verbigeration, or glossolalia is not confined to the biomedical disciplines, but extends into business, the trades, government, and all professions.' Lois then spotlights a term which she and her sister coined to label this epidemic, admittedly in a problematic way for today's readers:

> I call this disabled language 'Medicant.' Ironically, the malady seems to be pedogogenic, induced by our educational institutions. It's highly contagious, passing freely from teacher to student, speaker to listener, and writer to reader. Language is largely derivative. We mimic the expressions of those to whom we are exposed, and the faulty models we have are abundant and ubiquitous.

The sisters' invention and consistent use of this blending of the words 'medic' and 'can't' – a notably capitalised portmanteau – was humorous and pivotal: they used 'Medicant' to poke fun at professionals who despite being known for their ability to do challenging work, used their own professional language (too often inappropriately and with professional short-sightedness, Lois and Selma argued) to define their community and scope of practice. This shaped their own professional identity and credibility in the eyes of these professionals. 'Medicant' also gave currency to the sisters' very identity as communication experts and change agents, helping to cushion and simplify their arguments humorously. Moreover, 'Medicant' helped to form their unique voices in the media, providing a focus for discussions of their work.

With her focus clear, Lois proceeds carefully to offer several other examples of 'Medicant', notably 'all from reputable publications' whose authors she intentionally does not identify in order to avoid harming their reputations which she ultimately wishes to improve, not ruin.[24] She then dedicates the remaining forty-two minutes of her video to further description of such 'Medicant' punctuated with humorous cartoons intended to illustrate its absurdity and pervasiveness. Lois and Selma had been developing and deploying this visual technique in their work for over a decade, commissioning cartoons from various artists. Over time, it became a prominent feature of their work.

The DeBakeys' visual culture

The 1970 article 'Every careless word that men utter', authored by Lois and published in two parts by *Anesthesia and Analgesia*, is one of the sisters' earliest uses of humorous cartoons to focus and advance their advocacy.[25] 'Careless words are costly', Lois began, and continued sarcastically and provocatively by appealing to the vanity, ego and professional self-image of her largely male readers: 'Friendships have been severed, elections lost, fortunes dissolved, marriages disrupted, men murdered, and peaceful international relations exploded by verbal bungling.' Despite such implications, she explains inclusively and therefore disarmingly, 'most of us continue to treat language indifferently or casually'. Moreover, she argued tactfully, 'some who take infinite care to display good manners, impeccable taste, and attractive grooming are curiously unmindful of their speech and writing'. Appealing further to the physicality of her audience, Lois continued:

> Although they would not think of being seen with disheveled hair, dusty shoes, soiled tie, or wrinkled shirt, they seem insensitive to crude expressions, slovenly speech, and disordered language. Careless language is particularly hazardous in scientific disciplines, where precision is paramount. Yet scientists who work tirelessly to perfect a laboratory or clinical technic sometimes neglect the medium through which they communicate their observations and discoveries to the world.[26]

Simultaneously, critical and respectful to both correct and support her audience, Lois pointed to several examples of such costly written communication, including 'cramming writing with clichés' which, she explains, is 'a sure way to devitalize literary style' and 'distract your reader from the subject if they evoke amusing mental images'.[27] To underscore her argument, Lois presented three cartoons drawn in pen and ink wash by 'Nakashima' (Figure 8.3). *He Turned the Floor Over to the Chairman* depicts a man angrily throwing a collection of wooden planks toward another man who is aghast at the action. *The Volume Fills an Important Gap* shows a man of short stature looking up to a taller man pointing to a stack of

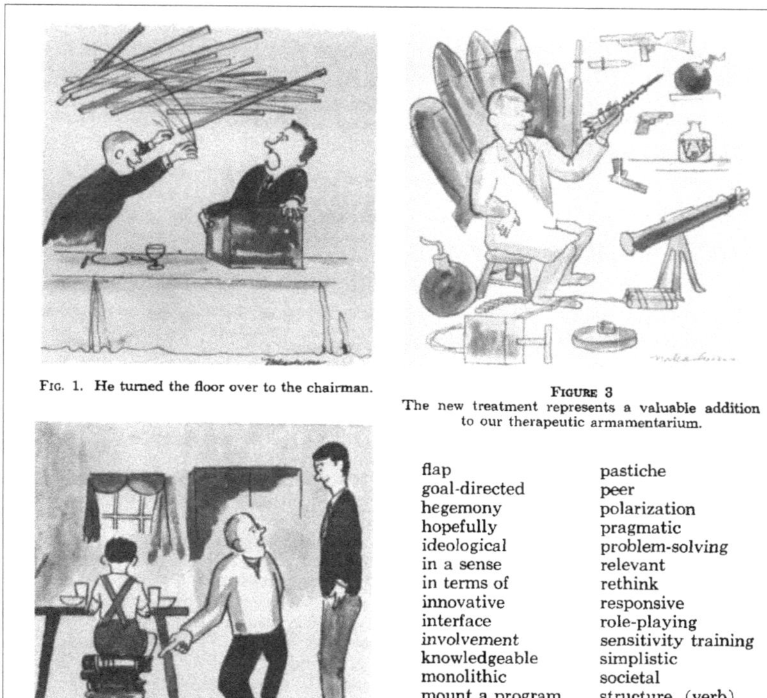

FIG. 1. He turned the floor over to the chairman.

FIGURE 3
The new treatment represents a valuable addition to our therapeutic armamentarium.

FIG. 2. This volume fills an important gap.

VOGUE-WORDS

People are notorious mimics, and scientists are no exception. They hear or read a novel expression and cannot wait to use it themselves, repeating it so often that it quickly loses its original force. Most vogue-words enjoy transient popularity only, and those that continue to be used become clichés. Some current vogue-words and expressions that are avoided by careful writers are:

ambivalence	confrontation
ambience	conglomerate
area	dialogue
bizarre	ecological doom
commitment	expertise
flap	pastiche
goal-directed	peer
hegemony	polarization
hopefully	pragmatic
ideological	problem-solving
in a sense	relevant
in terms of	rethink
innovative	responsive
interface	role-playing
involvement	sensitivity training
knowledgeable	simplistic
monolithic	societal
mount a program	structure (verb)
move forward	thrust
mystique	viable
negotiable	vis-a-vis

EUPHEMISMS

Softening of the language and emphasis on egalitarianism have led to a profusion of euphemisms. A bookie calls himself a *commission agent*, a hairdresser a *cosmetologist*, a bartender a *mixologist*, an undertaker a *mortician*, a newsman an *information scientist*, a personnel officer a *social engineer*, a garbage collector a *sanitation engineer*, a janitor a *custodian*, and a watchman a *security officer*. We call a graveyard a *memorial park*, and education is now a *learning experience*. Backward nations are *underdeveloped*, the victims of *deprivation*; juvenile delinquents are exceptional or *underpriviliged*; and the unemployable are *underskilled* or *disadvantaged*. Scientific writing is largely literal, so that objectivity and precision are paramount, and euphemisms have little place in literal writing.

Figure 8.3 Excerpt from 'Every careless word that men utter. II. The language of science'. *Anesthesia and Analgesia* 49:5 (1970), 827–34; 830, featuring cartoons by 'Nakashima'.

large books upon which a young boy sits so that he is able to reach a work desk. *The New Treatment Represents a Valuable Addition to our Therapeutic Armamentarium* presents a physician sitting on a stool, wearing a white coat, and holding a rocket while surrounded by bombs, dynamite, guns and missiles. The third of these cartoons is notable because its visual messaging reappears a decade later in the 'Doctor, Are You Speaking in Tongues?' video, drawn by a different artist. More than mere repetition, this fact testifies to Lois and Selema evolving their visual aids over time, understanding the need for enhancements to hone their arguments about 'Medicant' toward achieving greater impact.[28] As Lois herself once explained: 'We experimented with cartoons graphically depicting mental images of flawed writing, and fortunately for us, they were effective didactic tools. As physicians in our classes laughed heartily at the cartoons, they became relaxed, and their minds were open to the serious instruction we wished to impart.'[29] This explanation points to a key understanding Lois and Selma valued in their work, namely the power of laughter to disarm a potentially hostile, largely male audience, and educate them to improve in ways they could not see for themselves.

Within a year after the appearance of 'Every careless word that men utter', Lois published 'Medical gobbledygook and writer's gookledygobb' in the *Illinois Medical Journal*. Directed at 'the medical journalist', the article explained that 'as a liaison between the medical profession and the public', this individual has responsibilities to both. Achieving well-crafted prose without 'medical gobbledygook' should be the goal, Lois concluded, and such work should meet many and important expectations, including 'maintain[ing] the highest standards of accuracy and objectivity … not misus[ing] or falsify[ing] science by writing cheap, sensational, or inaccurate stories … secur[ing] … information through ethical, reliable sources and … not stoop[ing] to improper methods and activities'.[30] To help make these arguments palatable to readers, and ultimately to encourage change, Lois featured two humorous pen-and-ink cartoons (Figure 8.4). One depicts a man, presumably a medical journalist, wearing a shirt and tie and holding his finger to his chin pensively. The opposing cartoon depicts a two-headed worm. The caption, *Which end is UP?*, reveals what the bewildered

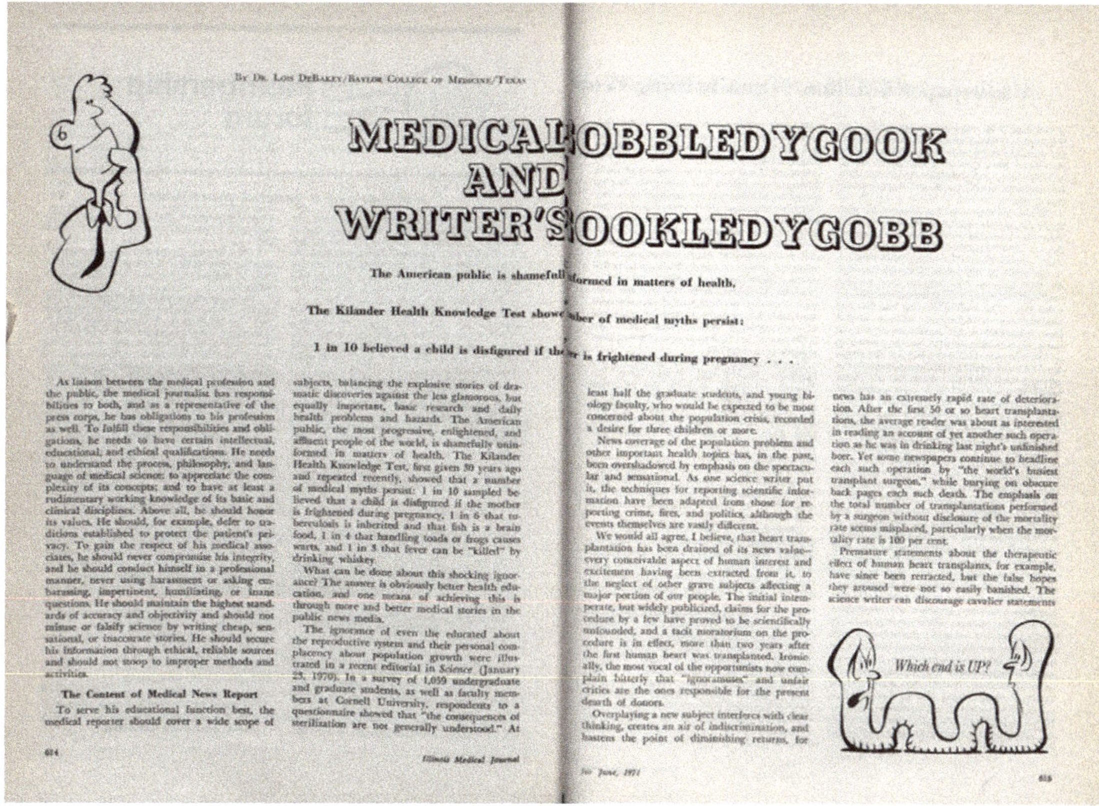

By Dr. Lois DeBakey/Baylor College of Medicine/Texas

MEDICAL GOBBLEDYGOOK AND WRITER'S GOOKLEDYGOBB

The American public is shamefull formed in matters of health.

The Kilander Health Knowledge Test show ber of medical myths persist:

1 in 10 believed a child is disfigured if th r is frightened during pregnancy . . .

As liaison between the medical profession and the public, the medical journalist has responsibilities to both, and as a representative of the press corps, he has obligations to his profession as well. To fulfill these responsibilities and obligations, he needs to have certain intellectual, educational, and ethical qualifications. He needs to understand the process, philosophy, and language of medical science; to appreciate the complexity of its concepts; and to have at least a rudimentary working knowledge of its basic and clinical disciplines. Above all, he should honor its values. He should, for example, defer to traditions established to protect the patient's privacy. To gain the respect of his medical associates, he should never compromise his integrity, and he should conduct himself in a professional manner, never using harassment or asking embarrassing, impertinent, humiliating, or inane questions. He should maintain the highest standards of accuracy and objectivity and should not misuse or falsify science by writing cheap, sensational, or inaccurate stories. He should secure his information through ethical, reliable sources and should not stoop to improper methods and activities.

The Content of Medical News Report

To serve his educational function best, the medical reporter should cover a wide scope of subjects, balancing the explosive stories of dramatic discoveries against the less glamorous, but equally important, basic research and daily health problems and hazards. The American public, the most progressive, enlightened, and affluent people of the world, is shamefully uninformed in matters of health. The Kilander Health Knowledge Test, first given 30 years ago and repeated recently, showed that a number of medical myths persist: 1 in 10 sampled believed that a child is disfigured if the mother is frightened during pregnancy, 1 in 6 that tuberculosis is inherited and that fish is a brain food, 1 in 4 that handling toads or frogs causes warts, and 1 in 3 that fever can be "killed" by drinking whiskey.

What can be done about this shocking ignorance? The answer is obviously better health education, and one means of achieving this is through more and better medical stories in the public news media.

The ignorance of even the educated about the reproductive system and their personal complacency about population growth were illustrated in a recent editorial in *Science* (January 23, 1970). In a survey of 1,059 undergraduate and graduate students, as well as faculty members at Cornell University, respondents to a questionnaire showed that "the consequences of sterilization are not generally understood." At least half the graduate students, and young biology faculty, who would be expected to be most concerned about the population crisis, recorded a desire for three children or more.

News coverage of the population problem and other important health topics has, in the past, been overshadowed by emphasis on the spectacular and sensational. As one science writer put it, the techniques for reporting scientific information have been adapted from those for reporting crime, fires, and politics, although the events themselves are vastly different.

We would all agree, I believe, that heart transplantation has been drained of its news value—every conceivable aspect of human interest and excitement having been extracted from it, to the neglect of other grave subjects affecting a major portion of our people. The initial intemperate, but widely publicized, claims for the procedure by a few have proved to be scientifically unfounded, and a tacit moratorium on the procedure is in effect, more than two years after the first human heart was transplanted. Ironically, the most vocal of the opportunists now complain bitterly that "ignoramuses" and unfair critics are the ones responsible for the present dearth of donors.

Overplaying a new subject interferes with clear thinking, creates an air of indiscrimination, and hastens the point of diminishing returns, for news has an extremely rapid rate of deterioration. After the first 50 or so heart transplantations, the average reader was about as interested in reading an account of yet another such operation as he was in drinking last night's unfinished beer. Yet some newspapers continue to headline each such operation by "the world's busiest transplant surgeon," while burying on obscure back pages each such death. The emphasis on the total number of transplantations performed by a surgeon without disclosure of the mortality rate seems misplaced, particularly when the mortality rate is 100 per cent.

Premature statements about the therapeutic effect of human heart transplants, for example, have since been retracted, but the false hopes they aroused were not so easily banished. The science writer can discourage cavalier statements

Figure 8.4 Excerpt from 'Medical gobbledygook and writer's gookledygobb' featuring two unattributed cartoons, *Illinois Medical Journal* 139:6 (1971): 614–17; 614–15.

head on the left is asking the equally bewildered head on the right. The message to readers: failure of the medical journalist in the duty to understand medical practices and terminologies and communicate them clearly contributes to the confusion and rot of medical journalism, and, thereby, medical education.

The late 1970s marked a new chapter in the sisters' ongoing use of humorous cartoons to convey the central messages of their work. They departed from and enhanced the visual work of previous artists to engage Dick Putney, a talented artist in his own right who was working in the marketing department of the *Houston Post*. The sisters had selected Putney after approaching a few of the newspaper's editorial cartoonists.[31] However, none of them could oblige due to their association with the news enterprise of the paper, which limited the scope of their official work and did not allow them to freelance. Putney, however, could freelance, and he proceeded to do so for the DeBakeys. He met regularly with them in their Houston Methodist Hospital office to discuss their ideas and intended audience, received from them lists of terms and phrases they wanted him to illustrate and over time shared with them pencil sketches for their feedback as he worked on final versions. 'They were very cordial', Putney recalled. 'They knew what they were trying to do, and they had a pretty good idea of the ideas they wanted to present to their audience.' They also had a good sense of humour, Putney recalled further. There was 'a lot of chuckling' along the way as they discussed their ideas and worked with Putney to bring them into focus visually.[32]

Putney completed his cartoons in multi-coloured pen and ink. Ten appeared in the sisters' seminal 1978 article 'Medicant: Nothing hinders communication as much as words – when they are used badly or incorrectly'.[33] This article reflected their ongoing embrace of a combination of playful and even childish verbiage and visuals to convey the silliness of physicians and others using 'Medicant', and to temper the underlying, assertive message to these professionals that they needed to improve their communication. Herein were a variety of interrelated themes, from light-hearted challenges to the authority of, and language used by, medical professionals to upending orderliness and turning the hospital environment upside down. Through these humorous images and their associated captions targeted to their largely male audience of physicians, the sisters conveyed their fundamental argument: words matter. Those used carelessly create disorder and do a disservice to patients. Those used carefully serve to support quality care for patients and to maintain an ordered, responsible and responsive healthcare environment.

Putney's cartoons depicted precisely the variety of 'Medicant' identified by Lois and Selma. Among the many examples of his work was *The Patient Was Throwing Emboli* which featured a male patient sitting upright in his hospital bed tossing blood clots at a doctor and a nurse, hitting both of them repeatedly. Another, *Bucking the Medicant Barrier*, presented a female patient banging on a wall of specialised medical terms while a bewildered male doctor stands on the opposite side of the terms. Through such imagery developed in close cooperation with the sisters, Putney literally animated their approach and arguments, highlighting humorous words and phrases spoken in commonplace medical situations to make them a focus of communication lessons to be learned.

Lois and Selma's 'Medicant' article paved the way to their 'Doctor, Are You Speaking in Tongues?' video, informing the script directly, with several areas almost verbatim. Throughout this production, Lois featured twenty-one cartoons by Putney, five of which she and Selma modified from earlier versions through abbreviation, lengthening, shortening or a combination of these approaches. In total, three cartoons appeared as they had previously, and thirteen were new, demonstrating the depth and breadth of the sisters' collaboration with Putney. Among the new cartoons were *Autopsied Men Who Ate More Than 33% of the Experimental Meals*, depicting a coroner in a morgue feeding the corpse of a man while holding up his head; *A Large Body of Information*, featuring an obese man with specialised medical terms tattooed across his arms, chest and stomach; and, as an example of medical impropriety like those discussed by Rebecca Whiteley in his volume, *The Patient was Unresponsive in Bed*, showing a woman pushing away a doctor as she lay propped up in a hospital bed (Figure 8.5).

Through the 1990s, more than a decade after the production of 'Doctor, Are You Speaking in Tongues?' and two decades since

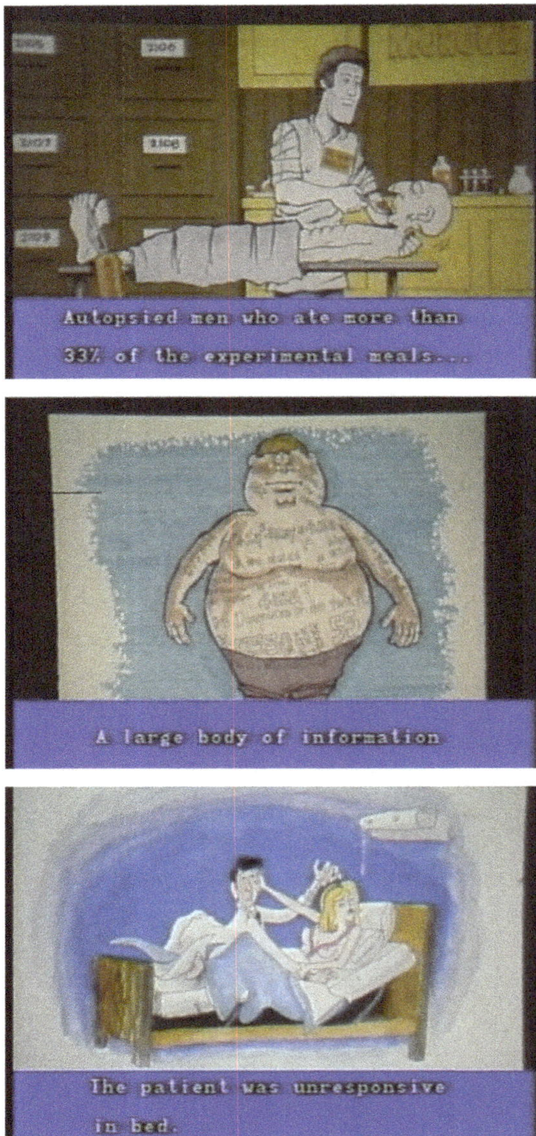

Figure 8.5 Selection of the cartoons by Dick Putney, created under commission of Lois and Selma DeBakey, appearing in 'Doctor, are You Speaking in Tongues?'.

they had begun working with Putney, the sisters continued to use and re-use many of his cartoons. Their co-authored 1992 article 'Medical writing: Inadvertent humor and other anomalies' featured five Putney cartoons. Notable among them were *Both the Patient and the Physician Were Blinded During the Experiments* and *The Group Was Composed of Half Men and Half Women* (Figure 8.6), which visualised incongruity, disrupted familiar language templates, provoked physicians to reflect on – and self-correct – their communication practices and conveyed succinctly Lois and Selma's fundamental argument: word choice matters, and when you are careless with your words, you are not merely creating absurdity at best, or, at worst, chaos, but you are also disrespecting yourselves as professionals, your professional environment and your colleagues and patients. The sisters' bottom-line message to their audiences of physicians and other medical professionals was: you owe it to yourself and everyone you serve to correct and improve your communication practices.

Reception

Lois and Selma were keenly aware that their advocacy had the potential to fall flat or offend. As Lois once conveyed to a physician colleague, 'Criticizing a physician's writing sometimes requires more tact than criticizing his grooming or personal hygiene.'[34] While further research is needed to determine if and under what circumstances any physicians were indeed affronted – perhaps during the early years of the sisters' work – available sources suggest genuine and widespread appreciation of their humour and expertise, albeit in the midst of a fear of being called out as a poor writer and adding to their many examples of poor writing. 'To put it simply, Dr Lois DeBakey has done more to bring literacy to medical writing than any other person in the country', said Robert Moser, a former editor of the *Journal of the American Medical Association*.[35] 'If you write well and are an honest person, she rewards you; but if not, she comes down on you like a ton of bricks.' Moser also characterised the sisters as the 'conscience of American Medical Letters'.[36] After he attended one of the sisters' classes, Donald Lindberg, director

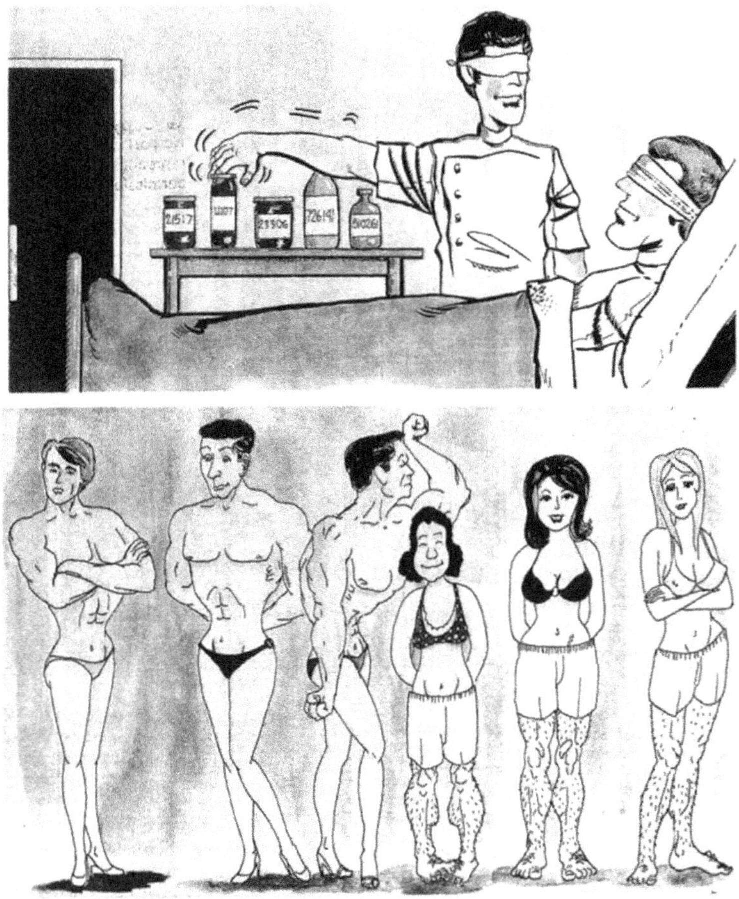

Figure 8.6 Selection of the cartoons by Dick Putney, created under commission of Lois and Selma DeBakey, appearing in 'Medical Writing: Inadvertent Humor and Other Anomalies', *International Angiology* 11:4 (1992), 272–80. Top: 'Both the patient and the physician were blinded during the experiments.' Bottom: 'The group was composed of half men and half women.'

of the National Library of Medicine, remarked that he and his colleagues 'were greatly entertained, and also lived in mortal fear we'd fall into that trap [of poor writing] – and into their collection [of poor writing]'.[37] Their courses, like the one Lindberg attended, were 'the most popular by far [at the annual meetings of the American College of Surgeons]', said C. Rollins Hanlon, former president of the organisation, who also praised the DeBakeys as 'renowned exemplars of clear, forceful writing'.[38] Testifying even further to the impact of the sisters, William Winters Jr, editor of the *Methodist DeBakey Cardiovascular Journal*, stated, 'I feel I have guardian angels looking over my shoulder ... Your suggestions are right on the mark. You are priceless gems to this community.'[39] With such appreciation, Winters suggested how he and his physician colleagues warmly received the sisters' humour and expertise dedicated unwaveringly to improving medical communication by the profession, and, by extension, for the patients and families it served.

The DeBakeys in the popular press

Lois and Selma DeBakey's distinctive work contributed not only to acceptance of their advocacy in physician circles but also to the widespread dissemination of news about them in the popular press. Some newspaper headlines characterised their work in medical terms, aligning with their own language play. 'DeBakey Sisters Cure "Medicalese"' and 'Patient Sisters Wield Knife on Words', *The Los Angeles Times* reported.[40] 'DeBakey Sisters Operate on Medical Jargon', declared the *Rapid City Journal*.[41] Other headlines dispensed with metaphor, clearly stating the sisters' intention to improve physicians' communication: 'Sick of Medical Lingo, Sisters Help Wordy Doctors', announced *The Courier-Journal*.[42] 'DeBakey Sisters Urge Doctors to Learn to Talk Straight', reported the *Pensacola News*.[43] 'Doctors Often Turn English into Latin', observed *The Central New Jersey Home News*.[44]

In addition to such regional press and much more, *Time* magazine, in its issue of 19 May 1980, spotlighted the sisters' work in an article entitled 'A Pox on "Medicant"'.[45] A cartoon by Putney, *The Patient Was Explored*, illustrated the piece, depicting three doctors and a nurse in 'Excavation Room 4', gathered around a patient lying on an operating table, each holding a shovel and wearing an explorer's pith helmet, and ready to begin their surgery. 'Lois DeBakey ... thinks that technical jargon not only alienates patients but masks fuzzy thinking', the article explained, and concluded: 'Says DeBakey: "Until society restores literacy to a position of esteem, there is no motivation for young people to learn to read and write."' Apropos of her view, she advised doctors to heed the words of Enlightenment-era poet and satirist Alexander Pope: 'Words are like leaves; and where they most abound/Much fruit of sense is rarely found.'[46] A dozen years after this national spotlight on the DeBakeys, the *Houston Post* featured a story about them with a photograph of Lois, smiling widely in front of Putney's cartoons displayed in her office, and reflecting her pride, as well as Selma's, in embracing these images and using them to advance their collaborative work.[47]

Legacy in the health humanities

With verbal and visual humour as diplomatic tools in their advocacy against 'Medicant', combined with their careful navigation through medical circles enabled by their mutual support as well as that of their brother, Lois and Selma recognised the broader relevance and implications of their work:

> [T]he deficiency in communicating effectively is not unique to medicine, but pervades all professions and occupations because teachers, and therefore students, are not taught critical reasoning and lucid language beginning in the early years and continuing throughout formal education. *Activating the pen or tongue before engaging the mind* is one of the most serious impediments to good writing and speaking. In other fields, drivel and faulty expression, especially if ponderous and vacuous, are known as *educationese, legalese, journalese, businessese*, and of course, the ever-present *politicalese*.[48]

Beyond this crisis of the professions, Lois spoke to the broader issue of growing illiteracy. In a *US News and World Report* article about 23 million Americans lacking the reading and writing skills needed to handle the minimal demands of daily life, she observed that 'What we are creating [in our society] is a kind of semiliteracy – a breakdown in the way we communicate with one another. Our regard for language has become so debased that it is destroying the ability even of educated people to evaluate ideas rationally.'[49] Thus, while Lois and Selma focused their work on the medical field, they were keenly aware of the broader scourge of badly communicated jargon like 'Medicant' in wider society.

Through these and many similar observations, as well as deliberate contributions to projects like *The American Heritage Guide to Contemporary Usage and Style*, on whose advisory panel Lois served, the sisters located their voices squarely within the contemporary chorus of individuals speaking about the failure of communication in various disciplines – ranging from medicine and science to the social sciences and humanities – and the importance and value of communicating more clearly to improve individual and public health, indeed to improve society as a whole.[50] In this broader context, their publications therefore deserve greater study in the ecosystem of contemporary style guides encouraging clearer communication, such as Theodore Bernstein's *The Careful Writer* (1965), Joseph M. Williams's *Style: Ten Lessons in Clarity and Grace* (1981) and William Strunk Jr and E.B. White's classic *The Elements of Style* (originally published privately in 1919 and reprinted many times due to its popularity). The aforementioned *Houston Post* article evoked this broader ecosystem as it quoted Lois testifying to the humanism that she and Selma embodied through their work: 'If everyone read more, watched less TV, thought independently, and communicated effectively, the world would be a better place.'[51] Excavating their voices and advocacy, and uncovering the unwavering relationships which informed their public work, allows us to appreciate the currency of their perspectives and efforts in their time, and our own.

Acknowledgements

The author thanks the editors of this volume for their critical feedback on earlier versions of this chapter, Richard Putney for his reflections on working with Lois and Selma DeBakey as a freelance illustrator, Paola Abrate of Edizioni Minerva Medica SpA for permission to reproduce images which originally appeared in *International Angiology*, Renée Cuthbert and the team of NIH Library for their interlibrary loan expertise, Debra Kay Kolah of Rice University for her valuable time and research expertise, Joyce Lee of the Houston Chronicle Library for permission to reproduce images which originally appeared in *The Houston Post* and Josh Smith of *Anesthesia and Analgesia* for permission to reproduce images which originally appeared in that journal.

Notes

1 The author is Senior Historian on the federal staff of the National Library of Medicine (NLM), National Institutes of Health (NIH). He authored this chapter with support from the NLM/NIH. His contribution is considered a Work of the United States Government, and the conclusions presented are his alone and do not necessarily reflect the views of the NIH or the US Department of Health and Human Services.

2 Ronda Wendler, 'DeBakey Sisters Teach Logic and Language of Medicine', *Texas Medical Center News*, 1 May 2008.

3 Michael Crichton, 'Medical Obfuscation: Structure and Function', *The New England Journal of Medicine* 293:24 (1975), 1257–9; Robert H. Moser, *Adventures in Medical Writing* (Thomas, 1970). See also Francis Crick, *The Astonishing Hypothesis: The Scientific Search for the Soul* (Simon & Schuster, 1994), and Ivan Illich, *Limits to Medicine – Medical Nemesis: The Exploration of Health* (Pantheon Books/Random House, 1975).

4 Annmarie Adams, 'Encountering Maude Abbott', *Feminist Encounters: A Journal of Critical Studies in Culture and Politics* 2:2 (2018), 323–49.

5 Craig Miller, *A Time for All Things: The Life of Michael E. DeBakey* (Oxford University Press, 2020) and William L. Winters Jr, with Betsy Parish, *Houston Hearts: A History of Cardiovascular Surgery and Medicine and The Methodist DeBakey Heart and Vascular Center Houston Methodist Hospital* (Elisha Freeman Publishing, 2014).

6 Selma DeBakey and Lois DeBakey, 'Michael E. DeBakey, MD, and the Collegial Family Triad', *CV Network Online: International Academy of Cardiovascular Sciences* 7:3 (2008), 6–9.

7 Miller, *Time for All Things*, pp. 24, 54, 79, 244. See also William L. Winters Jr, 'Selma and Lois DeBakey: Icons of Medical Communication: Selma DeBakey 12/3/1915–3/6/2013: Lois DeBakey, PhD, 7/6/1920–6/15/2016', *Methodist DeBakey Cardiovasc Journal* 12:3 (2016), 188–9.
8 'Local Women Named Medical Writers Magazine Editors', *Lake Charles American-Press* (27 November 1960), 5.
9 'Famed Doctor's Sister: Former Resident Develops Medical Writing Course', *Lake Charles American-Press*, 21 March 1965, 7.
10 DeBakey and DeBakey, 'Michael E. DeBakey, MD', 6.
11 DeBakey and DeBakey, 'Michael E. DeBakey, MD', 6.
12 DeBakey and DeBakey, 'Michael E. DeBakey, MD', 6.
13 Wendler, 'DeBakey Sisters', 2.
14 Wendler, 'DeBakey Sisters', 2.
15 Lois and Selma DeBakey, 'Michael E. DeBakey, MD: Beloved Brother, Master Mentor, Compatible Colleague, Professional Paragon', *Methodist DeBakey Cardiovascular Journal* 4:3 (2009), 50–1.
16 DeBakey and DeBakey, 'Michael E. DeBakey, MD', 51.
17 Fran Fawcett-Peterson, 'Family Affair: Selma and Lois DeBakey', *H-Texas Magazine* 14:1 (2008), 12–14.
18 Nicholas C. Chriss, '2 Other DeBakeys Do Word Surgery', *Des Moines Tribune*, 20 July 1977, 25.
19 Chriss, '2 Other DeBakeys', 25.
20 Phil R. Manning and Lois DeBakey, *Medicine: Preserving the Passion* (Springer-Verlag, 1987), p. xix.
21 Wendler, 'DeBakey Sisters', 6.
22 Winters Jr, 'Selma and Lois DeBakey', 189.
23 See Winters Jr, 'Selma and Lois DeBakey'; DeBakey and DeBakey, 'Michael E. DeBakey, MD and the collegial family triad'; and DeBakey and DeBakey, 'Michael E. DeBakey, MD: Beloved Brother', in which the sisters use 'The Durable Triad' to describe their relationship with their brother.
24 The passages read by Lois included selections from Michel Radomisli, 'The paper-writing function of the ego', *American Journal of Psychotherapy* 28:2 (1974), 278–81; C.K. Ogden and L.A. Richards (eds), *The Meaning of Meaning: A Study of the Influence of Language upon Thought and of the Science of Symbolism* (Harcourt, Brace & Co., 1923); and James A. Shannon (ed.), *Science and the Evolution of Public Policy* (Rockefeller University Press, 1975).
25 Lois DeBakey, 'Every careless word that men utter. I. The English language', *Anesthesia and Analgesia* 49:4 (1970), 567–74, and Lois

DeBakey, 'Every careless word that men utter. II. The language of science', *Anesthesia and Analgesia* 49:5 (1970), 827–34.

26 DeBakey, 'Every careless word that men utter. I', 567.

27 DeBakey, 'Every careless word that men utter. II', 830.

28 Feedback from students who enrolled in their classes likely influenced if and how Lois and Selma enhanced their visual aids. This aspect of their work, among many others, is ripe for future research.

29 DeBakey and DeBakey, 'Michael E. DeBakey, MD and the collegial family triad', 7.

30 Lois DeBakey, 'Medical gobbledygook and writer's gookledygobb', *Illinois Medical Journal* 139:6 (1971), 614.

31 R. Putney, Interview by Jeffrey S. Reznick [telephone], 4 March 2024.

32 R. Putney, Interview by Jeffrey S. Reznick [telephone], 4 March 2024. Following his work with the DeBakeys, Putney became an accomplished Creative Services Manager at the *Houston Post*, responsible for a team of artists, photographers and writers dedicated to various marketing products associated with the paper, such as subscriptions, posters and other materials involving special events. Putney held this position until his retirement.

33 Lois DeBakey and Selma DeBakey, 'Medicant: Nothing hinders communication as much as words – when they are used badly or incorrectly', *Forum on Medicine* 1:1 (1978), 38–40, 42–3, 80–1.

34 Lois DeBakey, as quoted in John O. Godden, 'The scientific paper as artefact (Guest editorial)', *Canadian Psychiatric Association Journal* 14:6 (1969), 535.

35 Moser, as quoted in Wendler, 'DeBakey Sisters', 2.

36 Moser, as quoted in Winters, 'Selma and Lois DeBakey', 189.

37 Lindberg, as quoted in Wendler, 'DeBakey Sisters', 3.

38 Hanlon, as quoted in Wendler, 'DeBakey Sisters', 3.

39 Winters, as quoted in Wendler, 'DeBakey Sisters', 3.

40 'Doctors Down the Logorrhea: DeBakey Sisters Cure "Medicalese"', *The Los Angeles Times* (17 July 1977), 29, and 'Patient Sisters Wield Knife on Words', *The Los Angeles Times* (29 March 1982), 2.

41 'DeBakey Sisters Operate on Medical Jargon', *Rapid City Journal* (31 March 1982), 49.

42 'Sick of Medical Lingo, Sisters Help Wordy Doctors', *The Courier-Journal* (17 July 1977), 3.

43 'DeBakey Sisters Urge Doctors to Learn to Talk Straight', *Pensacola News* (20 November 1977), 82.

44 'Doctors Often Turn English into Latin', *The Central New Jersey Home News* (28 September 1970), 2.

45 'A Pox on "Medicant"', *Time Magazine* (19 May 1980), 88. Notably, this spotlight on the work of the DeBakey sisters appears as part of a feature story entitled 'The Righting of Writing: From Kindergarten on Up, Americans are Wrestling with the Word'.
46 'A Pox on "Medicant"', 88.
47 While this photo could have been an opportunity for the *Houston Post* to promote the talent of Putney, that was unlikely due to his freelance collaboration with the sisters.
48 DeBakey and DeBakey, 'Michael E. DeBakey, MD', 7.
49 Stanley Wellborn, 'Ahead: A Nation of Illiterates?', *US News and World Report*, 17 May 1982, 53.
50 *The American Heritage Guide to Contemporary Usage and Style* (Houghton Mifflin, 2005), p. viii.
51 Leslie Loddeke, 'DeBakey Tells Doctors How to Communicate', *The Houston Post*, 26 May 1992, 1.

References

Adams, Annmarie. 'Encountering Maude Abbott'. *Feminist Encounters: A Journal of Critical Studies in Culture and Politics* 2:2 (2018), 323–49.

The American Heritage Guide to Contemporary Usage and Style. Houghton Mifflin, 2005.

Bernstein, Theodore. *The Careful Writer*. Atheneum, 1965.

Chriss, Nicholas. '2 Other DeBakeys Do Word Surgery'. *Des Moines Tribune*, 20 July 1977, 25.

Crick, Francis. *The Astonishing Hypothesis: The Scientific Search for the Soul*. Simon & Schuster, 1994.

Crichton, Michael. 'Medical Obfuscation: Structure and Function'. *The New England Journal of Medicine* 293:24 (1975), 1257–9.

DeBakey, Lois. 'Every careless word that men utter. I. The English language'. *Anesthesia and Analgesia* 49:4 (1970), 567–74.

DeBakey, Lois. 'Every careless word that men utter. II. The language of science'. *Anesthesia and Analgesia* 49:5 (1970), 827–34.

DeBakey, Lois, and Selma DeBakey. 'Medicant: Nothing hinders communication as much as words – when they are used badly or incorrectly'. *Forum on Medicine* 1:1 (1978), 38–40, 42–3, 80–6.

DeBakey, Lois, and Selma DeBakey. 'Michael E. DeBakey, MD, and the collegial family triad'. *CV Network Online: International Academy of Cardiovascular Sciences* 7:3 (2008), 6–9.

DeBakey, Lois, and Selma DeBakey. 'Michael E. DeBakey, MD: Beloved brother, master mentor, compatible colleague, professional paragon'. *Methodist DeBakey Cardiovascular Journal* 4:3 (2009), 49–56.
'DeBakey Sisters Operate on Medical Jargon'. *Rapid City Journal*, 31 March 1982, 49.
'DeBakey Sisters Urge Doctors to Learn to Talk Straight'. *Pensacola News*, 20 November 1977, 82.
'Doctors down the logorrhea: DeBakey Sisters cure "Medicalese"'. *The Los Angeles Times*, 17 July 1977, 29.
'Doctors Often Turn English into Latin'. *The Central New Jersey Home News*, 28 September 1970, 2.
'Famed Doctor's Sister: Former Resident Develops Medical Writing Course'. *Lake Charles American-Press*, 21 March 1965, 7.
Fawcett-Peterson, Fran. 'Family affair: Selma and Lois DeBakey'. *H-Texas Magazine* 14:1 (2008), 12–14.
Godden, John O. 'The scientific paper as artefact (Guest editorial)', *Canadian Psychiatric Association Journal* 14:6 (1969), 535–8.
'Local Women Named Medical Writers Magazine Editors'. *Lake Charles American-Press*, 27 November 1960, 5.
Loddeke, Leslie. 'DeBakey Tells Doctors how to Communicate'. *The Houston Post*, 26 May 1992, 1.
Manning, Phil R, and Lois DeBakey. *Medicine: Preserving the Passion*. Springer-Verlag, 1987.
Miller, Craig. *A Time for All Things: The Life of Michael E. DeBakey*. Oxford University Press, 2020.
Moser, Robert H. *Adventures in Medical Writing*. Thomas, 1970.
Ogden, C.K., and L.A. Richards (eds). *The Meaning of Meaning: A Study of the Influence of Language upon Thought and of the Science of Symbolism*. Harcourt, Brace & Co., 1923.
'Patient Sisters Wield Knife on Words'. *The Los Angeles Times*, 29 March 1982, 2.
'A Pox on "Medicant"'. *Time Magazine*, 19 May 1980, 88.
Putney, R. Interviewed by Jeffrey S. Reznick. 4 March 2024, telephone.
Radomisli, Michel. 'The paper-writing function of the ego'. *American Journal of Psychotherapy* 28:2 (1974), 278–81.
'The Righting of Writing: From Kindergarten on Up, Americans are Wrestling with the Word'. *Time Magazine*, 19 May 1980, 88.
Shannon, James A. (ed.). *Science and the Evolution of Public Policy*. Rockefeller University Press, 1975.
'Sick of Medical Lingo, Sisters Help Wordy Doctors', *The Courier-Journal*, 17 July 1977, 3.
Strunk Jr, William, and E.B. White. *The Elements of Style*. Privately printed, 1919.

Wellborn, Stanley. 'Ahead: A Nation of Illiterates?', *US News and World Report*, 17 May 1982, 53.

Wendler, Ronda. 'DeBakey Sisters Teach Logic and Language of Medicine', *Texas Medical Center News*, May 1 2008, pp. 1–8.

Williams, Joseph M. *Style: Ten Lessons in Clarity and Grace*. Addison-Wesley Educational Publishers, 1981.

Winters Jr, William L. 'Selma and Lois DeBakey: Icons of Medical Communication: Selma DeBakey, 12/3/1915–3/6/2013: Lois DeBakey, PhD, 7/6/1920–6/15/2016'. *Methodist DeBakey Cardiovasc Journal* 12:3 (2016), 188–9.

Winters Jr, William L., with Betsy Parish. *Houston Hearts: A History of Cardiovascular Surgery and Medicine and The Methodist DeBakey Heart and Vascular Center Houston Methodist Hospital*. Elisha Freeman Publishing, 2014.

9

Tough Shit Thomas and Peanut Pete: Harm reduction comics and British identities in the 1990s

Peder Clark

See note[1]

Sometime in the late 1730s, in the rue Saint-Severin, Paris, the 'funniest thing that ever happened' in the working life of one Nicolas Contat, an apprentice in a printing shop, was the riotous, bloody and somewhat ritualistic slaughter of the cats of the neighbourhood.[2] In the view of Contat and his fellow put-upon apprentices, these pampered felines had been treated far better than themselves, and their summary execution was richly deserved by their owners. The incident was re-enacted over the following days to peals of laughter, growing ever more humorous in the re-telling. Indeed, the hilarity of the episode was so pronounced that the worker would still be writing about the incident some twenty years later. To modern readers – especially in these ailurophilic times – the treatment of these poor animals seems barbaric and 'repulsive', not to say very 'unfunny'.[3] This episode is notably (although not exclusively) the subject of Robert Darnton's classic work of cultural history *The Great Cat Massacre, and Other Episodes in French Cultural History* (1984). Darnton shows us how 'jokes' – even, or in fact, especially, when we don't 'get' them – can open up lines of inquiry and understanding that otherwise may seem inaccessible.[4] Darnton encourages us to look at who is laughing, and for what reasons, suggesting that humour can illuminate our awareness of the worldviews of those in the past, as the apprentices invert the power relationship between them and their master. He also asks us to place these instances of hilarity in wider contexts in order to see the traditions and discourses in which the jokes are taking part, in short, to not only understand the joke, but to see what social function it plays.[5]

All this is by way of roundabout introduction to another cat – among other characters – some two and a half centuries later, in post-industrial Manchester rather than pre-industrial Paris. The feline in question went by the name of (excuse my French) Tough Shit Thomas. Thomas was a character drawn primarily by Michael Linnell, an illustrator who drew a series of comics for the Manchester-based drugs charity Lifeline during the 1980s through to the 2000s. Alongside Thomas, Linnell drew a number of other characters, most prominently Peanut Pete, who became a highly recognisable icon of rave culture. Lifeline had been formed in 1971 by psychiatrist Eugenie Cheesmond and former heroin user Rowdy Yates. Described by Yates as one of the 'field hospitals of the counter culture revolution' offering food and a '"place to crash" for drug users', Lifeline had expanded its services by the 1980s and was providing harm reduction advice.[6] Yates noted that the 'change and growth from such beginnings into an organization, almost – not quite, but almost – in the mainstream of voluntary sector welfare provision was … slow … [and] predictably painful'.[7] Its approach had evolved into one that was avowedly 'agnostic', working alongside drug users, believing their consumption to be neither 'altogether "good" nor "bad"'.[8] Lifeline aimed to address drug users on their own terms, and started using the medium of comics to do so in 1987.

This chapter uses Lifeline's pivot to this visual and vernacular method of communicating its harm reduction messages as a means of exploring wider social attitudes to various recreational drugs in 1990s Britain, and what role humour played in expressing and delineating different identities. The first half of the chapter concentrates on Lifeline's introduction of the comic book genre to their range of information literature and wider activities, via the cast of characters created for their publication *Smack in the Eye*, which ran for nine issues from 1987 to 1993.[9] Lifeline used humorous representations to address marginalised groups and discuss 'serious' and arguably unfunny social issues such as heroin addiction and the developing HIV/AIDS epidemic. The second half of the chapter looks at Peanut Pete, who first made an appearance in issue six of

Smack in the Eye, but would go on to become the charity's most recognisable and enduring character. The emergence of Peanut Pete marked both a shift in Lifeline's activities and tone towards a much more stridently articulated regional identity, but also the arrival of Ecstasy into widespread use and public consciousness. Following Darnton's example, a close reading of the humorous exploits and aesthetics of Peanut Pete, Tough Shit Thomas and other associated characters across standalone leaflets provide an insight into British regional, social, gender and subcultural identities in the 1990s.

Tough Shit Thomas, the AIDS crisis and the limits of humour

Tough Shit Thomas is not only an ungainly segue from Darnton's cat massacre in the introduction to this chapter, but also significant as the first character to appear in *Smack in the Eye*. This comic was a vehicle for Lifeline's harm reduction messaging, and took its cues from 1960s US underground comix such as Gilbert Shelton's *Fabulous Furry Freak Brothers*, which not only featured risqué counterculture humour and copious marijuana smoke, but also Fat Freddy's Cat.[10] Indeed, cats of literally all stripes were a key trope in comic book culture – for example, Garfield or Hobbes of *Calvin and* fame – perhaps mirroring the way that Darnton's cat massacre was in a tradition of feline-related mischief and practical jokes such as the German *Katzenmusic*.[11] Tough Shit Thomas's place in this longer lineage also pointed to how, in art historian Steve Baker's analysis, 'the animal operates as a flexible symbolic device within the everyday life of the culture'.[12] This also suggests the manner in which humour could sometimes function: anthropomorphised creatures could be stand-ins or conduits for expressing opinions or thoughts that their human equivalents left unspoken. For example, in his debut strip, Thomas comes close to losing the last of his nine lives by injecting heroin with a used syringe; a story with a near tragic ending that could be played for laughs, stealthily implanting the serious message about harm reduction in the reader's mind.[13]

Thomas's narrowly avoided demise would have been brought about by contracting HIV from shared hypodermic needles. It was the public health and governmental response to the burgeoning AIDS crisis that provided the resources for Lifeline's activities. People who injected drugs were, alongside men who had sex with men, viewed as the group most at risk of contracting HIV. The concern from official quarters, in Scotland for example, was that there was

> a serious risk that infected drug misusers will spread HIV beyond the presently recognised high risk groups and into the sexually active general population ... The gravity of the problem is such that on balance the containment of the spread of the virus is a higher priority in management than the prevention of drug misuse.[14]

From 1985 onwards, the British government published two major reports on 'AIDS and Drug Misuse', as well as assigning £17m (with a further £3m in 1988) to develop services for the needs of this particular constituency, including the introduction of needle exchanges in many areas.[15] Lifeline were the indirect beneficiaries of this focus, receiving £5,000 in 1987 from the North West Regional Health Authority specifically to address HIV prevention.[16]

For Lifeline, at least in presenting the work externally to the World Health Organization, *Smack in the Eye* was a 'Radical Departure from Standard Drugs and HIV Education'.[17] Although *Smack in the Eye* was certainly bracing to those of a sensitive disposition, this was also something of a deliberate overstatement. The comic book format was novel for Lifeline, but the use of humour was not. A documentary made for the BBC's *Open Door* series in September 1978 showed Lifeline's methods for disseminating their, at the time, solidly anti-drugs rhetoric. Street theatre alongside humorous ditties and songs were deployed, primarily to educate about the risks of prescription medication.[18] But the comic genre had not gone unexplored in health education circles either. The Health Education Council (HEC) had used Superman, albeit to target 'children aged 7–11-years-old' as part of an early 1980s anti-smoking drive.[19] A more adult audience was reached with the late 1980s *Look After Your Heart* campaign, which syndicated the popular Andy Capp character from the *Daily Mirror*'s comic pages.[20]

But if comics were not new to health education more broadly, where Lifeline's approach did break largely new ground was in its approach to sexually transmitted infections (STIs) and illegal drugs (although Lifeline themselves acknowledged previous efforts in Merseyside and the Netherlands).[21] While the HEC and successor organisation the Health Education Authority (HEA) had had no problem with making light of such issues as cigarette smoking – their Saatchi and Saatchi commissioned adverts being another example – or heart attacks, their approach to AIDS and heroin was deadly serious.[22] The 1986 AIDS campaign Don't Die of Ignorance and the previous year's Heroin Screws You Up both favoured a largely monochrome palette and dark imagery, including tombstones in the former. Both were criticised at the time and subsequently for their scaremongering approach.[23]

Lifeline did indeed depart radically from this sombre tone and aesthetic with *Smack in the Eye*. Mark Gilman, who worked for Lifeline for the latter half of the 1980s and most of the 1990s in various roles, helped to develop *Smack in the Eye*, but also, importantly, to evaluate its impact. He described how, very deliberately, Lifeline sought to distinguish their approach from the official messaging of government-backed campaigns: 'we were consciously aiming for a style and tone that would make the comic stand out – that would make its readers remember both the medium and the message'.[24] Or as Gilman's colleague Mike Linnell more colourfully put it, '*Smack in the Eye* was tossed like a … hand grenade into the cobwebbed world of what passed for drugs education at the time.'[25]

Certainly, *Smack in the Eye* stood in stark contrast to the 'social advertising' produced by more conventional health educators. Lifeline explained that because of their 'negative emphasis, they are perceived as threatening by the audience', and missed the point of why people might engage in apparently 'risky' behaviours in the first place. 'This means that such advertising can induce anxiety … which prompts a dismissal of the message', while material such as *Smack in the Eye* and 'the humour of the comic book format clearly distances … from the standard serious messages which create such defensiveness'.[26] Humour was therefore a way to get alongside the intended audience: a way to speak with, rather than down to, them. In doing so, Lifeline drew on a different tradition of knowledge dissemination about the risks and pleasures of drugs, that of the underground comix of the 1960s and 1970s. As one contemporary observer noted, 'fifteen years ago there was a flourishing underground press that provided more concrete drug education than an army of drug educationalists'.[27] These were also fondly remembered by many readers of *Smack in the Eye*, who 'used to buy the "High Times" years ago and the "Home Grown" magazine'.[28] The periodical nature and ongoing narrative of comics was also significant, in contrast to the Don't Die of Ignorance campaign, which had been a single mailshot to every UK home. As Gilman explained, 'Unlike the one-off leaflet that can be perceived as a single exercise in inoculation against HIV, the comic format can be reproduced regularly to repeat and reinforce harm reduction messages using different characters and scenarios.'[29] Indeed, arguably it was both the episodic and sequential structure of the comic that made the format so appealing to Lifeline. The narrative advancement and visual repetition of the comic book meant that the characters quickly captured the reader's attention and provided familiarity from frame to frame and from issue to issue. In short, Lifeline believed comics to be the perfect medium for their concerns, echoing contemporary scholarship on the form that described 'cartooning as a form of amplification through simplification'.[30]

Consumers of the pilot issue seemed to appreciate these efforts, and the clear line that they drew, 'in direct contrast to the traditional use of "fear arousal"' employed by health education bodies.[31] Lifeline were taken aback by the level of animosity towards official messaging around HIV, which constituted 'standard official leaflets, television adverts and billboards'. A 29-year-old respondent suggested that 'a lot of my mates are convinced that the AIDS adverts are just propaganda from the government to stop us enjoying ourselves'. Lifeline characterised such instances of 'conspiracy theories' as on a 'continuum', indicating a deep-seated scepticism towards health education and harm reduction messages that were unshakeable by conventional means. Humour and 'naughtiness' was a way of disrupting these theories, demonstrating to people who used drugs that Lifeline was on their 'side'.[32] Their feedback suggested that those interviewed did indeed believe that Lifeline had got alongside them, and that *Smack in the Eye* served an useful dialogic function: 'Outreach and detached workers use the comic as a way of opening up a dialogue ... this is a particularly useful way of beginning discussion [about safer sexual practices] with a group whose primary concern relates to reducing the harm that can arise from drug use.'[33]

While *Smack in the Eye* was largely well received by its target audience, other interested parties were less appreciative of both its medium and message. The Crown Prosecution Service interviewed Lifeline staff twice following complaints by a director of social services, while a letter apparently from a tranquilliser addiction support group read:

> I think that you ... are a lot of dirty-minded, foul mouthed perverts unfit to associate with normal decent people ... I would not lift a finger to help the kind of scum to whom you [*sic*] the filth you have got together under the name of 'comic' is addressed. Their filthy habits [and] lack of self-respect ... has been responsible for [the] predicament in which they find themselves.[34]

Such epistolary missives may have been distressing (and perhaps a little amusing) to receive, but they also indicated the function of humour in sharply delineating between the 'normal decent people' that the correspondent presumably represented, and the 'scum' that Lifeline sought to reach. In this context, the shared jokes of *Smack in the Eye* operated as a way of establishing an 'us' and 'them' dynamic for a marginalised group, and reinforcing Lifeline's reputation as a reliable and trusted source.

Having sketched out the context and response to the first two issues of *Smack in the Eye*, it is now worth turning to its actual content, via a close reading of its third issue. This issue has been selected not only because it opens with an edited and abridged version of the above correspondence on its 'Readers' Letters Page', but also because it represents the comic in its mature form, as an established voice in harm reduction. Furthermore, *Smack in the Eye* was by this point being drawn by Michael Linnell, who would go on to produce all of Lifeline's visual material, after the commercial artist who had produced the pilot and second issues had moved on.[35] Linnell's contribution to the success of *Smack in the Eye* – and later to the character of Peanut Pete – should not be underestimated. Although much of the early content of *Smack in the Eye* appears to have been predicated on Gilman's research, from this point on Linnell was also crucial. While his contribution to the visual and aesthetic distinctiveness of the comics was apparent, he was equally as committed as Gilman in articulating the effectiveness of the comic book format, doing so at postgraduate thesis length.[36] As Linnell reflected later in his career, 'You have to communicate successfully with people if you're going to gain their trust ... There's no point bombarding people with facts if they don't think you're on their side.'[37]

Nonetheless, the reader wouldn't struggle to find advice and factual information in issue three.[38] At the bottom of the letters page was a short strip entitled 'The Wise Guys', itself indebted to a Dutch harm reduction comic, but in this rendering a pastiche of *Star Trek*.[39] In this comic, the spacecraft is an enormous hypodermic needle and Mr Smack (bearing a close visual resemblance to Dr Spock) dispenses accurate advice about the relative merits of using citric acid or lemon juice when injecting heroin (Figure 9.1).

The following strip in the issue saw Tough Shit Thomas being taken in by an apparently well-meaning grandmother with a well-stocked pharmacopeia. Thomas raids the medicine cupboard for its supply of temazepam, a medicine conventionally used to treat sleeping problems but commonly used at the time as a substitute for heroin or methadone. Unused to the drug's effects, Thomas ends up attempting to have sex with the vacuum cleaner (Figure 9.2). When the woman returned to the 'wreckage of her house', she brutally retaliated by dousing Thomas with petrol and lighting a

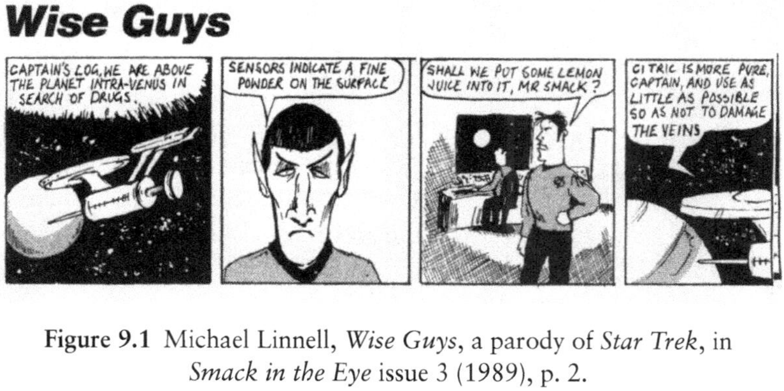
Wise Guys
CAPTAIN'S LOG, WE ARE ABOVE THE PLANET INTRA-VENUS IN SEARCH OF DRUGS.
SENSORS INDICATE A FINE POWDER ON THE SURFACE
SHALL WE PUT SOME LEMON JUICE INTO IT, MR SMACK?
CITRIC IS MORE PURE, CAPTAIN, AND USE AS LITTLE AS POSSIBLE SO AS NOT TO DAMAGE THE VEINS

Figure 9.1 Michael Linnell, *Wise Guys*, a parody of *Star Trek*, in *Smack in the Eye* issue 3 (1989), p. 2.

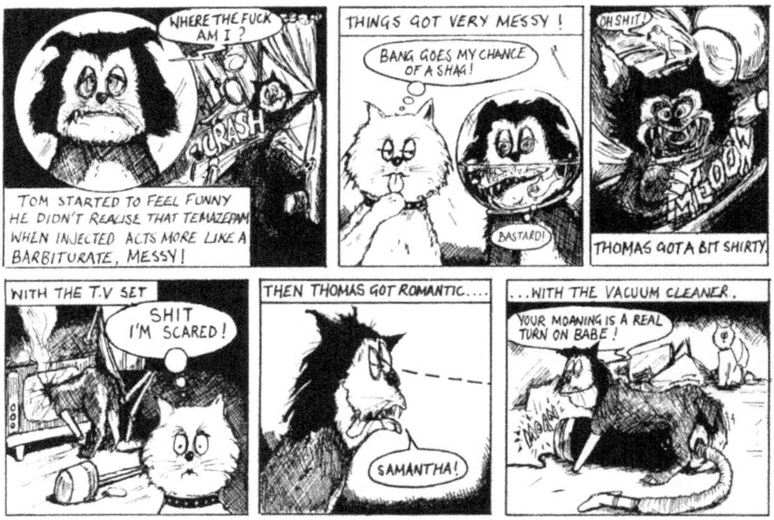
WHERE THE FUCK AM I ?
CRASH
TOM STARTED TO FEEL FUNNY HE DIDN'T REALISE THAT TEMAZEPAM WHEN INJECTED ACTS MORE LIKE A BARBITURATE, MESSY!
THINGS GOT VERY MESSY !
BANG GOES MY CHANCE OF A SHAG!
BASTARD!
OH SHIT!
MEOOW
THOMAS GOT A BIT SHIRTY
WITH THE T.V SET
SHIT I'M SCARED!
THEN THOMAS GOT ROMANTIC....
SAMANTHA!
...WITH THE VACUUM CLEANER.
YOUR MOANING IS A REAL TURN ON BABE !
MOAN

Figure 9.2 Michael Linnell, Tough Shit Thomas attempts to have sex with a vacuum cleaner, in *Smack in the Eye* issue 3 (1989), p. 4.

match, causing him to 'woof' like a dog, a fate not too far removed from the unfortunate victims of Darnton's cat massacre. The final two panels concluded with the comic's moral admonishment; 'it's a dog's life cranking temazepam', and 'it had not been one of Tom's best days'.

The next page contained a quiz which provided answers (more 'facts') to serious questions such as 'Can HIV be passed on through sharing water, spoons and filters?' Another short three-panel strip followed, offering a counterbalance to 'The Wise Guys': 'The Daft Bastards'. As their moniker might suggest, this regular feature illustrated drug-taking behaviour considered particularly risky or reckless. In this instance, it was the treatment of cellulitis; 'don't be a daft bastard[,] see your GP or go to hospital'. The following full-page strip addressed the burgeoning culture of weight-lifting and anabolic steroid use, with 'Pumping Iron' and the character Locker Room Lenny.[40] Portraying an homoerotic locker-room scene, it again offered a simple cautionary message: 'no matter what drug you are injecting never share injection equipment'. This was followed by a full-page instructional illustration of how to dispose of a used needle safely. The two middle pages of the comic were taken up by an A–Z of 'Safer Sex' full of British colloquialisms and slang ('G is for golden showers (water sports) or pissing on someone: low risk'; 'W is for wanking, try it on each other'), with a free condom provided at the end (Figure 9.3).

Page 10 provided the answers to the quiz, with a further iteration of 'The Wise Guys', with the key piece of information being: 'rotating injection places gives my veins a rest'. 'Prisoner: Cell Block A' grimly parodied the Australian television series of almost the same name which had run between 1979 and 1986, suggesting that life inside was much riskier in the era of AIDS than previously, with the protagonist concluding that 'if I do go down ... I'll stick to wanking and smoking drugs'. This was followed by a more romantic tale – that of Romeo and Juliet – in which the former serenaded the latter, before being rebuffed by his paramour with the stark message of 'No condom – no needle exchange – no way'. Finally, interspersed between two advertising pages featuring Mainline, a 'drug users union – run by users for users' and Lifeline's services, was another quintessential *Smack in the Eye* character, Grandpa 'Smackhead' Jones ('the oldest junkie in the world'). Two younger consumers of drugs sought out Jones's advice on 'crack', at this juncture sweeping through American inner cities.[41] Jones detailed his experiences ('very nice ... [but] this is getting expensive') before dispensing his judgement: 'it costs loads of money, is difficult to control and you could lose your shirt' (Figure 9.4).

For Lifeline, the humour of *Smack in the Eye* could 'be a very effective tool' but one that was 'very often a double-edged one as it often requires a target'. Lifeline was a balancing act, attempting to produce something funny that nonetheless stuck with the reader after the page had been turned: 'The problem is to create humour with a sting in its tail ... humour can be employed to attract attention yet leave behind a meaningful harm reduction message.'[42] The issue, however, was in how to do so in a way that neither valorised nor stigmatised the groups represented. For the former case, Lifeline did not want certain characters to become 'anti-heroes, proud of their kamikaze attitude and behaviour'.[43] On the other hand, one of the concerns that was raised with Lifeline, and

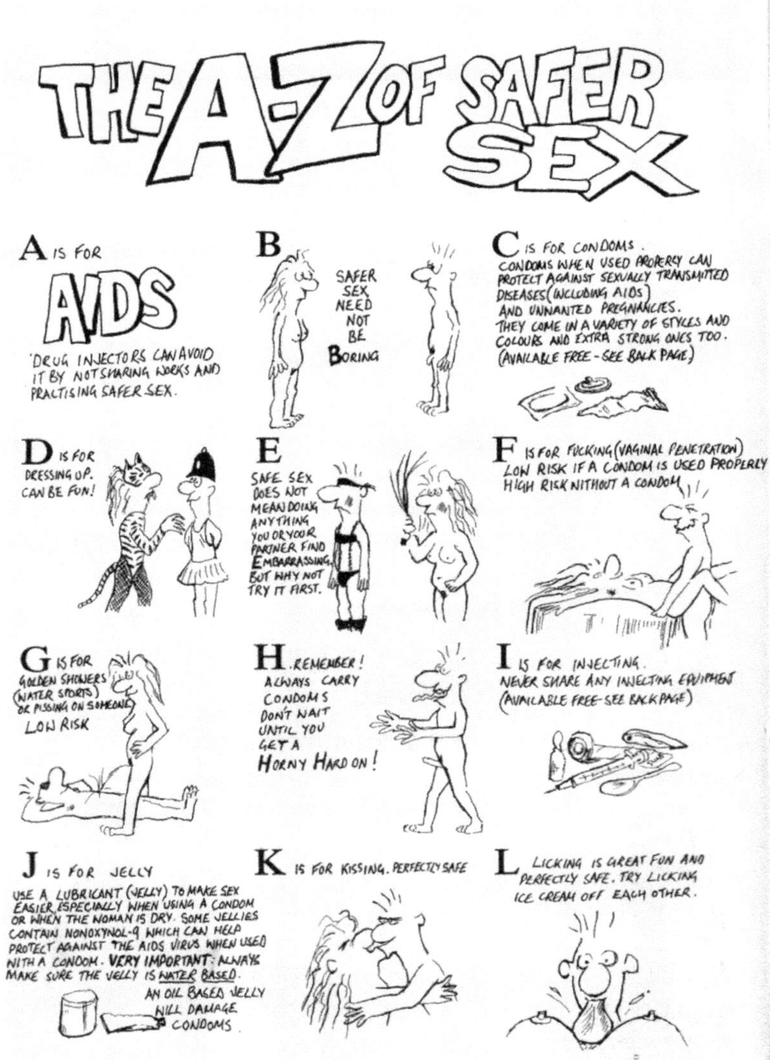

Figure 9.3 Michael Linnell, *The A–Z of Safer Sex*, in *Smack in the Eye* issue 3 (1989), p. 8.

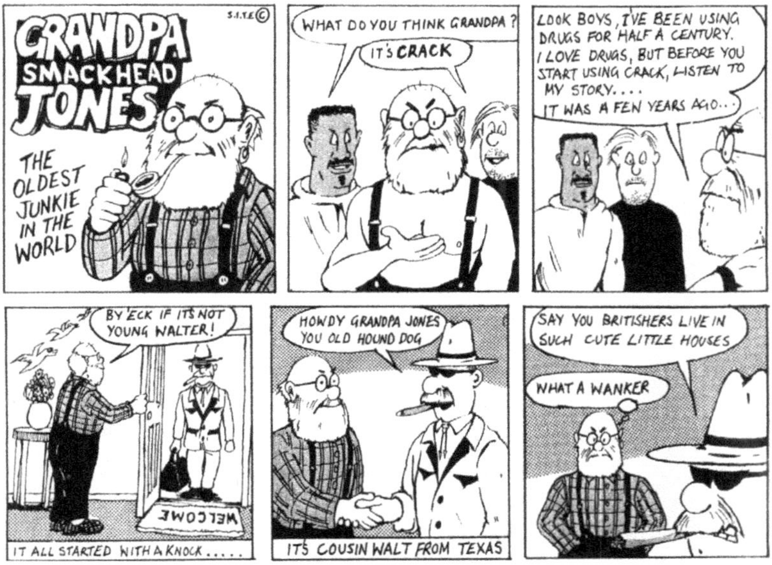
GRANDPA SMACKHEAD JONES
S.I.T.E©
THE OLDEST JUNKIE IN THE WORLD
WHAT DO YOU THINK GRANDPA ?
IT'S CRACK
LOOK BOYS, I'VE BEEN USING DRUGS FOR HALF A CENTURY. I LOVE DRUGS, BUT BEFORE YOU START USING CRACK, LISTEN TO MY STORY....
IT WAS A FEW YEARS AGO...
BY 'ECK IF IT'S NOT YOUNG WALTER!
WELCOME
IT ALL STARTED WITH A KNOCK.....
HOWDY GRANDPA JONES YOU OLD HOUND DOG
IT'S COUSIN WALT FROM TEXAS
SAY YOU BRITISHERS LIVE IN SUCH CUTE LITTLE HOUSES
WHAT A WANKER

Figure 9.4 Michael Linnell, Grandpa 'Smackhead' Jones dispenses advice about crack cocaine, in *Smack in the Eye* issue 3 (1989), p. 14.

that the staff spent considerable time wrestling with, was whether their depictions reified or resisted stereotypes of people who used drugs. Indeed, a significant minority believed *Smack in the Eye* failed in this endeavour: '13% of respondents felt that sections of the comic reinforced negative and inaccurate images of drug users as, "foul-mouthed idiots who screw around"'.[44] Nonetheless, many of the characters, most especially Tough Shit Thomas and Grandpa Smackhead Jones, resonated strongly with *Smack in the Eye*'s readership. Indeed, there was a sense among some of the readership that *Smack in the Eye*, while on the one hand presenting a highly caricaturised version of drug use, was in fact too accurate and realistic in its portrayal. One of the more interesting strands of Gilman's evaluation was the suspicion that some of the most vituperative criticism received was given by those 'quite shocked at its content rather than its style'. These critics were apparently embittered by the demystification of drug subcultures. A 'drug injector' confided to Lifeline that the comic made them feel 'a bit uncomfortable', as if they had been 'sussed ... a realisation that other people, "straights", actually had a good idea of drug using lifestyles'. This uneasy feeling manifested itself as an 'angry dismissal' of its contents, a malignancy that could only be addressed, in Lifeline's view, by repeated publications, closing the 'credibility gap' between the charity and their readership.[45]

In short, the contents of a typical *Smack in the Eye* were very diverse, with a range of humorous tactics employed, from slapstick to gallows to parody. But it was, despite Lifeline's rhetoric, also highly didactic, providing health education messages as explicit as the depictions of drug-taking and sexual practices. The language was robust, but so was the advice and the moral judgements, with readers neatly divided into 'wise guys' or 'daft bastards' depending on their attitude and compliance with the advice and information offered. Indeed, some of this messaging was also comparatively conservative. For example, the pastiche of 'Prisoner: Cell Block A' implied that abstention was the best form of prevention for the prison-dwelling population, a recommendation that ran counter to much of Lifeline's wider philosophy. Nonetheless, it was Gilman's contention that the development of *Smack in the Eye* had helped 'the Lifeline Project re-discover the "radical cutting-edge" which characterised the project at its inception in the 1970's'.[46] Despite the occasional boorish humour and moralising content of *Smack in the Eye*, this claim stood up to scrutiny.

Compared to official drug education campaigns such as 'Heroin Screws You Up', *Smack in the Eye* was radical, both in content and form.[47] As part of his evaluation of Lifeline, Gilman surveyed readers, and some respondents did protest that the comic taught them what they already knew, or that it 'tried to teach them to suck eggs', but in Lifeline's defence, they were often responding to a rapidly shifting environment.[48] They were contending not only with the emergence of a novel disease in the form of AIDS, but also the rapid emergence of apparently novel drugs. Crack cocaine was causing alarm for drug education agencies across the Atlantic, but, more consequentially for Lifeline, it was the arrival of Ecstasy in Britain that was most significant.

Peanut Pete, Ecstasy and regional identity

Ecstasy (or 3,4-methelynedioxymethamphetamine or MDMA), in combination with another American import – house music – fuelled an entirely new subculture of 'acid house' from the summer of 1988 onwards. Manchester became one of the epicentres of this 'rave' scene, with some of its nightclubs – especially The Haçienda on Whitworth Street West – becoming destinations for young people eager to hear new music and, it must be said, take new drugs. Many of these hotspots were a mere stone's throw from Lifeline's new office on Oldham Street, where associated subcultural outlets such as clothing emporium Affleck's Palace, record shop Eastern Bloc and The Haçienda's sister pub, the Dry Bar, were all neighbours. As Linnell put it, 'We basically had people out of their faces on the doorstep.'[49] This new class of drug consumer presented a puzzle for Lifeline. For the majority of ravers and clubbers who consumed Ecstasy, their 'drug use [was] an adjunct to fun and pleasure rather than the organising force of a lifestyle'.[50] Journalist Matthew Collin summarised this issue in a profile of Lifeline for the *Observer* newspaper:

> Ecstasy, LSD or speed were strictly weekend fun drugs. The ravers might occasionally feel rough if they'd overdone it, but they didn't see themselves as junkies or people with a problem … The problem, though, was how Lifeline could get them to take drug use seriously, and contact the agency if it became a problem. The ravers weren't keen to hang out in a place populated by what they perceived as sad, dirty smackheads.[51]

As the tabloid press were only too keen to direct attention to, Ecstasy consumption was not entirely without risk. Manchester's Haçienda was the venue at which 16-year-old Claire Leighton took Ecstasy in July 1989. She later collapsed and died, becoming the first widely reported fatality associated with the drug.[52] Unsure of the risks of the drug, medical opinion erred on the side of caution, with leading toxicologist John Henry warning consumers that they were engaging in a 'dance of death'.[53]

Against this backdrop, Lifeline largely stuck to their guns, using their tried and tested methods again with ravers, creating a new character for *Smack in the Eye* and subsequent solo adventures: Peanut Pete. Pete was based on a real-life individual who had engaged with Lifeline's counselling services: a laid-back young man with his baseball cap worn backwards, a 'vaguely' peanut-shaped head, and a 'bit of a big nose'.[54]

His first appearance, in 1990, did not in fact address Ecstasy, but rather LSD, in a booklet called *A Trip Around Manchester*. In the title and the images, 'trip' here has a humorous double meaning, encompassing both a hallucinogenic experience and a pleasant day out. Our protagonist ingests a Purple Ohm (an acid blotter with the symbol representing the Hindu sacred sound emblazoned on it) before 'feeling like a paranoid pineapple' as he walks around the metropolis.[55] Pete's jumbled thoughts were depicted in a visual style running back to Fritz Kahn's conception of the body as a mechanical machine, perhaps a further nod to the city's industrial heritage.[56] Significantly, *A Trip Around Manchester* was embedded in the world in which its putative audience moved, referencing Mancunian landmarks both real and fictional, with Pete confusedly stumbling into the Rover's Return, the pub of TV soap *Coronation Street* (Figure 9.5). Where characters such as Tough Shit Thomas or Grandpa 'Smackhead' Jones had been non-regionally specific British, the creation of Peanut Pete marked a shift in Lifeline's articulation of regional identity. Vernacular and cultural reference points were northern, and indeed a later comic, *In The Zone*, would document Pete and his friend Reg's attempts to navigate their way back from 'London's huge bustling metropolis', with the humour of the piece being derived equally from the substances (LSD and cannabis) that they consumed and the fish-out-of-water experience of northerners down south.[57]

As for Pete's intoxicant of choice in *A Trip Around Manchester*, while largely undocumented in popular histories of rave, LSD was widely used by ravers. Depending on who you listen to, acid house was so named because of the lysergic, trippy qualities of house music made using the Roland TB-303 bass synthesiser, most notably Phuture's 'Acid Trax', but also because LSD (or 'acid') was the drug of choice at the gay, Black clubs of Chicago where the music originated.[58] In Britain meanwhile, the popularity of LSD could at least partly be explained by its comparative cheapness.

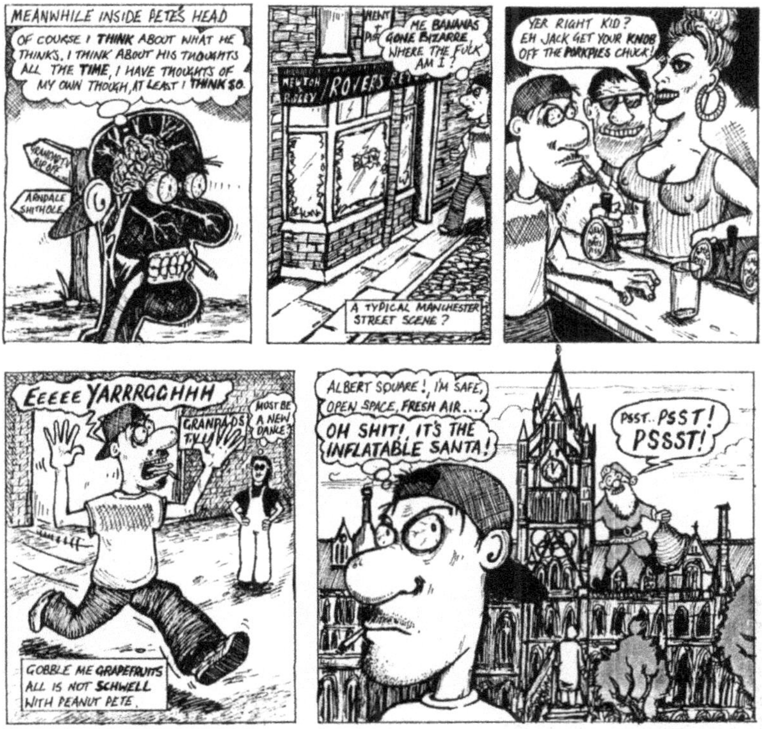
MEANWHILE INSIDE PETE'S HEAD
OF COURSE I THINK ABOUT WHAT HE THINKS. I THINK ABOUT HIS THOUGHTS ALL THE TIME, I HAVE THOUGHTS OF MY OWN THOUGH, AT LEAST I THINK SO.
ARNDALE SHITHOLE
ME BANANAS GONE BIZARRE, WHERE THE FUCK AM I?
ROVERS
A TYPICAL MANCHESTER STREET SCENE?
YER RIGHT KID? EH JACK GET YOUR KNOB OFF THE PORKPIES CHUCK!
EEEEE YARRRGGHHH
GRANDADS
MOST BE A NEW DANCE?
GOBBLE ME GRAPEFRUITS ALL IS NOT SCHWELL WITH PEANUT PETE.
ALBERT SQUARE!, I'M SAFE, OPEN SPACE, FRESH AIR....
OH SHIT! IT'S THE INFLATABLE SANTA!
PSST.. PSST! PSSST!

Figure 9.5 Michael Linnell, Peanut Pete in *A Trip Around Manchester* (1990), p. 2.

While a single Ecstasy pill could cost anything between £15 and £25, a tab of acid could be bought for a few pounds. Nonetheless, according to a former drug dealer at The Haçienda, approximately a quarter of drug-consuming ravers took acid compared to three-quarters on pills.[59] Furthermore, for the dealers themselves, the profits to be made from Ecstasy far exceeded the relatively paltry mark-up for LSD.

Next to be published was *E By Gum*, in which Pete, seeking respite from his low-paid job, wishes to go to a rave. A 'fairy godfather' appears, to grant his wishes for a mountain of Es, but also to warn him of the dangers of possession, and of taking too many at once (Figure 9.6). Again, the tone is flippant, but its narrative

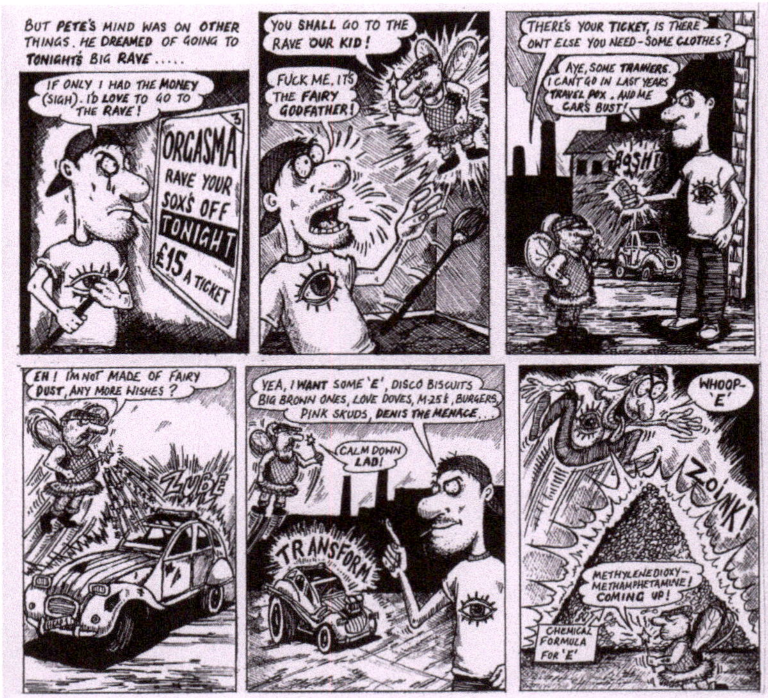
BUT PETE'S MIND WAS ON OTHER THINGS. HE DREAMED OF GOING TO TONIGHT'S BIG RAVE.....
IF ONLY I HAD THE MONEY (SIGH). I'D LOVE TO GO TO THE RAVE!
ORGASMA RAVE YOUR SOX'S OFF TONIGHT £15 A TICKET
YOU SHALL GO TO THE RAVE OUR KID!
FUCK ME, IT'S THE FAIRY GODFATHER!
THERE'S YOUR TICKET, IS THERE OWT ELSE YOU NEED - SOME CLOTHES?
AYE, SOME TRAINERS. I CAN'T GO IN LAST YEARS TRAVEL POX. AND ME CAR'S BUST!
EH! I'M NOT MADE OF FAIRY DUST, ANY MORE WISHES?
ZUBE
YEA, I WANT SOME 'E', DISCO BISCUITS BIG BROWN ONES, LOVE DOVES, M-25's, BURGERS, PINK SKUDS, DENIS THE MENACE...
CALM DOWN LAD!
TRANSFORM
WHOOP-'E'
ZOINK!
METHYLENEDIOXY-METHAMPHETAMINE! COMING UP!
CHEMICAL FORMULA FOR 'E'

Figure 9.6 Michael Linnell, Peanut Pete's fairy godfather grants him wishes in *E By Gum* (1990), p. 2.

was grounded in the issues facing young people: poor employment prospects, low wages, the desire for consumer goods and the generational divide, illustrated by the brusque exchanges between Pete and his father.[60]

The humour of these comics came not only from Pete's fantastical adventures, but also from the industrial language and, more importantly, the post-industrial setting. Peanut Pete parodied clichés about northern Britain, with its references to Corrie, flat caps and of course the titular 'E By Gum'. 'E by Gum', more usually phoneticised as 'ee by gum' in a regional and euphemistic variation of exclamations such as 'oh my god' or 'I swear by god!' here has double meaning, with 'E' also being shorthand for Ecstasy. While a phrase perhaps more associated with Yorkshire and the city across the Pennines (after all, as ravers used to say, you can't spell Leeds without two Es and LSD), it played and made fun of the versions of the North that were held by London-centric policymakers, drug workers and music press alike. The phrase appeared in Coronation Street, and was also frequently uttered by Andy Capp, the *Daily Mirror*'s cartoon character whose use by the HEA was contemporaneous with Lifeline's comics.[61] This was about who was laughing, and what they were laughing about, with Lifeline attempting to tap into regional and civic pride to connect with their audience. Indeed, reflecting on the success of Peanut Pete in a recent oral history interview, Gilman and his former colleague Alan Haughton revealed that the comics had been primarily addressed and intended for their geographically proximal peers, and that its wider reception, while welcome, was largely unexpected.[62]

Peanut Pete also chimed perfectly with the visual culture of the rave scene, namely its club flyers and fanzines.[63] *Smack in the Eye* and Peanut Pete were both influenced by *Viz*, a satirical and foul-mouthed magazine that was reaching the heights of its popularity in the mid-1980s.[64] *Viz* itself had been influenced by punk fanzines, and the rave zines followed in the lineage, with comic strips and short articles discussing and mocking the latest fashions in music, clothing and intoxicants. One such example was the unofficial zine of The Haçienda, *Freaky Dancing*, and Lifeline capitalised on this loose affiliation, publishing *E by Gum* in a special edition with The Haçienda.

The death of Claire Leighton had brought significant scrutiny on the nightclub and the drug culture surrounding it. Tony Wilson, the club's impresario, commented in 2004 that 'none of us knew about ecstasy deaths then – the idea that somebody's body boils'.[65] Leighton's death was the third Ecstasy-related fatality in Britain by that point; what Wilson was referring to was the emergent evidence that these deaths may have been caused by heatstroke and dehydration. Contributing factors included a chemically induced imperative to dance non-stop and clubs that were so packed with bodies that sweat dripped down the walls. But many clubs had also taken to turning off the water taps, forcing ravers to buy bottled water from the bar if they wanted to replace fluids. As Wilson noted elsewhere, The Haçienda and clubs like it were not profitable enterprises, despite the 'huge crowds and great atmosphere', which was all 'fuelled by ecstasy, not alcohol'.[66] The loss of these bar receipts meant that some clubs took extraordinary (and highly dangerous) measures to claw back income. Lifeline produced a Peanut Pete comic on the subject with the title *Too Damn Hot*, advising ravers to 'DRINK A PINT OF WATER OR SOFT DRINK EVERY HOUR' and 'HAVE A REST FROM DANCING REGULARLY.'[67]

Further Peanut Pete comics addressed other potentially challenging aspects of Ecstasy or LSD consumption, from paranoia and psychosis (*Paranoia and the Don't Care Bears*), come-downs (*Where's Me Slippers*) and panic attacks (*In the Zone*). While dealing with serious topics, Peanut Pete maintained the same self-admitted 'gratuitous swearing and gratuitous violence' that *Smack in the Eye* had introduced.[68] Football was a common reference, while *Too Damn Hot*, *Paranoia and the Don't Care Bears* and *Where's Me Slippers* included literal toilet humour with depictions of urination, defecation and exclamatory excrement. Lisa, Pete's long-suffering girlfriend, was also a constant presence, patiently putting up with his self-inflicted misadventures.

Despite Peanut Pete's success, selling over a million copies in 1992 to 'buyers from local authorities to the Boy Scout movement', Lifeline suspected that both the medium, and Pete's laddish antics, were not reaching the real-life equivalents of Lisa, the significant numbers of female ravers.[69] Lifeline responded by producing a series of postcards, intended to 'mimic the glossy fashion magazine style popular with young women'.[70] These postcards' implicitly feminine aesthetic, devoid of the gritty humour of Lifeline's other publications, however, ultimately failed to chime with its intended audience, and Peanut Pete was in fact just 'as popular with women as much as men'. Without the apparently vital ingredient of humour, Lifeline's communications came across as self-conscious and stilted.

Two female characters were subsequently developed by Linnell. Described as 'female version[s] of Peanut Pete', Claire and Jose's adventures featured across three comics, which I have discussed elsewhere at greater length. These comics depicted women as 'variously, at risk of intoxication to the point of overdose, [as] easy sexual quarry for predatory men, and reminded that ecstasy could provide only temporary respite for both the social and biological travails of being a young woman'.[71]

The moral implications of these depictions subtly differed from Peanut Pete's experiences. Although Pete's misadventures were presented in a gonzo style in which the harms that he suffered were often self-inflicted, he was never in any serious jeopardy. Claire and Jose, on the other hand, were frequently in harm's way because of their gender, and their misfortunes had an altogether darker tone. Again, this illustrates that humour carries all sorts of assumptions: comedy that appears to be edgy or transgressive can also perpetuate conservative, gender normative values. In this instance, the unspoken inference was that male protagonists such as Peanut Pete could engage in 'risky' behaviours without serious consequence, whereas the same was not true of female characters such as Claire and Jose. But we should also be careful of projecting back our contemporary judgements on historical actors; the topics contained in the leaflets were suggested by focus groups of young women, and the characters developed in collaboration with them. An evaluation deemed that the leaflets were 'informative, funny and have some good storylines'.[72]

Conclusion

Despite the qualified success of Claire and Jose, Peanut Pete would remain the character most associated with Lifeline. Indeed, according to journalist Matthew Collin's assessment, the 'pop-eyed scally perennially buzzing off his nut, pulling on a spliff while simultaneously dispensing no-nonsense advice ... [helped Lifeline] become as much a part of the fabric of club culture as DJs and its propagation of self-preservation rituals through the dance music media would undoubtedly save lives'.[73] His comics were highly influential on other harm reduction groups, most notably Edinburgh's Crew 2000 organisation and their two informational comics *Jellytime* and *Dunt*.[74] Although the flurry of Peanut Pete comics released in the early 1990s would slow, he would continue to be the face of future informational leaflets on newly popular drugs such as ketamine (2000), a collaboration with Greater Manchester Council for the *Safer Dancing* initiative (1995) and Lifeline's collaboration with youth radio station BBC Radio 1, *The Big Blue*

Book of Dance Drugs (1992).[75] The latter was the highest profile appearance of Pete, and Linnell was conscious of how the images produced could be used to delineate between those that Lifeline wished to communicate with, and those who didn't 'get it': 'on the cover of "The Big Blue Book of Dance Drugs" … a man's brain is seen exploding from his head as a result of the drug he has taken. This can be viewed as the terrible consequences of drug abuse or alternatively as the desired "buzz" from the drug of choice.'[76]

Again, this demonstrated how Lifeline successfully deployed apparently shocking and transgressive humour to speak to their core audience. Darnton's suggestions for how we might usefully analyse humour in the archive are useful starting points for getting at wider issues, even if we think, because of the shorter passage of time, that we 'get' the joke. Jokes are funny because of their context, their reference points, who is laughing and at whom. Jokes, especially transgressive ones, can be used to delineate between social groups, between those that understand the context, and those that do not. Peanut Pete revealed how drug consumption in the north of Britain was situated in the material realities of – and an escape from – everyday life, while Claire and Jose doubled down on long-held gender stereotypes of intoxication. Meanwhile, *Smack in the Eye* used anthropomorphic characters and parodies of popular culture to speak to a disenfranchised and marginalised social group, in the process revealing (and perhaps normalising) for a wider audience some of the practices and philosophies of people who used drugs.

Notes

1 This work was supported by the Wellcome Trust [223559/Z/21/Z].
2 Robert Darnton, *The Great Cat Massacre and Other Episodes in French Cultural History* (Vintage Books, 1985), p. 75.
3 Darnton, *The Great Cat Massacre*, p. 77.
4 Darnton, *The Great Cat Massacre*, p. 78.
5 While highly influential, *The Great Cat Massacre* also attracted some robust criticism. For example, Harold Mah, 'Suppressing the text: The metaphysics of ethnographic history in Darnton's *Great Cat Massacre*',

History Workshop 31 (1991), 1–20. For a wider discussion, see James Fernandez, 'Historians tell tales: Of Cartesian cats and Gallic cockfights', *Journal of Modern History* 60:1 (1998), 113–27.

6 Wellcome Library SA/DRS/B/1/244, Mark Gilman, *Telling the Truth about Drugs* (Lifeline, 1995); Alex Mold and Virginia Berridge, *Voluntary Action and Illegal Drugs: Health and Society in Britain Since the 1960s* (Palgrave Macmillan, 2010), p. 63.

7 Rowdy Yates, *If it Weren't for the Alligators: A History of Drugs, Music and Popular Culture in Manchester* (Lifeline, 1992), p. iii.

8 Kellie Sherlock, *Claire and Jose: An Evaluation of Three Leaflets aimed at Young Women Drug Users* (Lifeline, 1994), p. 6.

9 *Smack in the Eye* worked as a pun on a number of levels, but perhaps most obviously, 'smack' is a street name for the opiate heroin. The phrase is also an idiom for a snub or a rejection.

10 Gilbert Shelton, *The Fabulous Furry Freak Brothers Omnibus* (Knockabout, 2008). The term 'comix', which emerged in the late 1960s, differentiated such underground publications from their mainstream counterparts, while the 'x' 'emphasize[d] the ... X-rated'. These were 'basically an American phenomenon, which was then imitated in Britain'. Roger Sabin, *Comics, Comix and Graphic Novels: A History of Comic Art* (Phaidon, 1996).

11 Darnton, *The Great Cat Massacre*, p. 83.

12 Steve Baker, *Picturing the Beast: Animals, Identity, and Representation* (Manchester University Press, 1993), p. 9.

13 Anon., *Smack in the Eye*, 1 (1987), 3–5, https://michaellinnell.org.uk/michael_linnell_archive/smack_in_the_eye/pdf/A1/A1%20SITE%201.pdf (accessed 23 December 2023). Physical copy also available to view at the Science Museum 'Smack in the Eye', issue 1, 1992–199/4 Science Museum Group Collection Online (accessed 15 April 2025), https://collection.sciencemuseumgroup.org.uk/objects/co8608489/smack-in-the-eye-issue-1.

14 Scottish Home and Health Department, *HIV Infection in Scotland: Report of the Scottish Committee on HIV Infection and Intravenous Drug Misuse* (Scottish Home and Health Department, 1986), no pagination, quoted in Virginia Berridge, *AIDS in the UK: The Making of Policy, 1981–1994* (Oxford University Press, 1996), p. 96.

15 Virginia Berridge, 'AIDS and British Drug Policy: History Repeats Itself ...?' in David K. Whynes and Philip T. Bean (eds), *Policing and Prescribing: The British System of Drug Control* (Palgrave Macmillan, 1991), pp. 176, 189.

16 Wellcome Library SA/DRS/B/1/244, Mark R. Gilman, 'Comics as a Strategy in Reducing Drug Related Harm' (Lifeline, 1989), 11.
17 Wellcome Library SA/DRS/B/1/244, Mark R. Gilman, 'A Radical Departure from Standard Drugs and HIV Education' (Lifeline, 1989).
18 BBC *Open Door: Swallowing is Believing*, episode aired 18 September 1978, https://www.imdb.com/title/tt14706364/ This documentary was viewable as part of the exhibition *People Make Television* at Raven Row, London, 28 January to 26 March 2023, https://ravenrow.org/exhibitions/people-make-television (accessed 6 November 2023).
19 Alex Mold and Hannah Elizabeth, 'Superman vs. Nick O'Teen: anti-smoking campaigns and children in 1980s Britain', *Palgrave Communications* 5:116 (2019), https://doi.org/10.1057/s41599-019-0326-6.
20 Health Education Authority, *Look After Your Heart!: Report on the First Four Years of Advertising and Publicity for the Look After Your Heart! Programme 1987–1990* (Health Education Authority, 1992), p. 111. For background on Reg Smythe's character Andy Capp, see Mark Bryant, *Dictionary of Twentieth-Century British Cartoonists and Caricaturists* (Ashgate, 2000), pp. 210–11.
21 Wellcome Library SA/DRS/B/1/244, Gilman, 'A Radical Departure', 5; Wellcome Library SA/DRS/B/1/244, Gilman, 'Comics as a Strategy', 20.
22 Virginia Berridge and Kelly Loughlin, 'Smoking and the new health education in Britain 1950s-1970s', *American Journal of Public Health* 95:6 (2005), 956–64.
23 Matt Cook, '"Archives of Feeling": the AIDS Crisis in Britain 1987', *History Workshop Journal* 83:1 (2017), 51–78; Nicholas Dorn, 'Media Campaigns', *Druglink*, July/August 1986, 8–9; Alex Mold, 'Just say know: Drug education and its publics in 1980s Britain', *International Journal of Drug Policy* 88 (2021), 103029.
24 Wellcome Library SA/DRS/B/1/244, Gilman, 'A Radical Departure', 5.
25 Mike Linnell, 'Flushing out the truth about drugs', *Druglink*, September/October 2005, 13.
26 Wellcome Library SA/DRS/B/1/244, Gilman, 'Comics as a Strategy', 18.
27 Wellcome Library SA/DRS/B/1/244, R. Lewis, 'Selling Smack and Chasing Dragons', *Emergency* 3 (1985), no pagination. Quoted in Gilman, 'Comics as a Strategy', 12.
28 Wellcome Library SA/DRS/B/1/244, Gilman, 'Comics as a Strategy', 47. *High Times*, founded in 1974, is and was an American periodical focused on cannabis culture. Alongside its news, comment and opinion articles, it also included comix from 1976. See High Times Editors (ed.), *High Times: A 40-year History of the World's Most Infamous*

Magazine (Powerhouse Books, 2014). *Home Grown* meanwhile was a British publication surveying drugs culture (mainly marijuana and LSD), published between 1977 and 1982.

29 Wellcome Library SA/DRS/B/1/244, Gilman, 'A Radical Departure', 4.

30 Scott McCloud, *Understanding Comics: The Invisible Art* (Harper Perennial, 1993), p. 32.

31 Mark R. Gilman, 'A smack in the eye for standard drugs and HIV education', *British Journal of Addiction* 85 (1990), 1661–3.

32 Gilman, 'Comics as a Strategy', 43.

33 Gilman, 'A Radical Departure', 7.

34 Anon, letter to North West Regional Drug Training Unit, 15 April 1989, https://michaellinnell.org.uk/michael_linnell_archive/smack_in_the_eye/pdf/A3/shocked_of_surrey_850.jpg (accessed 14 December 2023).

35 Anon, *Smack in the Eye: Issue 1* (the pilot issue), https://michaellinnell.org.uk/michael_linnell_archive/smack_in_the_eye/smack_in_the_eye_issue_1.html (accessed 14 December 2023).

36 Michael Linnell, 'SMACK IN THE EYE: An evaluation of a harm reduction comic for drug users' (MSc thesis, Leeds Metropolitan University, 1993).

37 Annie Kelly, 'NEWSMAKER: Wrong side of the law – Michael Linnell, Director of communications, Lifeline', *Third Sector*, 4 September 2002, https://www.thirdsector.co.uk/newsmaker-wrong-side-law-michael-linnell-director-communications-lifeline/article/611616 (accessed 13 December 2023).

38 Lifeline, *Smack in the Eye*, issue 3, 1989, https://michaellinnell.org.uk/michael_linnell_archive/smack_in_the_eye/pdf/A3/A3%20SITE3.pdf (accessed 16 December 2023). Physical copy also available to view at Science Museum, 'Smack in the Eye' comic, issue 3, 1992–199/5, Science Museum Group Collection Online, https://collection.sciencemuseumgroup.org.uk/objects/co8608490/smack-in-the-eye-comic-issue-3 (accessed 15 April 2025).

39 See Gilman, 'Comics as a Strategy', 20, for further detail on the Dutch comics.

40 For an account of this culture in a US context, see Daniel Rosenke, 'Dawn of the War on Steroids', *The International Journal of the History of Sport* 40:10–11 (2023), 877–926.

41 For an authoritative history, see David Farber, *Crack: Rock Cocaine, Street Capitalism, and the Decade of Greed* (Cambridge University Press, 2019).

42 Gilman, 'Comics as a Strategy', 15.

43 Gilman, 'Comics as a Strategy', 16
44 Gilman, 'Comics as a Strategy', 47.
45 Gilman, 'Comics as a Strategy', 76.
46 Gilman, 'Comics as a Strategy', 75.
47 Mold, 'Just say know: Drug education and its publics in 1980s Britain'.
48 Gilman, 'Comics as a Strategy', 44.
49 Matthew Collin, 'Alternative comics', *The Observer*, 23 October 1994, 46.
50 Wellcome Library SA/DRS/B/1/244, Lifeline 'The New Drug Takers 2: Application Form' (1992).
51 Collin, 'Alternative comics', 46.
52 Andrew Loudon, 'Nightclub girl died on first Ecstasy "trip"', *Daily Mail*, 18 July 1989, 4.
53 John A. Henry, 'Ecstasy and the Dance of Death', *British Medical Journal* 305 (1992), 5–6.
54 Exchange Supplies, 'The Birth of Peanut Pete', 19 December 2011, https://www.youtube.com/watch?v=ve_BN1IU_2k (accessed 18 December 2023).
55 Lifeline, *A Trip Around Manchester* (Lifeline, 1990). For a recent exploration of so-called blotter art, see Erik Davis, *The Untold Story of an Acid Medium* (MIT Press, 2024).
56 See Michael Sappol, *Body Modern: Fritz Kahn, Scientific Illustration, and the Homuncular Subject* (University of Minnesota Press, 2017).
57 Lifeline, *In the Zone* (Lifeline: 1992).
58 Andy Thomas, 'House of Revolution', *Wax Poetics* 45 (January/February 2011), 54–61, https://magazine.waxpoetics.com/connections/pride/article/ron-hardy-house-of-revolution/ (accessed 11 April 2025). For the wider context of Chicago house, see Micah Salkind, *Do You Remember House?: Chicago's Queer of Color Undergrounds* (Oxford University Press, 2019).
59 Nick Chester, 'I Was the Haçienda's Resident Acid Dealer', *Vice*, 10 May 2016, https://www.vice.com/en/article/hacienda-acid-house-drug-dealer-interview/ (accessed 23 May 2019).
60 Lifeline, *E By Gum* (Lifeline, 1991).
61 Anon, 'Ee bah gum, it's in t' dictionary', *BBC News*, 9 June 1999, http://news.bbc.co.uk/1/hi/uk/364517.stm (accessed 2 December 2024).
62 Interview between the author and Mark Gilman and Alan Haughton, 7 January 2025.
63 Phil Beddard (ed.), *Highflyers: Clubravepartyart* (Booth-Clibborn Editions, 1995), p. 9.
64 Gilman, 'Comics as a Strategy', 77.

65 Gibby Zobel, 'Chemical Reaction', *Druglink* (July/August 2009), 7.
66 Luke Bainbridge, *Acid House: The True Story* (Omnibus Press, 2013), p. 227.
67 Lifeline, *Too Damn Hot!* (Lifeline, 1992).
68 Lifeline Chief Executive Alan Haughton, quoted in Louisa Saunders, 'The heat is on', *Guardian*, 7 September 1993, A2.
69 Saunders, 'The heat is on', A2–3; Angela McRobbie, *Postmodernism and Popular Culture* (Routledge, 1994), 163–4.
70 Sherlock, *Claire and Jose*, 10.
71 Peder Clark, 'Claire and Jose get off their cake: Ecstasy, raving and women's pleasure in 1990s Britain', *Cultural and Social History* 20:1 (2023), 125.
72 Kellie Sherlock, *Clare and Jose: An Evaluation of Three Leaflets aimed at Young Women Drug Users* (Lifeline, 1994). p. 19.
73 Matthew Collin, *Altered State: The Story of Ecstasy Culture and Acid House* (Serpent's Tail, 1997), p. 309.
74 Anon., *Jelly Time* (Crew 2000, 1992); Wellcome Library SA/DRS/B/1/115, Anon., *Dunt* (Crew 2000; 1995).
75 Lifeline, *The Big Blue Book of Dance Drugs* (Lifeline, 1992); Lifeline, *Planet Ketamine 2000* (Lifeline, 2000).
76 Linnell, 'SMACK IN THE EYE', p. 40.

References

Anon. *Smack in the Eye* 1 (Lifeline, 1987), 3–5. https://michaellinnell.org.uk/michael_linnell_archive/smack_in_the_eye/pdf/A1/A1%20SITE%201.pdf (accessed 23 December 2023).

Anon. Letter to North West Regional Drug Training Unit, 15 April 1989. https://michaellinnell.org.uk/michael_linnell_archive/smack_in_the_eye/pdf/A3/shocked_of_surrey_850.jpg (accessed 14 December 2023).

Anon. 'Ee bah gum, it's in t' dictionary' *BBC News*, 9 June 1999. http://news.bbc.co.uk/1/hi/uk/364517.stm (accessed 2 December 2024).

Bainbridge, Luke. *Acid House: The True Story*. Omnibus Press, 2013.

Baker, Steve. *Picturing the Beast: Animals, Identity, and Representation*. Manchester University Press, 1993.

Beddard, Phil (ed.). *Highflyers: Clubravepartyart*. Booth-Clibborn Editions, 1995.

Berridge, Virginia. 'AIDS and British Drug Policy: History Repeats Itself …?' In David K. Whynes and Philip T. Bean (eds), *Policing and Prescribing: The British System of Drug Control*. Palgrave Macmillan, 1991.

Berridge, Virginia. *AIDS in the UK: The Making of Policy, 1981–1994*. Oxford University Press, 1996.
Berridge, Virginia, and Kelly Loughlin, 'Smoking and the new health education in Britain 1950s–1970s'. *American Journal of Public Health* 95:6 (2005), 956–64.
Bryant, Mark. *Dictionary of Twentieth-Century British Cartoonists and Caricaturists*. Ashgate, 2000.
Chester, Nick. 'I Was the Haçienda's Resident Acid Dealer' *Vice*, 10 May 2016. https://www.vice.com/en/article/hacienda-acid-house-drug-dealer-interview/ (accessed 23 May 2019).
Clark, Peder. 'Claire and Jose get off their cake: Ecstasy, raving and women's pleasure in 1990s Britain'. *Cultural and Social History* 20:1 (2023), 117–32.
Collin, Matthew. 'Alternative Comics'. *The Observer*, 23 October 1994.
Collin, Matthew. *Altered State: The Story of Ecstasy Culture and Acid House*. Serpent's Tail, 1997.
Cook, Matt. '"Archives of Feeling": the AIDS Crisis in Britain 1987'. *History Workshop Journal* 83:1 (2017), 51–78.
Darnton, Robert. *The Great Cat Massacre and Other Episodes in French Cultural History*. Vintage Books, 1985.
Davis, Erik. *The Untold Story of an Acid Medium*. MIT Press, 2024.
Dorn, Nicholas. 'Media Campaigns'. *Druglink*, July/August 1986, 8–9.
Exchange Supplies. 'The Birth of Peanut Pete'. 19 December 2011. https://www.youtube.com/watch?v=ve_BN1IU_2k (accessed 18 December 2023).
Farber, David. *Crack: Rock Cocaine, Street Capitalism, and the Decade of Greed*. Cambridge University Press, 2019.
Fernandez, James. 'Historians tell tales: Of Cartesian cats and Gallic cock-fights'. *Journal of Modern History* 60:1 (1998): 113–27.
Gilman, Mark R. 'A smack in the eye for standard drugs and HIV education'. *British Journal of Addiction*, 85 (1990), 1661–3.
Health Education Authority. *Look After Your Heart!: Report on the First Four Years of Advertising and Publicity for the Look After Your Heart! Programme 1987–1990*. Health Education Authority, 1992.
Henry, John A. 'Ecstasy and the Dance of Death'. *British Medical Journal* 305 (1992), 5–6.
Kelly, Annie. 'NEWSMAKER: Wrong side of the law – Michael Linnell, Director of communications, Lifeline'. *Third Sector*, 4 September 2002. https://www.thirdsector.co.uk/newsmaker-wrong-side-law-michael-linnell-director-communications-lifeline/article/611616 (accessed 13 December 2023).
Lifeline. *Smack in the Eye: Issue 3*, 1989. https://michaellinnell.org.uk/michael_linnell_archive/smack_in_the_eye/pdf/A3/A3%20SITE3.pdf (accessed 16 December 2023).

Lifeline. *A Trip Around Manchester*. Lifeline, 1990.

Lifeline. *E By Gum*. Lifeline, 1991.

Lifeline. *The Big Blue Book of Dance Drugs*. Lifeline, 1992.

Lifeline. *Too Damn Hot!* Lifeline, 1992.

Lifeline. *In The Zone*. Lifeline, 1992.

Lifeline. *Planet Ketamine 2000*. Lifeline, 2000.

Linnell, Michael. 'SMACK IN THE EYE: An evaluation of a harm reduction comic for drug users'. MSc thesis, Leeds Metropolitan University, 1993.

Linnell, Mike. 'Flushing out the truth about drugs'. *Druglink*, September/October 2005.

Loudon, Andrew. 'Nightclub Girl Died on first Ecstasy "trip"'. *Daily Mail*, 18 July 1989.

Mah, Harold. 'Suppressing the text: The Metaphysics of ethnographic history in Darnton's *Great Cat Massacre*'. *History Workshop* 31 (1991), 1–20.

McCloud, Scott. *Understanding Comics: The Invisible Art*. Harper Perennial, 1993.

McRobbie, Angela. *Postmodernism and Popular Culture*. Routledge, 1994.

Mold, Alex, and Virginia Berridge, *Voluntary Action and Illegal Drugs: Health and Society in Britain Since the 1960s*. Palgrave Macmillan, 2010.

Mold, Alex, and Hannah Elizabeth. 'Superman vs. Nick O'Teen: anti-smoking campaigns and children in 1980s Britain'. *Palgrave Communications* 5:116 (2019). https://doi.org/10.1057/s41599-019-0326-6.

Mold, Alex. 'Just say know: Drug education and its publics in 1980s Britain'. *International Journal of Drug Policy* 88 (2021), 103029.

Rosenke, Daniel. 'Dawn of the War on Steroids'. *The International Journal of the History of Sport* 40:10–11 (2023), 877–926.

Sabin, Roger. *Comics, Comix and Graphic Novels: A History of Comic Art*. Phaidon, 1996.

Shelton, Gilbert. *The Fabulous Furry Freak Brothers Omnibus*. Knockabout, 2008.

Sherlock, Kellie. *Claire and Jose: An Evaluation of Three Leaflets aimed at Young Women Drug Users*. Lifeline, 1994.

Saunders, Louisa. 'The heat is on'. *Guardian*, 7 September 1993.

Thomas, Andy. 'House of Revolution'. *Wax Poetics* 45 (January/February 2011), 54–61.

Wellcome Library SA/DRS/B/1/244, Mark R. Gilman, 'Comics as a Strategy in Reducing Drug Related Harm'. Lifeline, 1989.

Wellcome Library SA/DRS/B/1/244, Mark R. Gilman, 'A Radical Departure from Standard Drugs and HIV Education'. Lifeline, 1989.

Wellcome Library SA/DRS/B/1/244, Mark R. Gilman, 'Telling the Truth about Drugs'. Lifeline, 1995.
Wellcome Library SA/DRS/B/1/115, Anon., *Dunt*. Crew 2000; 1995.
Yates, Rowdy. *If it Weren't for the Alligators: A History of Drugs, Music and Popular Culture in Manchester*. Lifeline, 1992.
Zobel, Gibby. 'Chemical Reaction'. *Druglink* (July/August 2009).

10

Pandemic funnies: Humour in COVID-19 comics

Soha Bayoumi

Visual humour during the early years of the COVID-19 pandemic found a home in a variety of platforms, media and genres: from internet memes on social media to TikTok videos to lighthearted public health posters demonstrating masking etiquette or instructing the public on how to keep a safe distance and properly wash their hands. This chapter, however, analyses the visual humour of COVID-19 by placing itself within recent scholarship on graphic medicine that focuses on the intersection between the medium of comics and the discourse of healthcare.[1] It centres a variety of English-language comics, published in books, edited anthologies, comics magazines and online (on personal blogs and websites, on comics websites and on social media) about the COVID-19 pandemic in order to examine the forms of humour they contain.

COVID-19 prompted an explosion of comics produced by both professional and amateur creators on a variety of platforms.[2] The comics I chose for this chapter were mostly created at the height of the pandemic in 2020 and 2021 and cover many facets of the public health crisis, going beyond the biomedical aspects of COVID-19 to also shed light on some of the social, cultural and political impacts of the pandemic, in what has been described by Sweetha Saji, Sathyaraj Venkatesan and Brian Callender as 'covidity'.[3] I argue that the collective crisis, loss and grief brought about by COVID-19 enabled a new form of humour in the field of graphic medicine by virtue of the intertwining of the personal and collective. I analyse the different functions of humour in a selection of comics that I cite as representative of the varied uses of humour in relation to COVID-19.

Relying on a functional theory to understand both comics and the humour they contain, this chapter begins by contrasting the didactic and cathartic functions of the humour in COVID-19 comics. I then examine what is known as 'gallows humour', particularly in comics produced by healthcare workers who had to deal with a unique set of challenges and stressors at the height of the pandemic. I then discuss a new sub-genre of comics that I refer to as 'cosy comics', which highlights domestic themes and tropes of comfort in the search for a semblance of normality during an extraordinary time. In the final section, I document the use of humour in comics as a vehicle for political and social commentary before concluding with a discussion of the limits of humour in early COVID-19 comics and the ways in which the use of humour in those comics was perhaps an affordance of a too-often white, middle-class privilege. My discussion features examples of how humour did not centrally feature in comics produced by creators of colour about underserved and marginalised communities facing additional challenges – challenges that were not commonly featured in the mainstream media and in general discourses around COVID-19.

By analysing all of these pandemic-era functions of humour, this chapter contributes to our understanding of the ways in which visual culture, especially comics, helped us at both the individual and collective levels to process, manage and cope with some of the extraordinary pressures exerted by the COVID-19 pandemic. Inversely, this chapter shows how the pandemic enabled different forms of visual expression and allowed for the emergence of new forms of humour and new forms of comics – notably what I describe as 'cosy comics' – and how that can be analysed as one of the effects of the COVID-19 pandemic in the field of graphic medicine.

Functions of humour in graphic medicine: Didactic vs. cathartic

The plethora of comics about COVID-19 lends itself to various criteria of categorisation and examination, based on genres and themes, artistic styles, length and format, modes of creation, publication platforms and so on. In this chapter, I propose a functional approach to analysing comics. By this, I mean that I categorise these comics by the function of the humour they contain. In his functional analysis of comics, comics studies scholar Paul Fisher Davies explains that 'Comics have long been used to do a wide range of the things language does: tell stories, record memoirs, recount histories, and even to instruct and advise, or argue, promote and explain ideas. Comics incorporate verbal language to those ends, as well as using images to serve and support those purposes.'[4] I argue that this functional approach – focusing on the uses of humour in these pieces – enables the analysis of very different comics across a wide spectrum: comics of various lengths and formats, produced by professional and amateur creators, published online and in books.

Comics have been described as involving a more intense level of collaboration between creator and reader than many other art forms. Comics require readers to both contribute to setting the pace of the comic and to 'read between the gutters' (the space between comic panels) – that is, to bring a lens of active interpretation to what they are reading/viewing in a more engaging way than other storytelling genres.[5] In fact, renowned Italian filmmaker Federico Fellini (1920–93), who is less known for the comics he created than for films such as *La Dolce Vita* (1960), is credited as once saying, 'Comics, more than film, benefits from the collaboration of the readers: one tells them a story that they tell to themselves; with their particular rhythm and imagination in moving forward and backward.'[6] Readers' intense involvement is a factor that must be taken into account when thinking about the functions of comics and how they are received by their readers.

Adopting a functional analysis of the comics explored here, I propose the two primary functional categories of didactic versus cathartic humour. This categorisation is by no means clear-cut. In many comics, there is a significant overlap between these two categories. However, my inquiry relies on what I consider to be the dominant function of the humour contained in the comics under analysis, taking into account the role of the reader as an active collaborator in interpreting the comics and defining their functions.

I use the term 'didactic humour' to refer to humour used for educational purposes. Ample scholarship has discussed the role of humour in education as creating a relaxed atmosphere for learning, increasing retention and recall of information and enhancing critical thinking through highlighting paradoxes and ironies.[7] I use the term 'cathartic humour' to refer to the use of humour as a coping mechanism, as a way of processing trauma or making sense of difficult life experiences. This form of humour serves a cathartic function for the creator but often for the reader as well. This function can be complex; a recent qualitative study discussed how engaging in humour can sometimes trigger a renewed sense of grief in bereaved individuals despite also serving as an effective coping mechanism to manage grief.[8] The next two sections expand on these concepts and apply them to a selection of COVID-19 comics to explore the ways in which their creators used humour.

Didactic humour

Humour has long been used in informational graphic medicine comics as a way of conveying facts about diseases and health conditions in a light-hearted manner – a way of discussing difficult subjects in a palatable and digestible format. Medical cartoonist Cathy Leamy is known for her contributions to this genre. Some of her comics, produced in collaboration with the Massachusetts General Hospital Diabetes Self-Management Education & Support Program, humorously explain facts about diabetes and diabetes care. For instance, her webcomic titled 'Diabetes is After Your Dick' starts with this catchy title and relies on humorous/risqué language to explain the physiological mechanisms of diabetes and to draw attention to how uncontrolled diabetes can lead to erectile dysfunction.[9] The humour in this comic relies on satirising fragile masculinity and the cliché that cis-men are more likely to pay attention to their health once it pertains somehow to their sexual function and virility.

As Carol Tilley points out, comics have been used for educational purposes for more than a century. In the early twentieth century, when tuberculosis was the leading cause of death in the United States, in addition to instructional comics, there were proposals 'to have students draw comics to highlight hygienic practices related to the disease' as an important instructional strategy.[10] Sarah McNicol explains that educational comics can support individuals to deal with various health conditions by improving their 'understanding of factual information' as well as helping them manage their feelings towards their health conditions.[11] They can also be a useful educational resource for a patient's family members, caregivers and loved ones. Cilléin Kearns and Nethmi Kearns specifically discuss the educational and communicative role of comics in public health during the COVID-19 pandemic and argue that comics have been used as a vehicle to present scientific narratives, 'harnessing the power of visuals, text, and storytelling in an engaging format' and enabling public engagement with the science of the pandemic.[12] I offer this background to preface my following analysis with the note that the use of comics for educational purposes is not a new phenomenon. I focus here, though, on the role played by humour in these COVID-related educational comics.

Early on in the pandemic, in March 2020, as members of the public were exhorted to carefully wash their hands to reduce the risk of COVID-19 infection, cartoonist Ellen Forney, author of by-now graphic medicine classics such as *Marbles: Mania, Depression, Michelangelo, and Me* (2012) and *Rock Steady: Brilliant Advice From My Bipolar Life* (2018), and curator of the online and travelling National Library of Medicine exhibition *Graphic Medicine: Ill-Conceived & Well-Drawn*, created a comic for *The Washington Post* to explain what twenty seconds of handwashing look like (Figure 10.1).[13] The short comic relied on funny metaphors to teach the proper techniques of handwashing, from rubbing one's palms while snickering like a villain, to spiders on piggyback (rubbing backs of hands) and spiders kissing (rubbing palm to palm while interlacing fingers), to kung fu grip (rubbing backs of fingers), to motorcycle throttle (rubbing thumbs), to mortar and pestle (rubbing fingertips against opposite palm). Forney invents a hilariously nonsensical story of villain versus spiders both because 'mumbling [it] at a leisurely pace' takes a little over twenty seconds and because it serves as a mnemonic device by which to remember these different handwashing techniques in sequence: 'The villain gets angry because the spiders are all happy, spider-piggybacking & spider-kissing… so picks a kung fu fight, but loses & flees on a motorcycle, & the spiders celebrate with dinner at a nice restaurant that uses

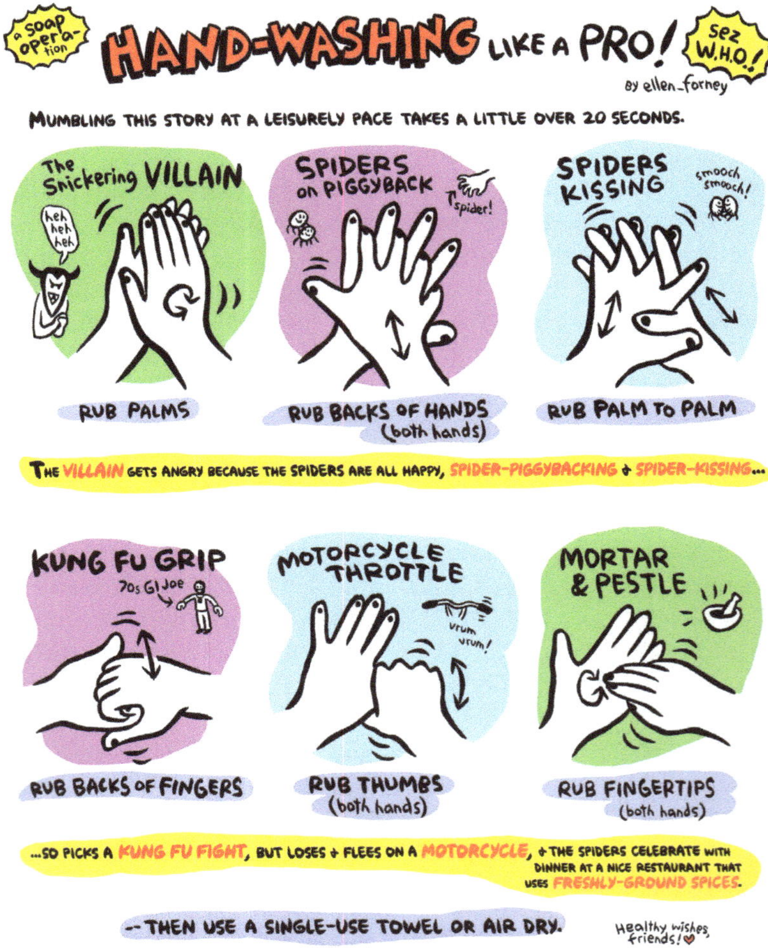
a soap opera-tion
HAND-WASHING LIKE A PRO!
sez W.H.O.!
BY ellen_forney
MUMBLING THIS STORY AT A LEISURELY PACE TAKES A LITTLE OVER 20 SECONDS.
The Snickering VILLAIN
heh heh heh
RUB PALMS
SPIDERS on PIGGYBACK
spider!
RUB BACKS OF HANDS (both hands)
SPIDERS KISSING
smooch smooch!
RUB PALM TO PALM
THE VILLAIN GETS ANGRY BECAUSE THE SPIDERS ARE ALL HAPPY, SPIDER-PIGGYBACKING + SPIDER-KISSING...
KUNG FU GRIP
70s GI Joe
RUB BACKS OF FINGERS
MOTORCYCLE THROTTLE
vrum vrum!
RUB THUMBS (both hands)
MORTAR & PESTLE
RUB FINGERTIPS (both hands)
...SO PICKS A KUNG FU FIGHT, BUT LOSES + FLEES ON A MOTORCYCLE, + THE SPIDERS CELEBRATE WITH DINNER AT A NICE RESTAURANT THAT USES FRESHLY-GROUND SPICES.
--THEN USE A SINGLE-USE TOWEL OR AIR DRY.
Healthy wishes, friends!

Figure 10.1 Ellen Forney, 'Hand-Washing Like a Pro', *The Washington Post*, 20 March 2020.

freshly ground spices.' This comic, titled 'Hand-Washing Like a Pro: A Soap Opera-tion' (2020), is tantamount to a Public Service Announcement (PSA) about the importance of handwashing and the proper techniques for it. It relies on spoof as an aide-memoire to teach hygienic practices to a panicking public. The comic circulated widely on social media, with users appreciating the humour it relies on for conveying such a simple yet critical public health message.

In late November 2020, successful Phase 3 clinical trials of multiple SARS-CoV-2 vaccines were underway. As Americans anticipated authorisation by the US Federal Drug Administration of a number of COVID vaccines, physician and cartoonist Mike Natter posted a comic on his Instagram account. In the comic, Natter used his signature style to explain the basic biology of how the COVID-19 mRNA vaccine works and to dispel some of the myths surrounding the vaccine (Figure 10.2).[14] The comic describes how the virus's genetic code included in the vaccine amounts to a set of instructions that the vaccine relays to muscle cells. Those cells are then expected to reproduce the SARS-CoV-2 spike protein that is ultimately used to train immune cells to create antibodies that would then fight the actual virus in case of the body's exposure to it. In its depiction of a complex biological subject, the comic employs a burlesque style of humour, which relies on parody or mimicry to represent subjects in an ironic or ludicrous way. In one panel, it anthropomorphises a muscle cell receiving the vaccine, depicted as overwhelmed by the task at hand and in the face of

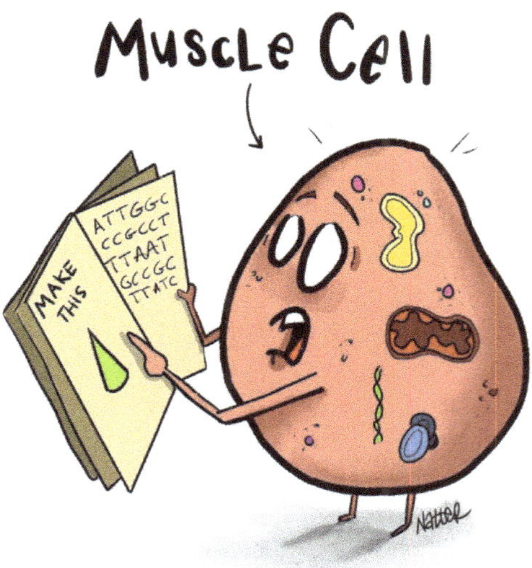

Figure 10.2 Mike Natter, 'Muscle Cell', *Instagram*, 23 November 2020.

information overload (Figure 10.2). In the same comic, the virus is depicted as a villain, and the immune cells are depicted, following the classic trope, as soldiers defending the body against attack.[15] This simple style of humour uses anthropomorphism as a humoristic device and mimics children's comics. It was an effective way of explaining complex biological information and allowed the comic to circulate widely at the time, garnering more than 12,000 likes on Instagram. The humour successfully served to ease many a layperson's anxieties about the vaccine, while the fact that the comic was created by a physician reassured many readers about the accuracy of the information depicted humorously in the comic.

As confinement gradually eased and many folks started negotiating what levels of being outside or being with others felt safe to them, many had questions about what the evolving science said about virus transmission modes. Parents of small children who needed to be outside to play were wondering if public playgrounds were safe spaces for children to use. In December 2020, *NPR* published a cartoon by cartoonist Malaka Gharib, author of the graphic memoir *I Was Their American Dream* (2019), illustrating an informational story about how to use a playground during the pandemic.[16] The comic starts by explaining what scientists understood at the time about virus transmission and how the likelihood of SARS-CoV-2 transmission from surfaces is lower than initially assumed (Figure 10.3). The comic then illustrates the precautions parents should take to minimise the risk of infection when accompanying their children to a public playground, including masking, handwashing, avoiding crowds and using disinfecting wipes to sanitise playground equipment. Using simple drawings and subtle gross-out humour, including a child licking playground equipment and another picking their nose, the comic addresses with levity parents' concerns while sharing specific precautions based in the science of the time. This humour carries a sentimental dimension as well, as parents may perceive the comic with a blend of wry amusement and affection, recognising their own child and family dynamic within the depicted scenes. It exemplifies a form of humour that fosters a sense of shared belonging, particularly among parents with small children.

As we see from these comics, humour plays an effective role in communicating ideas about health and safety during the pandemic.

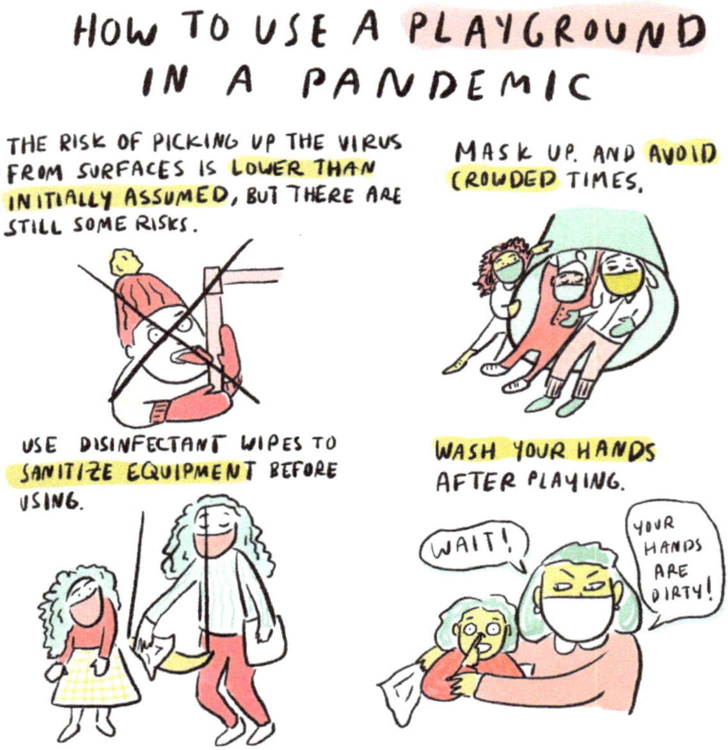

Figure 10.3 Malaka Gharib, 'How to Use a Playground in a Pandemic', *NPR*, 3 December 2020.

As Kearns and Kearns show, 'comics can bend the rules of reality to more clearly communicate ideas'.[17] The abstraction of comics can facilitate communication. As comics creator and theorist Scott McCloud argues in *Understanding Comics: The Invisible Art* (1993), 'When we abstract an image through cartooning, we're not so much eliminating details as we are focusing on specific details. By stripping down an image to its essential "meaning," an artist can amplify that meaning in a way that realistic art can't.'[18] It is, in part, thanks to these artistic strategies that comics can serve a powerful didactic function. Additionally, the visual humour included in these COVID-19 comics relies on familiar iconography (spoof, anthropomorphism, mimicry, etc.) that can ease tension, introduce levity and communicate ideas effectively.

Cathartic humour

Humour is often used as a way to escape, manage and/or cope with grief and stress. In fact, humour is often described as a self-help or self-care technique.[19] Engaging in jokes while anxious or grieving can manifest in dark humour – as a way of whistling past the metaphorical graveyard. This form of cathartic humour can be entertaining; it can make overwhelming stress feel more manageable; it can help relieve heavy emotional baggage and even shift outlooks and perspectives on a difficulty or a crisis.

This humour was the most prevalent form employed in the comics created about the COVID-19 pandemic and its social impacts. In April 2020, *New Yorker* cartoonist Jason Chatfield published a comic diary on his website about his experience contracting COVID-19.[20] A *Washington Post* article was soon written about it, and the comic started circulating widely on both social and traditional media.[21] Later on, the comic appeared in the *Covid Chronicles* comics anthology published as part of the Penn State University Press's Graphic Mundi series.[22] In this comic (Figure 10.4), Chatfield chronicles the onset of his illness and traces its course over the following twelve days. Even though (or perhaps because) he thought at the time that 'it was the end for me', Chatfield started drawing up his symptoms in a cartoon every day 'in the hopes that it might be useful to people as an anecdotal reference'.[23]

Doubtless, Chatfield meant the comic to serve as an educational PSA, aligning in part with the 'didactic' function of COVID-19 comics. He said in an interview with *The Washington Post*, 'I've been curtailing my exposure to social media since the beginning of the pandemic for my mental health, but when I did my daily check-in, I'd become increasingly upset at seeing people not take the virus seriously.'[24] He decided to create the comic to show people that contracting the virus was a serious matter.

However, his reliance on humour was also a way of easing his own anxiety about his mortality and a way of facilitating

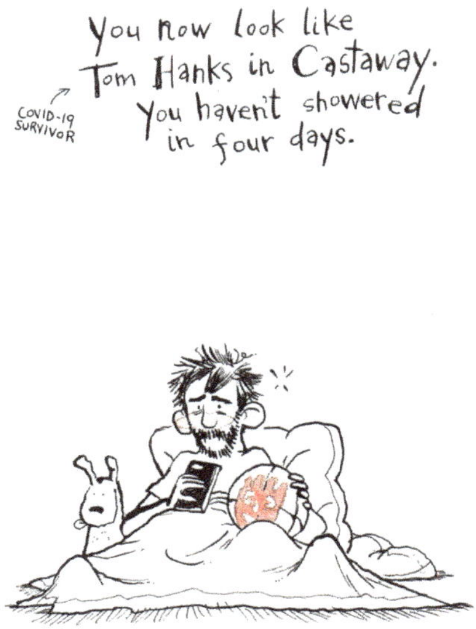
You now look like
Tom Hanks in Castaway.
You haven't showered
in four days.
COVID-19
SURVIVOR

Figure 10.4 Jason Chatfield, *COVID-19 Diary*, https://www.jasonchatfield.com/coronavirus, 2020.

communication about a difficult, and potentially traumatic, experience. From references to pop culture, movie plots such as that of *Cast Away* (2000) and sitcoms, to colourful puns ('Netflix and the Chills'), the humour in the Chatfield comic aims to lighten the mood while discussing bodily fluids, feverish hallucinations about dying in a basketball stadium – recalling the movie *Contagion* (2011) – and the freneticism of contact tracing.

Likewise, author Colleen AF Venable and her collaborator, artist Ellen T. Crenshaw, relied on a similar form of humour when chronicling Venable's experience with COVID-19 and her prolonged symptoms. Venable and Crenshaw's comic humorously documents Venable being in denial in late April 2020 about having contracted COVID-19 in New York City.[25] It then goes on to describe her symptoms: she depicts losing her sense of smell as a blessing, given her inability to shower and take care of the litter of rabbits she was fostering. Venable and Crenshaw use levity in this COVID visual chronicle through, for example, likening the image created by Venable's 'boob sweat' on her shirt to 'Deadpool's face'

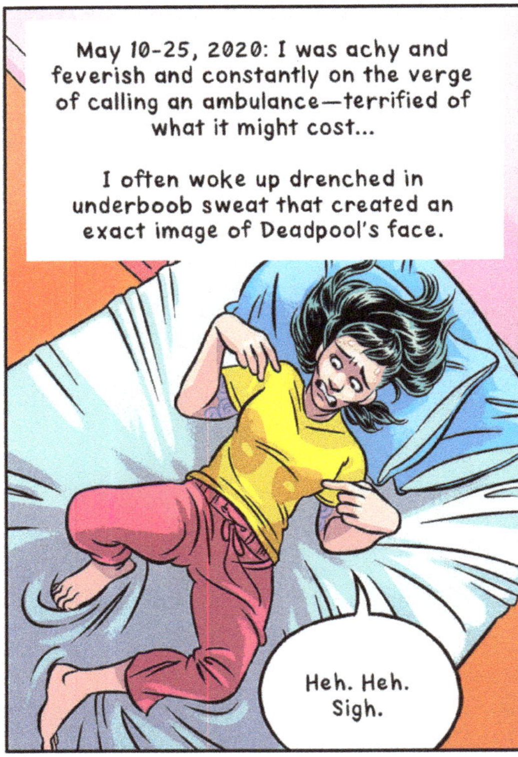
May 10-25, 2020: I was achy and feverish and constantly on the verge of calling an ambulance—terrified of what it might cost...
I often woke up drenched in underboob sweat that created an exact image of Deadpool's face.
Heh. Heh. Sigh.

Figure 10.5 Colleen AF Venable and Ellen T. Crenshaw, 'The New Normal', *The Nib*, 31 May 2021.

(Figure 10.5) and describing how she kept herself entertained while bedridden by watching pigeon drama unfold outside her window – an activity she dubbed 'Pigeon TV' – and rooting for her newfound pigeon friend Phyllis.

In the examples discussed here, we see how these comics creators who had serious COVID-19 symptoms in the early days of the pandemic used humour as a way of cathartically processing their difficult experience, making meaning of it and packaging it for others to partake in their experiences, which were relatable to many. The humour here made what would have been a difficult and grim topic to read about more digestible and easier to consume. Even though some of these comics had a secondary educational function,

I argue that they served a primarily cathartic function, whereby both creators and audiences approached these comics as a way of managing and coping with these experiences, often making light of them using dark comedy. I also argue that the exceptional nature of the pandemic made the use of grotesque, morbid and sometimes gross-out humour in these cathartic comics (and in some didactic comics, such as the one by Malaka Gharib) more palatable and mainstream, as even scientific discussions of the pandemic normalised mentions of droplets, spit, coughing, sneezing, smell (or lack thereof) and other bodily functions. Some of these comics capitalised on that moment by mainstreaming discussions of bodily effluvia and how these creators managed them as they fought COVID infections. The use of humour allowed these discussions to shift from the realm of 'TMI' ('too much information') to the realm of relatability.

Gallows humour

The field of graphic medicine includes many comics created by healthcare providers. Healthcare workers have long used comics as a way to process difficult experiences or to contemplate the interactions of their personal and professional lives. Examples of this genre include M.K. Czerwiec's *Taking Turns: Stories from HIV/AIDS Care Unit 371* (2017), where she documents her experience as a nurse and the devastating loss of life she witnessed in the early days of the AIDS epidemic in the first specialised AIDS/HIV unit in Chicago.[26] Physician and comics creator Ian Williams's semi-autobiographical *The Bad Doctor: The Troubled Life and Times of Dr Iwan James* (2014) chronicles, among other things, how Williams's obsessive compulsive disorder interacted with his medical studies and medical practice.[27] Grace Ferris, in a series of comics on her Instagram and in the *Annals of Internal Medicine* titled 'Dr Mom', depicts facets of life as a parent and physician.[28]

Comics by healthcare workers have served, among other functions, as a window into clinical spaces that are often not accessible to the wider public, either because of privacy norms or, more recently, during the pandemic, for fear of contagion. Many of the comics created by healthcare workers about said clinical spaces during the pandemic do not employ humour, but rather depict or contemplate the solemn reality they were dealing with and their proximity to death, dying and bodily suffering. However, many others employ a kind of gallows humour that touches upon the tensions they have to face navigating their responsibilities towards their patients and their anxieties about their own mortality and about their physical and mental health.[29]

For example, in one of his comics, Ian Williams documents the tail end of a telemedicine encounter with a patient who expresses gratitude for healthcare and frontline workers. In the last two panels, Williams asks the patient, 'Listen ... shall I book you in for a follow-up call in a month?' To which the patient responds, 'Oh, yes, please ... If we're both still around!'[30]

Gallows humour in comics can be a bridge between didactic and cathartic forms of humour. These comics are often created by healthcare workers whose access to death and bodily suffering allows them to point out some of the incongruities they encounter in their work and offer wider audiences access to otherwise closed-off clinical spaces. Therefore, these comics, and the humour they contain, can educate, but they can also be a vehicle for healthcare workers to process their own difficult experiences. Wider audiences are allowed and encouraged to share in this humour, and to see these healthcare workers in their full humanity, vulnerability and contradictions, thereby enabling both understanding and empathy.[31]

Cardiologist Shirlene Obuobi, then an internal medicine resident, published many comics during the early months of the pandemic, most of which deal with the stressors and anxieties placed on healthcare providers. In a series she first published on her Instagram, she satirises the adaptations healthcare providers made to their clothing, illustrating them as fashion choices. Examples include the 'hoarder', a patient-facing hospital worker who accumulates excessive amounts of personal protective equipment (PPE), and a telemedicine doctor rocking pyjamas from home under their white coat.[32] In these comics, Obuobi creates empathetic images of her colleagues' varying anxieties about their own mortality and mental health in their changed (and dangerous) work environment, while mocking them gently.

Gallows humour can vary in levity. In another comic by Obuobi, she contrasts the light-heartedness with which doctors express their anxiety around the lack of PPE with the actual fear and despair they are feeling (Figure 10.6).[33] In this comic, the contrast between how doctors are presenting and what they are jokingly saying 'on the outside' versus what they are thinking and feeling 'on the inside' is a perfect illustration of how gallows humour operates. The comic also serves as a meta-commentary on how the cathartic function of humour works in comics created by

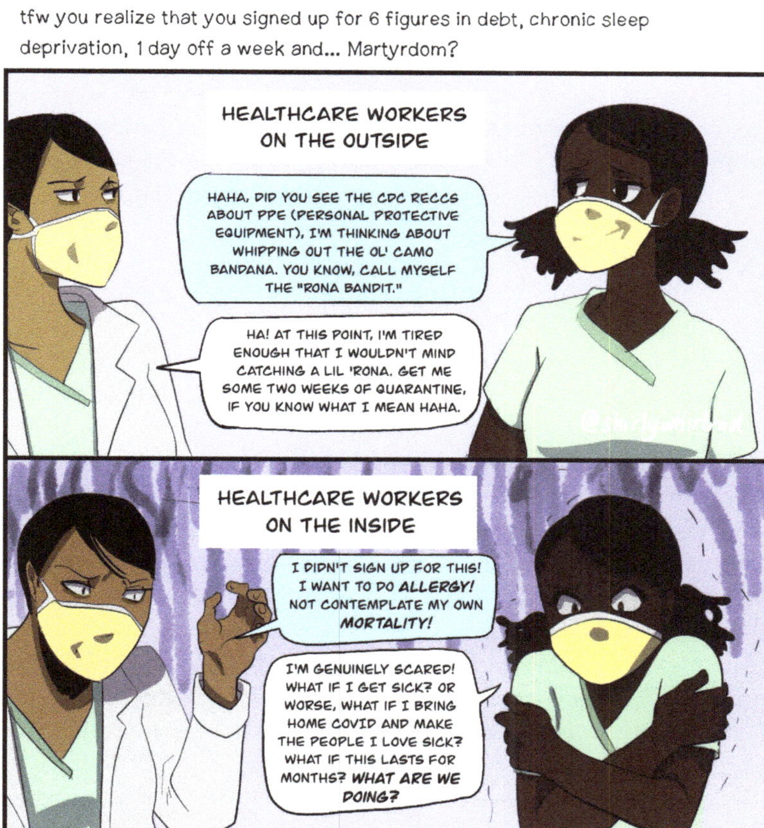
tfw you realize that you signed up for 6 figures in debt, chronic sleep deprivation, 1 day off a week and... Martyrdom?
HEALTHCARE WORKERS ON THE OUTSIDE
HAHA, DID YOU SEE THE CDC RECCS ABOUT PPE (PERSONAL PROTECTIVE EQUIPMENT), I'M THINKING ABOUT WHIPPING OUT THE OL' CAMO BANDANA. YOU KNOW, CALL MYSELF THE "RONA BANDIT."
HA! AT THIS POINT, I'M TIRED ENOUGH THAT I WOULDN'T MIND CATCHING A LIL 'RONA. GET ME SOME TWO WEEKS OF QUARANTINE, IF YOU KNOW WHAT I MEAN HAHA.
HEALTHCARE WORKERS ON THE INSIDE
I DIDN'T SIGN UP FOR THIS! I WANT TO DO ALLERGY! NOT CONTEMPLATE MY OWN MORTALITY!
I'M GENUINELY SCARED! WHAT IF I GET SICK? OR WORSE, WHAT IF I BRING HOME COVID AND MAKE THE PEOPLE I LOVE SICK? WHAT IF THIS LASTS FOR MONTHS? WHAT ARE WE DOING?

Figure 10.6 Shirlene Obuobi, 'tfw you realize that you signed up for …', *Instagram*, 22 March 2020.

both healthcare providers and ordinary people. The dissonance, or incongruity, between the negative thoughts and feelings we experience and the comical ways in which we express them captures an essential function of humour, as illustrated by this comic by Obuobi.

These uses of humour in COVID comics by healthcare workers illustrate the forms of coping afforded by gallows humour. Though controversial in some medical circles because it can be flippant or potentially expressive of a lack of empathy for patients, many have described gallows humour in medicine as ubiquitous, and sometimes even necessary. Physician and medical humanities and ethics scholar Katie Watson defends gallows humour, arguing that, under the right circumstances, it is acceptable to 'advocate for the humanity of patients without denying the humanity of those who treat them'.[34] The humour in the comics discussed here demonstrates the humanity and vulnerability of healthcare workers while not mocking patients or making light of their suffering.

Cosy comics

The COVID-19 pandemic spurred an explosion of comics that portray aspects of what Saji, Venkatesan and Callender term 'covidity', a concept they coined to denote 'both individual and collective philosophical, material, and wide-ranging emotional responses to the COVID-19 pandemic'.[35] Comics about COVID-19 were not just preoccupied with explaining the biology of the disease (as in the case of didactic comics), the documentation of symptoms and the processing of the experience of contracting the disease (as in the case of cathartic comics) or discussing clinical settings (as in the case of gallows comics). The fact that the pandemic upended many (most? all?) aspects of social life meant that a large number of what I describe here as COVID comics were interested in poking fun at the social anxieties surrounding the disease, coping with social isolation and humorously describing the new realities imposed by the pandemic (from 'Zoom dates' to parents' juggling working from home with online schooling for their children, among many other changes).

I call this sub-genre of COVID comics 'cosy comics', a riff on cosy video games and the cosy mystery novel genre (and, more recently, cosy fantasy).[36] These cosy comics highlight socially intimate situations or centre household settings and domestic themes consistent with pandemic lockdown or shelter-in-place orders. In his study of the video game *Animal Crossing: New Horizons* (2020), released in the early days of the pandemic and considered the prototypical cosy video game, media studies scholar Chris Comerford invokes the concept of 'comfort' as a way of explaining the appeal of the soothing visual aesthetics of the game during an otherwise tumultuous time.[37] Relying on this concept of visual comfort during the pandemic, Camilla Sestito, a student at Ryerson University in Toronto in 2021, created a series of comics that rely on humour 'as a counter-visual tactic that subverts the sensationalist imagery that bombards society during these already turbulent times'.[38] The pastel-coloured comics include depictions of a student, Rosie, 'in class' over Zoom, while at her desk at first, then in the kitchen in front of an open fridge and finally in bed under her covers. Sestito hopes that the humorous visuals soften the blow for the reader of what she otherwise describes as the feelings of alienation and isolation brought on by online schooling during the pandemic.[39] I argue that the element of 'comfort' in Sestito's comics, which I file under the 'cosy comics' label, relies on 'cosy' visuals that employ pastel colours, big eyes for the characters and a general dose of 'cuteness', all within a domestic setting.

In *Quarantine Comix: A Memoir of Life in Lockdown* (2021), British comics artist Rachael Smith offers what amounts to a graphic diary during pandemic lockdown.[40] Originally published on her Instagram, the comics offer a window into an honest and raw experience of loneliness, self-doubt and depression during the COVID-19 lockdown in the UK. Smith relies on humour as a way to introduce levity and light-heartedness to an otherwise heavy subject. In one strip, which might resonate with many readers, Smith contrasts her aspirational goals for lockdown time (getting in shape, developing healthy habits, being active) with what she actually ends up doing for much of the time (binge-watching Netflix while eating junk food and drinking wine).[41] The comics included in the book range from the contemplative to the whimsical, but most of them incorporate an element of humour that varies from self-deprecation to dark comedy. Many of Smith's comics in the book centre on her mood, her mental health, her fear of contagion, being isolated from loved ones and connecting with nature. She explains in the book that her best friend encouraged her to create these comics and share them with the world, which she did through her Instagram.[42]

Quarantine expectations versus quarantine reality, which centre the incongruity theory of humour, was a common motif in many 'cosy comics'.[43] From Brooklyn-based Kendra Wells's aspirational baking and yoga to US-based British cartoonist Gemma Correll's contrast between what she thinks she will do during the 'shelter-in-place order' and what she actually ends up doing, we see the themes of domesticity, isolation, light-heartedness and self-deprecation that are characteristic of this sub-genre of comics.[44] Correll, who generally shares comics on her social media about anxiety, mental health, reproductive health and millennials' attitudes created many comics during the pandemic. Some of Correll's cosy comics include 'video conference call bingo' with panels satirising common video call scenes, from surprise appearances by children and pets to technology failures, and *How to WFH Like a Pro* (2020) on recreating 'the real office experience at home'.[45] The latter illustrates workers at home microwaving fish to 'stink up the whole place' and leaving passive-aggressive notes on everything in the fridge. In these comics, Correll turns her readers' individual experiences of work and social life intruding into their private domestic spaces into light-hearted, collective jokes. At the end of 2020, Correll reflected on how pandemic experiences had become newly habitual in her comic *Twelve Days of COVID Christmas*. Correll's Twelve Days includes domestic scenes like eight hours a-zooming (video conferencing), and five 'maskne scars' (an acne-like rash caused by prolonged mask wearing) and '2 up-nose swabs'.[46]

Pandemic-flavoured holidays were a ubiquitous theme in cosy COVID comics. In one of his comics, writer and cartoonist Mark Zukor shares a number of 'pandemic-inspired Halloween costumes', including 'Work-from-Home Werewolf' and 'Zoom Meeting Zombie'.[47] The humour in these 'cosy comics' invokes household and domestic themes relatable to many readers, positioning new pandemic experiences alongside familiar holiday traditions. Unlike some of the previous sub-genres, most of these comics deal with more light-hearted issues that many people experienced during the pandemic. Unlike cathartic comics, for example, many of which also take place in domestic settings, the 'cosy' in cosy comics comes from a choice to focus on more playful and light-hearted themes. Touching on feelings of boredom, the humour is used here, for example, to self-deprecate or to satirise perceived individual failures, rather than to help process traumatic life experiences. The 'domestic' here is not simply a physical setting but a theme invoking ideas of relative safety and comfort and attempts to replicate normality, all while honouring feelings of anxiety, ennui or general malaise characteristic of the COVID experience for many, especially middle-class individuals staying at home.

Who tells jokes? Humour as political and social commentary in COVID comics

The early months of the pandemic in 2020, characterised by (individual) isolation, soon gave way to a summer of (collective) revolt against racial injustice in the United States, and other parts of the world, following the murder of George Floyd at the hands of a white police officer in Minneapolis, Minnesota. Some comics creators became cognisant of the apparent tension imposed by the syndemic, also known as the twin pandemic, of COVID-19 and racial injustice, as well as how it manifested in the lives of many who did not have the choice of staying home. These individuals could not stay home and partake in the 'cosiness' discussed because they were frontline or essential workers, or else because they chose to take to the streets to protest police brutality, facing a heightened risk of exposure to both police violence and COVID infections.

Cartoonist Zukor, who is based in Minneapolis, admitted that he 'always loved cartoons but never really made [his] own' before the pandemic and explained that drawing cartoons during the pandemic started for him as a 'creative way to entertain himself'.[48] He described his choice to create comics during the pandemic as a way to 'have a little fun during dark times' and 'to blow off some steam'.[49] Speaking to the idea that the pandemic touched many aspects of life, Zukor described how the cartoons he produced during the early period of the pandemic cover many subjects 'from current events, to politics, to everyday life', but that they are all still 'about the pandemic in some way'. Characterising his humour as 'cynical and sarcastic', Zukor wrote that 'looking for the humor in the darkness keeps me laughing at things that would otherwise be too depressing to deal with'.[50] For Zukor, this includes commentary on the syndemic of COVID-19 and racism. In one comic, for example (Figure 10.7), Zukor satirised the use of the mask, placed once on a person's mouth and nose with the word 'COVID-19' emblazoned on it, and one on the eyes with the word 'RACISM' on it.[51] He urges the reader to 'cover your mouth, not your eyes'. Here, the surgical or procedural mask, an everyday technology of the pandemic, becomes a tool of political commentary on the other pandemic that was not receiving as much attention: white supremacy and systemic racism. Relying on that simple element of satire serves as a poignant way of poking (fun) at society's ills.

Other comics creators used humour in their comics to make political and social commentary, such as cartoonist Matt Bors, who satirised Donald Trump's dismissive attitude towards COVID-19,

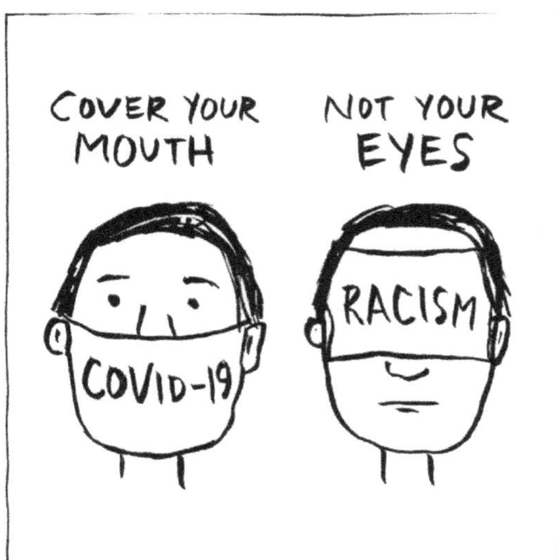

Figure 10.7 Mark Zukor, 'Cover Your Mouth, Not Your Eyes', *Instagram*, 30 May 2020.

even after he contracted the virus.[52] Political cartoonist Jen Sorensen used humour in one of her comic strips to describe how toxic masculinity exacerbated the pandemic, fomenting in some men's reluctance to get vaccinated or wear masks – a phenomenon that political scientists Carl Palmer and Rolfe Peterson have described as 'toxic mask-ulinity'.[53] These kinds of political critiques were not new or unique to comics. They were made by many others in other formats, with and without the use of humour. However, I argue here that comics offered a different venue, perhaps for different audiences, to be exposed to these critiques and that humour can be an effective way to poignantly open society's wounds without making light of the situation.

It is critical, however, throughout this discussion of humour in COVID comics, to be aware of who was telling jokes at the height of the pandemic, and who was getting them published and shared. Discussions about inclusivity (or rather lack thereof) in the field of graphic medicine have garnered attention in the last few years. I argue elsewhere that the COVID-19 pandemic had a diversifying effect on graphic medicine, as a result of the collective nature of the pandemic that eases the traditional (double) stigma – of illness and identity – experienced by minoritised individuals who find themselves faced with the choice to engage in a confessional narrative about their often stigmatised and/or tokenised experiences of illness.[54] However, it is noteworthy that comics produced by BIPOC and other minoritised artists about COVID-19 and its social impact have rarely relied on humour. They have instead used a rather sombre tone to convey the struggles of different individuals and communities. Take, for instance, Arigon Starr and Kalle Benallie's comic, which tells the story of Navajo phlebotomist Lilly Tsosie, who died of COVID-19 in the summer of 2020.[55] The comic aims to show the devastating impact of COVID-19 on the Navajo nation by centring the story of Tsosie and ending with a plea for masking.

Another example is Filipino-American queer creator Niccolo Pizarro's comic about Elmhurst Hospital in Queens, NY, which serves a mostly BIPOC, migrant and formerly incarcerated population. Pizarro's comic shows how underfunding and a lack of resources contributed to dismal outcomes at Elmhurst during the COVID-19 pandemic. Despite the praise heaped on (then) New

York Governor Andrew Cuomo for his handling of the pandemic, comics like Pizarro's shed light on the ways in which policies like Cuomo's had left the city, and especially the most impoverished and marginalised segments of it, unprepared for the scourges of the virus.[56] I discuss several of these comics elsewhere as I argue that the COVID-19 pandemic allowed for the emergence of a diversity of voices in comics in a field that had hitherto mostly centred white middle-class narratives.[57]

The fact that the preponderance of humour in COVID-related comics was produced by white, middle-class creators should give us pause to think through the limits of who experienced the luxury of joking in COVID-19 comics. The syndemic of COVID-19 and structural racism spelled the gravity of the issues facing BIPOC individuals and communities and was reflected in a dearth of humorous comics about the pandemic in comics made by certain groups or by people with certain experiences. As mentioned, there were many COVID comics that did not rely on humour as a narrative tool or as a tool for education, catharsis or the creation of a cosy domestic atmosphere. Whether they were comics by healthcare workers describing harrowing clinical experiences or comics by individuals who lost loved ones, or who captured heartwarming experiences in an otherwise trying time, many COVID comics adopted a sombre tone that eschewed humour altogether.

Conclusion

From the didactic to the cathartic, to gallows humour, to what I have described as 'cosy comics', to the use of humour for social and political commentary through comics during the pandemic, this chapter has aimed to offer an analysis of the uses of humour in a selection of COVID-19 comics across a variety of creators and platforms. Throughout the chapter, humour and its various devices have been discussed as important tools for communicating scientific information, processing difficult experiences, depicting clinical settings, coping with the daily difficulties imposed by pandemic realities and offering political critiques. The chapter has also discussed the limits of humour in COVID-19 comics and the relative privilege it takes to rely on levity in discussing some of the grim realities created or exacerbated by the pandemic. While this chapter has focused specifically on COVID-19 comics, it is worth noting that these works are part of a much longer tradition of humour serving didactic, cathartic and social commentary functions in both graphic medicine and (visual) humour, as evidenced throughout other chapters in this volume. What the pandemic offered was not so much new functions for humour, but rather a unique global context that amplified these existing traditions, while giving rise to new forms like 'cosy comics' that responded to the unique domestic confinement experiences of this global health crisis.

The chapter ultimately argues that the COVID-19 pandemic had an invigorating effect on the uses of humour in comics, especially in the field of graphic medicine. It argues that, although some graphic medicine works have traditionally relied on humour, many did not and focused instead on analysing and processing difficult personal experiences with illness. The collective nature of the pandemic, which impacted the lives of everyone on the planet (to varying degrees), allowed for an intermixing of the private and the public, the personal and the political and the individual and the collective. This, in turn, facilitated a new kind of engagement with health and illness narratives that allowed for the individual to be more collectively relatable and for the intimate and private to feel more publicly relevant. This translated into comics narratives choosing to be less self-conscious or less self-important and espousing humour more readily for catharsis, education or both. Whether this effect is transient or more permanent remains to be seen, but it is nevertheless noteworthy.

Notes

1 M.K. Czerwiec, Ian Williams, Susan Merrill Squier, Michael J. Green, Kimberly R. Myers and Scott T. Smith, *Graphic Medicine Manifesto* (Penn State University Press, 2015).

2 Soha Bayoumi, 'COVID Comics: Decentering White Narratives in Graphic Medicine During the COVID-19 Pandemic', https://videocast.nih.gov/watch=48675 (accessed 17 November 2023).

3 Sweetha Saji, Sathyaraj Venkatesan and Brian Callender, 'Comics in the time of a Pan(Dem)Ic: COVID-19, graphic medicine, and metaphors', *Perspectives in Biology and Medicine* 64:1 (2021), 136–54, https://doi.org/10.1353/pbm.2021.0010.
4 Paul Fisher Davies, *Comics as Communication: A Functional Approach* (Springer International Publishing, 2019), p. vi.
5 Scott McCloud, *Understanding Comics: The Invisible Art* (William Morrow Paperbacks, 1994), pp. 60–3.
6 Thierry Groensteen, *The System of Comics* (University Press of Mississippi, 2007), p. 11.
7 John A. Banas, Norah Dunbar, Dariela Rodriguez and Shr-Jie Liu, 'A review of humor in educational settings: Four decades of research', *Communication Education* 60:1 (2011), 115–44, https://doi.org/10.1080/03634523.2010.496867.
8 Donna M. Wilson, Michelle Knox, Gilbert Banamwana, Cary A. Brown and Begoña Errasti-Ibarrondo, 'Humor: a grief trigger and also a way to manage or live with your grief', *OMEGA – Journal of Death and Dying* 89:2 (2022), 514–29, https://doi.org/10.1177/00302228221075276.
9 Cathy Leamy, 'Metrokitty | Comics | Diabetes Is After Your Dick!', http://www.metrokitty.com/comics/webcomics/diabdick/ (accessed 20 November 2023).
10 Carol L. Tilley, 'Educating with Comics', in Matthew Smith and Randy Duncan (eds), *The Secret Origins of Comics Studies* (Routledge, 2017), p. 25.
11 Sarah McNicol, 'The potential of educational comics as a health information medium', *Health Information & Libraries Journal* 34:1 (2017), 20–31, https://doi.org/10.1111/hir.12145.
12 Ciléin Kearns and Nethmi Kearns, 'The role of comics in public health communication during the COVID-19 pandemic', *Journal of Visual Communication in Medicine* 43:3 (2020), 139–49, https://doi.org/10.1080/17453054.2020.1761248.
13 Ellen Forney, 'Perspective | Hand-Washing like a Pro', *The Washington Post*, 20 March 2020, https://www.washingtonpost.com/graphics/2020/opinions/amp-stories/outlook-coronavirus-hand-washing/ (accessed 20 November 2023). Ellen Forney, *Marbles: Mania, Depression, Michelangelo, and Me: A Graphic Memoir* (Gotham Books, 2012) and Ellen Forney, *Rock Steady: Brilliant Advice from My Bipolar Life*, illustrated edition (Fantagraphics Books, 2018).
14 Mike Natter (@mike.natter), 'The COVID-19 Vaccine!' *Instagram*, 23 November 2021, https://www.instagram.com/p/CH74YA-l1Fe/ (accessed 20 November 2023).

15 For literary and scholarly discussions of metaphors surrounding certain diseases and human immunity, see Susan Sontag, *Illness as Metaphor and AIDS and Its Metaphors* (Doubleday, 1990); and Emily Martin, *Flexible Bodies: Tracking Immunity in American Culture from the Days of Polio to the Age of AIDS* (Beacon Press, 1994).

16 Malaka Gharib, *I Was Their American Dream: A Graphic Memoir* (Clarkson Potter, 2019); Pranav Baskar, 'Coronavirus FAQs: Are playgrounds too risky? Do I need a mask for outdoor exercise?' *NPR*, 4 December 2020, sec. Coronavirus, Illustrated, https://www.npr.org/sections/goatsandsoda/2020/12/04/943252636/coronavirus-faqs-are-playgrounds-too-risky-do-i-need-a-mask-for-outdoor-exercise (accessed 20 November 2023).

17 Kearns and Kearns, 'The role of comics in public health communication during the COVID-19 pandemic'.

18 McCloud, *Understanding Comics*, p. 30.

19 Wilson et al., 'Humor: A Grief Trigger and Also a Way to Manage or Live With Your Grief.'

20 Jason Chatfield, 'My COVID-19 Diary', https://www.jasonchatfield.com/coronavirus (accessed 21 November 2023).

21 Michael Cavna, 'A New Yorker cartoonist got Covid-19. So he drew this public warning', *The Washington Post*, 25 April 2020, https://www.washingtonpost.com/arts-entertainment/2020/04/25/jason-chat/ (accessed 21 November 2023).

22 Kendra Boileau and Rich Johnson (eds), *COVID Chronicles: A Comics Anthology* (Graphic Mundi, 2021).

23 Chatfield, 'My COVID-19 Diary'.

24 Cavna, 'A New Yorker cartoonist Got Covid-19'.

25 Colleen AF Venable and Ellen T. Crenshaw, 'The New Normal', *The Nib*, 31 May 2021, https://thenib.com/the-thing/ (accessed 16 February 2023).

26 M.K. Czerwiec, *Taking Turns: Stories from HIV/AIDS Care Unit 371* (Penn State University Press, 2017).

27 Ian Williams, *The Bad Doctor: The Troubled Life and Times of Dr. Iwan James* (Penn State University Press, 2015).

28 See, for instance, Grace E. Farris, 'Annals Graphic Medicine – Dr. Mom: Doing It All', *Annals of Internal Medicine* 170:3 (5 February 2019), W41–42, https://doi.org/10.7326/G18-0042.

29 Katie Watson, 'Gallows humor in medicine', *The Hastings Center Report* 41:5 (2011), 37–45.

30 Brian Callender, Shirlene Obuobi, M.K. Czerwiec and Ian Williams, 'COVID-19, comics, and the visual culture of contagion', *The Lancet*

396:10257 (10 October 2020), 1061–3, https://doi.org/10.1016/S0140–6736(20)32084–5.

31 Patricia F. Anderson, Elise Wescom and Ruth C. Carlos, 'Difficult doctors, difficult patients: Building empathy', *Journal of the American College of Radiology*, Special Issue: Patient- and Family-Centered Care, 13:12 (1 December 2016), 1590–8, https://doi.org/10.1016/j.jacr.2016.09.015.

32 Shirlene Obuobi (@shirlywhirlmd), *Instagram*, 29 March 2020, https://www.instagram.com/p/B-U9JlCBQBp/ (accessed 17 February 2024).

33 Shirlene Obuobi (@shirlywhirlmd), *Instagram*, 22 March 2020, https://www.instagram.com/p/B-BmNqWBila/ (accessed 17 February 2024).

34 Watson, 'Gallows humor in medicine', 38.

35 Saji, Venkatesan and Callender, 'Comics in the Time of a Pan(Dem)Ic: COVID-19, graphic medicine, and metaphors'.

36 On the 'cosy' phenomenon in video games and literature, see Bettina Bódi, 'The duality of cozy games: Cozy agency, neoliberalism, and affect', *Replay. The Polish Journal of Game Studies* 11:1 (2024), 51–64, https://doi.org/10.18778/2391-8551.11.04; and Phyllis M. Betz (ed.), *Reading the Cozy Mystery: Critical Essays on an Underappreciated Subgenre* (McFarland & Company, 2021).

37 Chris Comerford, 'Coconuts, custom-play, and COVID-19: Social isolation, serious leisure, and personas in "Animal Crossing: New Horizons"', *Persona Studies* 6:2 (2021), 101–17, https://doi.org/10.21153/psj2020vol6no2art970.

38 Camilla Sestito, 'Comfort comics: Using humour to counter the pandemic's visual culture of fear', *Studies in Visual Culture* (blog), 23 April 2021, https://visualculture.blog.torontomu.ca/comfort-comics-using-humour-to-counter-the-pandemics-visual-culture-of-fear/ (accessed 17 February 2024).

39 Sestito, 'Comfort comics'.

40 Rachael Smith, *Quarantine Comix: A Memoir of Life in Lockdown* (Icon Books, 2021).

41 Smith, *Quarantine Comix*.

42 Rachael Smith (@flimsy_kitten), *Instagram*, https://www.instagram.com/flimsy_kitten (accessed 17 February 2024).

43 Michael Clark, 'Humor and Incongruity', in John Morreall (ed.), *The Philosophy of Laughter and Humor* (State University of New York Press, 1987), pp. 139–55.

44 Kendra Wells, 'Quarantine Expectation vs. Reality', *The Nib*, 17 April 2020, https://thenib.com/quarantine-expectation-vs-reality/ (accessed 17 February 2024); Gemma Correll, 'Creativity in Captivity', *The Nib*,

19 March 2020, https://thenib.com/creativity-in-captivity/ (accessed 17 February 2024).

45 Gemma Correll, 'Play Along at Home!' *The Nib*, 9 April 2020, https://thenib.com/video-conference-call-bingo/ (accessed 17 February 2024) and Gemma Correll, 'How to WFH Like a Pro', *The Nib*, 23 April 2020, https://thenib.com/how-to-wfh-like-a-pro/ (accessed 17 February 2024).

46 Gemma Correll, 'The 12 Days of COVID Christmas', *The Nib*, 30 November 2020, https://thenib.com/the-12-days-of-covid/ (accessed 17 February 2024).

47 Mark Zukor (@mazukor), *Instagram*, 29 June 2020, https://www.instagram.com/p/CCBXu_-AXRi/?img_index=1 (accessed 17 February 2024).

48 Mark Zukor, 'I draw pandemic-related comics to laugh at things that would otherwise be too depressing to deal with', *Bored Panda*, 25 May 2022, https://www.boredpanda.com/coronavirus-comics-pandemic-humor-mark-zukor/ (accessed 17 February 2024).

49 Zukor, 'I draw pandemic-related comics'.

50 Zukor, 'I draw pandemic-related comics'.

51 Mark Zukor (@mazukor), *Instagram*, 30 May 2020, https://www.instagram.com/p/CA0eqragjRx/ (accessed 17 February 2024).

52 Matt Bors, 'COVID patient Trump: possible outcomes', *The Nib*, 6 October 2020, https://thenib.com/covid-patient-trump-possible-outcomes/ (accessed 17 February 2024).

53 Jen Sorensen, 'Man Up', *The Nib*, 29 September 2021, https://thenib.com/pandemic-weaklings/ (accessed 17 February 2024). Carl L. Palmer and Rolfe D. Peterson, 'Toxic mask-ulinity: The link between masculine toughness and affective reactions to mask wearing in the COVID-19 era', *Politics & Gender* 16:4 (December 2020), 1044–51.

54 Bayoumi, 'COVID comics'.

55 Arigon Starr and Kalle Benallie, 'The Navajo nation was hit especially hard by COVID-19. Here's Just One Story', *The Nib*, 15 April 2021, https://thenib.com/navajo-nation-covid/ (accessed 17 November 2023).

56 Niccolo Pizarro, 'Center of gravity', *The Nib*, 9 April 2021, https://thenib.com/center-of-gravity/ (accessed 17 November 2023).

57 Bayoumi, 'COVID comics'.

References

Anderson, Patricia F., Elise Wescom and Ruth C. Carlos. 'Difficult doctors, difficult patients: Building empathy'. *Journal of the American College of Radiology*, Special Issue: Patient- and Family-Centered Care, 13:12 (1 December 2016), 1590–8. https://doi.org/10.1016/j.jacr.2016.09.015

Banas, John A., Norah Dunbar, Dariela Rodriguez and Shr-Jie Liu. 'A review of humor in educational settings: Four decades of research'. *Communication Education* 60:1 (2011), 115–44. DOI: 10.1080/03634523.2010.496867

Baskar, Pranav. 'Coronavirus FAQs: Are playgrounds too risky? Do I need a mask for outdoor exercise?' *NPR*, 4 December 2020, sec. Coronavirus, Illustrated. https://www.npr.org/sections/goatsandsoda/2020/12/04/943252636/coronavirus-faqs-are-playgrounds-too-risky-do-i-need-a-mask-for-outdoor-exercise (accessed 20 November 2023).

Bayoumi, Soha. 'COVID comics: Decentering white narratives in graphic medicine during the COVID-19 pandemic', 30 March 2023. https://videocast.nih.gov/watch=48675 (accessed 17 November 2023).

Betz, Phyllis M. (ed.). *Reading the Cozy Mystery: Critical Essays on an Underappreciated Subgenre* (McFarland & Company, 2021).

Bódi, Bettina. 'The duality of cozy games: Cozy agency, neoliberalism, and affect'. *Replay. The Polish Journal of Game Studie*, 11:1 (2024), 51–64. https://doi.org/10.18778/2391–8551.11.04.

Boileau, Kendra, and Rich Johnson (eds). *COVID Chronicles: A Comics Anthology*. Graphic Mundi, 2021.

Bors, Matt. 'COVID patient Trump: Possible outcomes'. *The Nib*, 6 October (2020). https://thenib.com/covid-patient-trump-possible-outcomes/ (accessed 17 February 2024).

Callender, Brian, Shirlene Obuobi, M.K. Czerwiec and Ian Williams. 'COVID-19, comics, and the visual culture of contagion'. *The Lancet* 396:10257 (10 October 2020), 1061–3, DOI: 10.1016/S0140–6736(20)32084–5.

Cavna, Michael. 'A *New Yorker* cartoonist got Covid-19. So he drew this public warning'. *The Washington Post*, 25 April 2020. https://www.washingtonpost.com/arts-entertainment/2020/04/25/jason-chatfield covid-diary-cartoon-comic/ (accessed 21 November 2023).

Chatfield, Jason. 'My COVID-19 Diary'. *New Yorker* Cartoonist Jason Chatfield, (2020). https://www.jasonchatfield.com/coronavirus (accessed 21 November 2023).

Clark, Michael. 'Humor and Incongruity'. In John Morreall (ed.), *The Philosophy of Laughter and Humor*, pp. 139–55. State University of New York Press, 1987.

Comerford, Chris. 'Coconuts, custom-play, and COVID-19: Social isolation, serious leisure, and personas in "Animal Crossing: New Horizons"', *Persona Studies* 6:2 (2021), 101–17. DOI: 10.3316/informit.963753190548669.

Correll, Gemma. 'Creativity in Captivity'. *The Nib*, 19 March 2020. https://thenib.com/creativity-in-captivity/ (accessed 17 February 2024).

Correll, Gemma. 'Play Along at Home!' *The Nib*. 9 April 2020. https://thenib.com/video-conference-call-bingo/ (accessed 17 February 2024).

Correll, Gemma. 'How to WFH Like a Pro'. *The Nib*, 23 April 2020. https://thenib.com/how-to-wfh-like-a-pro/ (accessed 17 February 2024).

Correll, Gemma. 'The 12 Days of COVID Christmas'. *The Nib*, 30 November 2020. https://thenib.com/the-12-days-of-covid/ (accessed 17 February 2024).

Czerwiec, M.K. *Taking Turns: Stories from HIV/AIDS Care Unit 371*. Penn State University Press, 2017.

Czerwiec, M.K., Ian Williams, Susan Squier, Michael J. Green, Kimberly R. Myers and Scott T. Smith. *Graphic Medicine Manifesto*. Penn State University Press, 2015.

Davies, Paul Fisher. *Comics as Communication: A Functional Approach*. Springer International Publishing, 2019.

Farris, Grace E. 'Annals graphic medicine – Dr Mom: Doing it all'. *Annals of Internal Medicine* 170:3 (February 5 2019), W41–42, DOI: 10.7326/G18–0042.

Forney, Ellen. *Marbles: Mania, Depression, Michelangelo, and Me: A Graphic Memoir*. Gotham Books, 2012.

Forney, Ellen. *Rock Steady: Brilliant Advice from My Bipolar Life*. Illustrated edition. Fantagraphics Books, 2018.

Forney, Ellen. 'Perspective | Hand-washing like a pro'. *The Washington Post*, 20 March 2020. https://www.washingtonpost.com/graphics/2020/opinions/amp-stories/outlook-coronavirus-hand-washing/ (accessed 20 November 2023).

Gharib, Malaka. *I Was Their American Dream: A Graphic Memoir*. Clarkson Potter, 2019.

Green, Michael J., and Kimberly R. Myers. 'Graphic medicine: Use of comics in medical education and patient care', *BMJ* 340 (1 January 2010), c863, DOI: 10.1136/bmj.c863.

Groensteen, Thierry. *The System of Comics*. University Press of Mississippi, 2007.

Kearns, Ciléin, and Nethmi Kearns. 'The role of comics in public health communication during the COVID-19 pandemic'. *Journal of Visual Communication in Medicine* 43:3 (2020), 139–49, DOI: 10.1080/17453054.2020.1761248.

Leamy, Cathy. 'Metrokitty | Comics | Diabetes Is After Your Dick!' https://www.metrokitty.com/comics/webcomics/diabdick/ (accessed 20 November 2023).

Martin, Emily. *Flexible Bodies: Tracking Immunity in American Culture from the Days of Polio to the Age of AIDS*. Beacon Press, 1994.

McCloud, Scott. *Understanding Comics: The Invisible Art*. William Morrow Paperbacks, 1994.

McNicol, Sarah. 'The potential of educational comics as a health information medium', *Health Information & Libraries Journal* 34:1 (2017), 20–31. DOI: 10.1111/hir.12145.

Natter, Mike (@mike.natter). 'The COVID-19 Vaccine!' *Instagram*, 23 November 2020. https://www.instagram.com/p/CH74YA-l1Fe/ (accessed 20 November 2023).

Obuobi, Shirlene (@shirlywhirlmd). *Instagram*, 22 March 2020. https://www.instagram.com/p/B-BmNqWBila/ (accessed 17 February 2024).

Obuobi, Shirlene (@shirlywhirlmd). *Instagram*, 29 March 2020. https://www.instagram.com/p/B-U9JlCBQBp/ (accessed 17 February 2024).

Palmer, Carl L., and Rolfe D. Peterson. 'Toxic mask-ulinity: The link between masculine toughness and affective reactions to mask wearing in the COVID-19 era'. *Politics & Gender* 16:4 (December 2020), 1044–51.

Pizarro, Niccolo. 'Center of Gravity'. *The Nib*, 9 April 2021. https://thenib.com/center-of-gravity/ (accessed 17 November 2023).

Saji, Sweetha, Sathyaraj Venkatesan and Brian Callender, 'Comics in the time of a pan(dem)ic: COVID-19, graphic medicine, and metaphors'. *Perspectives in Biology and Medicine*, 64:1 (2021), 136–54. DOI: 10.1353/pbm.2021.0010.

Sestito, Camilla. 'Comfort Comics: Using Humour to Counter the Pandemic's Visual Culture of Fear'. *Studies in Visual Culture* (blog), 23 April 2021. https://visualculture.blog.torontomu.ca/comfort-comics-using-humour-to-counter-the-pandemics-visual-culture-of-fear/ (accessed 17 February 2024).

Smith, Rachael. *Quarantine Comix: A Memoir of Life in Lockdown*. Icon Books, 2021.

Smith, Rachael (@flimsy_kitten). *Instagram*, https://www.instagram.com/flimsy_kitten (accessed 17 February 2024).

Sontag, Susan. *Illness as Metaphor and AIDS and Its Metaphors*. Doubleday, 1990.

Sorensen, Jen. 'Man Up'. *The Nib*, 29 September 2021. https://thenib.com/pandemic-weaklings/ (accessed 17 February 2024).

Starr, Arigon, and Kalle Benallie. 'The Navajo nation was hit especially hard by COVID-19. Here's Just One Story'. *The Nib*, 15 April 2021. https://thenib.com/navajo-nation-covid/ (accessed 17 November 2023).

Tilley, Carol L. 'Educating with Comics'. In Matthew Smith and Randy Duncan (eds), *The Secret Origins of Comics Studies*. Routledge, 2017.

Venable, Colleen AF, and Ellen T. Crenshaw. 'The New Normal'. *The Nib*, 31 May 2021. https://thenib.com/the-thing/ (accessed 16 February 2023).

Watson, Katie. 'Gallows humor in medicine', *The Hastings Center Report* 41:5 (2011), 37–45.

Wells, Kendra. 'Quarantine expectation vs. reality'. *The Nib*, 17 April 2020. https://thenib.com/quarantine-expectation-vs-reality/ (accessed 17 February 2024).

Williams, Ian. *The Bad Doctor: The Troubled Life and Times of Dr Iwan James*. Penn State University Press, 2015.

Wilson, Donna M., Michelle Knox, Gilbert Banamwana, Cary A. Brown and Begoña Errasti-Ibarrondo. 'Humor: A grief trigger and also a way to manage or live with your grief', *OMEGA – Journal of Death and Dying* 89:2 (2022), 514–29, DOI: 10.1177/00302228221075276.

Zukor, Mark (@mazukor). *Instagram*, 30 May (2021). https://www.instagram.com/p/CA0eqragjRx/ (accessed 17 February 2024).

Zukor, Mark (@mazukor). *Instagram*, 29 June 2020. https://www.instagram.com/p/CCBXu_-AXRi/?img_index=1 (accessed 17 February 2024).

Zukor, Mark. 'I draw pandemic-related comics to laugh at things that would otherwise be too depressing to deal with'. *Bored Panda*, 25 May 2022. https://www.boredpanda.com/coronavirus-comics-pandemic-humor-mark-zukor/ (accessed 17 February 2024).

Index

EU authorised representative for GPSR:
Easy Access System Europe, Mustamäe tee 50,
10621 Tallinn, Estonia
gpsr.requests@easproject.com

www.ingramcontent.com/pod-product-compliance
Ingram Content Group UK Ltd.
Pitfield, Milton Keynes, MK11 3LW, UK
UKHW020035180926
8718IPUK00003B/7
* 9 7 8 1 5 2 6 1 8 7 9 7 0 *